COLITIS

Edited by **Masayuki Fukata**

Colitis
Edited by Masayuki Fukata

Published by InTech
Janeza Trdine 9, 51000 Rijeka, Croatia

Publishing Process Manager Vedran Greblo

Technical Editor Teodora Smiljanic

Cover Designer InTech Design Team

Additional hard copies can be obtained from orders@intechopen.com

Colitis, Edited by Masayuki Fukata
p. cm.
ISBN 978-953-307-799-4

For EU product safety concerns:
IN TECH d.o.o., Prolaz Marije Krucifikse Kozulić 3, 51000 Rijeka, Croatia,
info@intechopen.com or visit our website at intechopen.com.

Meet the editor

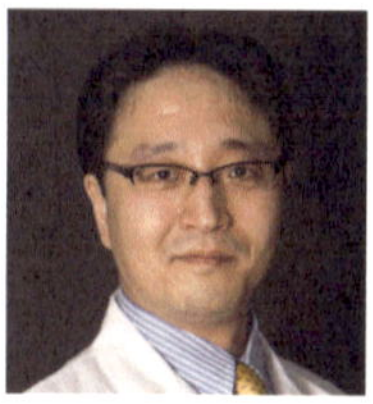

Dr. Masayuki Fukata MD, PhD is a physician and scientist in the field of gastroenterology and immunology. He graduated from the Jikei University School of Medicine in Tokyo Japan in 1994, and completed his residency in Internal Medicine in the Jikei University Hospital. During his fellowship in gastroenterology, Dr Fukata received basic science training at the Department of Anatomy in the Jikei University. After obtaining his PhD degree in 2003, Dr Fukata came to the United States as a post-doctoral fellow for the Inflammatory Bowel Disease Center at Cedars-Sinai Medical Center in Los Angeles. He then moved to the Mount Sinai School of Medicine in New York in 2004 and was promoted to Research Assistant Professor of Medicine in 2007. Since 2008, he is the Assistant Professor of Medicine at University of Miami Miller School of Medicine in Florida. Dr. Fukata's research interests are Toll-like receptor-mediated host-microbial interactions in intestinal mucosal interface, especially in the pathogenesis of colitis.

Contents

Preface

Colitis is a group of illnesses causing inflammation in the colon. It normally causes abdominal pain and diarrhea that sometimes contains blood and/or pus. As systemic manifestations, colitis may present dehydration, general fatigue, and fever. Many colitis cases are self-limited. However, in the cases of infants or elder individuals, it may lead to severe dehydration and malnutrition raising risk of death if proper treatments are not provided and symptoms continue or worsen over time. In idiopathic inflammatory bowel disease (IBD), colitis can be sustained or cycles of remission and relapse can occur during the course of treatment. Treatment of IBD includes immunosuppressive drugs, biologic agents, and sometimes requires surgical interventions, which differs from the treatments for other types of colitis. Therefore, providing effective treatments based on the correct diagnosis is important for managing colitis.

Understanding of the pathogenesis in each case of colitis is essential to identify the types of colitis, however, the causes of colitis vary. For example, it can be microbial infections or a side effect of chemical and/or radiological treatments. Particularly, the exact cause of IBD has not been identified. Difficulty in understanding exact pathogenesis of colitis is associated with the unique nature of the intestine which houses commensal microorganisms. Intestinal mucosa needs to maintain barrier complex in the host-commensal interface in order to keep homeostasis. Disruption of commensal bacterial composition by broad-spectrum antibiotics may result in colitis. Therefore, commensal bacteria serve as one of the key components of the barrier. The acquisitions of antimicrobial resistance in some of the enteric pathogens and the overgrowth of Clostridium difficile have become serious issues in hospital medicine. Amebic colitis is another worldwide public health issue. It has also become a critical concern in immunocompromised patients. Fulminant cases of amebic colitis are highly fatal, but we are currently unable to predict such cases upon diagnosis. Nevertheless, recent extensive studies have revealed some of the key molecular mechanisms underlying the pathogenesis of several types of colitis. Many books have provided detailed information about molecular pathogenesis of particular groups of colitis, yet there is a gap to translate the knowledge to clinical benefits for the management of colitis in daily practice.

This book aims to provide comprehensive knowledge of colitis that covers from general pathogenesis, mechanism of resolution, and treatment strategies, to recent advances in colitis research. We have four sections in this book. Section one is regarding pathophysiology of colitis. Complex mechanisms of host-commensal mutualism, development of mucosal barrier functions, and regulation of inflammatory signaling are discussed. The second section targets infectious colitis especially amebic colitis and *C. difficile* associated colitis. Expertise of this area of research provides very useful information for the pathogenesis and management of these unique types of colitis. The third section is regarding drug-induced colitis. This section particularly describes the pathogenesis and management of chemotherapy-associated colitis. Demand of treating this type of colitis may increase along with development of stronger chemotherapy agents. Thefinal section focuses on novel therapeutic targets and strategies for treating and/or preventing colitis. Individual chapters in these sections are contributed by renowned experts. Knowledge provided in this book will be beneficial for not only physicians and pathologists, but also medical students, nurses, and researchers that are interested in colitis. As a result, I hope this book will lead to better management of patients with colitis across the globe.

Masayuki Fukata
Assistant Professor of Medicine,
Division of Gastroenterology,
University of Miami Miller School of Medicine,
USA

Part 1

Pathophysiology of Colitis

1

The Role of Intestinal Barrier Function in Early Life in the Development of Colitis

R.C. Anderson[1], J.E. Dalziel[1], P.K. Gopal[2], S. Bassett[1], A. Ellis[3] and N.C. Roy[1,3]
[1]*Food Nutrition & Health Team, AgResearch Grasslands*
[2]*Fonterra Co-operative Group Limited*
[3]*Riddet Institute, Massey University*
New Zealand

1. Introduction

The human intestine has the dual role of allowing absorption of nutrients while also acting as a barrier to prevent pathogens and toxins from entering the body and potentially causing disease. In the immature infant intestine this barrier is underdeveloped and large quantities of macromolecules cross the epithelium into systematic circulation. Consequently infants are susceptible to conditions such as infectious diarrhoea, necrotising enterocolitis and allergic gastroenteropathy (Schreiber & Walker, 1988). It is essential that the infant intestinal barrier matures appropriately because barrier dysfunction in adulthood is a critical factor in predisposition to intestinal diseases (Groschwitz & Hogan, 2009) and is associated with autoimmune diseases in other parts of the body (Cereijido et al., 2007).

Illnesses associated with intestinal barrier dysfunction are more common in adults that were formula-fed as infants than in those that were breast-fed (Verhasselt, 2010). This shows that breast milk promotes intestinal barrier maturation (Schreiber & Walker, 1988) and illustrates the need for "humanised" infant formulas so that infants that are not able to breast-fed still obtain the benefits associated with breast milk. However, to achieve this, more knowledge is required about intestinal barrier development and maturation, the roles of various breast milk components, and the mechanisms of action of active ingredients in infant formula.

This review describes the role of intestinal barrier function in the pathogenesis of a range of colitis types and discusses how maturation of the intestinal barrier in infants is critical to healthy intestinal function throughout life.

2. The intestinal barrier

The intestinal barrier, with a surface area of 300-400 m^2, is the largest interface between the body and external environment. The intestinal barrier is a complex structure made up of four main components (Fig 1): the physical, chemical, immunological and microbiological barriers. The following sections describe the role of each barrier component in maintaining intestinal barrier function and discusses the link between motility and barrier function.

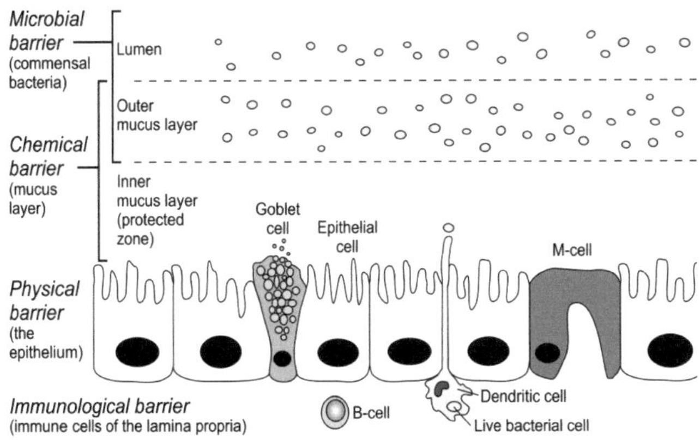

Fig. 1. Four components of the intestinal barrier.

2.1 Physical barrier

The physical barrier is made up of a layer of columnar epithelial cells that forms the first line of defence between the intestinal lumen and inner milieu. Of these cells, greater than 80% are enterocytes with the rest being enteroendocrine, goblet, and Paneth cells (Van Der Flier & Clevers, 2009). Between the epithelial cells are intercellular junctional complexes including tight junctions, adherens junctions, desmosomes and gap junctions (Fig 2) (Farquhar & Palade, 1963). These junctions allow the passage of fluids, electrolytes, and small macromolecules, but inhibit passage of larger molecules. Of the junctional complexes, tight junctions are the most apical and are primarily responsible for controlling permeability of the paracellular pathway. The adherens junctions and desmosomes are involved in cell-cell adhesion, whereas the gap junctions are involved in intracellular communication.

Tight junctions are formed by protein dimers that span the space between adjacent cell membranes (Fig 2). There are over 40 proteins with well recognised roles in tight junction formation. These proteins can be divided into three functional categories: 1) transmembrane proteins that form bridges between adjacent cell membranes; 2) scaffolding proteins that anchor transmembrane proteins to the actin cytoskeleton; and 3) dual location proteins that are not continuously associated with the tight junctions and also act as transcription factors.

2.2 Chemical barrier

The chemical barrier is primarily the layer of mucus that covers the intestinal epithelium. This mucus acts as a diffusion barrier against unwanted substances and also as a lubricant to minimise sheer stress on the physical barrier. The main component of mucus are the secreted mucins, which are heavily glycosylated proteins. Mucins consist of a peptide backbone containing alternating glycosylated and nonglycosylated domains, with O-linked glycosylated regions comprising 70–80% of the polymer (Deplancke & Gaskins, 2001).

The mucus layer is a dynamic defence barrier containing antimicrobial peptides (immunological barrier) that helps prevent contact between bacteria and the epithelial layer. The outer loose mucus layer contains a limited number of intestinal microbes; whereas the inner adherent mucus layer contains very few microbes (Fig 1). Numerous studies show that mucin gene expression, mucus composition and secretion are altered by intestinal microbiota and host-derived inflammatory mediators (Deplancke & Gaskins, 2001).

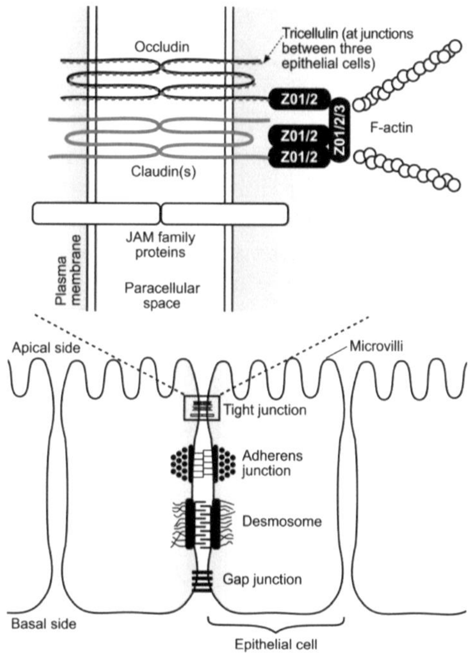

Fig. 2. The protein complexes between intestinal epithelial cells include tight junctions, adherens junctions, desmosomes and gap junctions. The tight junctions control paracellular permeability and consist of transmembrane (e.g., occludin, claudins and junctional adhesion molecules), scaffolding (e.g., zonula occludens, Crumbs group, Par group) and dual-location (e.g., cold shock domain protein A and cyclin-dependent kinase 4) proteins. Figure adapted from Ulluwishewa et al. (2011).

2.3 Immunological barrier

The immunological barrier's first line of defence is secretory IgA which binds to antigenic substances. These IgA-antigen complexes bind to IgA receptors on microfold M cells and the antigens are transferred to the lamina propria for presentation to dendritic cells. Antigen-presenting cells in the lamina propria receive immunostimulatory antigens from the lumen, which they process and present to T cells. The antigen-presenting cells also secrete interleukin (IL)-12 leading T cells to produce a T_H1 immune response. This results in T cell secretion of interferon (IFN)-γ, which in turn activates macrophages to secrete tumour necrosis factor (TNF)-α. IL-10 is also released from antigen-presenting cells, which feedbacks to limit the T_H1 response.

The intestinal immune system must fulfil the dual tasks of tolerance to dietary antigens and immune defence (Rautava & Walker, 2008). To avoid reacting to dietary antigens and the intestinal microbiota, the mucosal immune system exists in a predominantly immune-suppressed (tolerant) state involving antigen-presenting dendritic cells and T cells (Bienenstock et al., 2010). Non-pathogenic bacteria, however, induce a mild immune reaction that contributes to a normal low level inflammation (defence) of the intestine (Bibiloni & Schiffrin, 2010).

2.4 Microbial barrier

The microbial barrier is an essential component of intestinal barrier function that influences epithelial metabolism, proliferation and survival (Neish, 2009). These symbiotic microbes limit pathogen colonisation by competing for adherence to epithelial surfaces, producing antimicrobial compounds, and stimulating increased mucin production. They can also secrete chemicals that allow communication between bacterial species, which can suppress pathogens by optimising the numbers of beneficial microbes (Neish, 2009). The intestinal microbiota provides other crucial functions for the host such as nutrient acquisition and energy regulation (Palmer et al., 2007), and influences processes such as predisposition to obesity, immune homeostasis, inflammation, repair and angiogenesis (Kelly et al., 2007).

The adult gastrointestinal tract is comprised of more than 10^{14} microbes ranging from 10^{11} cells/g content in the ascending colon to 10^{7} - 10^{8} cells/g content in the distal ileum and 10^{2} - 10^{3} cells/g content in the proximal ileum and jejunum. Comprised of 500-1000 species, the microbiota of each adult human colon is unique and remains stable over time (Eckburg et al., 2005). In contrast, the infant intestinal microbiota composition is variable and less stable over time (Palmer et al., 2007), rapidly expanding to over 300 species within the first postnatal week (Park et al., 2005).

The microbiota also produces metabolites such as short chain fatty acids (acetate, propionate and butyrate) that result from fermentation (Kien, 1996). As well as a major energy source for epithelial cells, butyrate affects cellular proliferation and differentiation, increases intestinal blood flow, and may also aid in the strengthening of tight junctions (Neu, 2007; Sanderson, 2004). In addition, butyrate increases intestinal motility (Fukumoto et al., 2003).

2.5 The role of motility in intestinal barrier function

Intestinal motility can influence intestinal barrier function in a number of ways (Fig 3). Motility is one of the most influential determinants of intestinal microbiota growth (Kim & Lin, 2007). In conjunction with fluid/mucus secretion it propels bacteria and toxins (DeMeo et al., 2002) through the lumen, maintaining turnover and providing another defence mechanism for the epithelial barrier. Conversely, the composition of the intestinal microbiota can influence colonic neuromotor function (Verdu, 2009) through release of substances that influence intestinal motility (Kim & Lin, 2007). For example, supernatant from the probiotic, *Escherichia coli* Nissle 1917 (Mutaflor – used in the treatment of colitis) can increase colonic motility in isolated muscle strips from humans (Bar et al., 2009).

There are many neuromodulators in the colon that affect motility, including neurotransmitters: adrenergic (-), cholinergic (+), serotonergic (+), dopaminergic, GABAergic, neuropeptides. These may be released from neurons or other cell types and act on receptors located on a variety of cells including smooth muscle and enteric neurons. Factors that affect neuromodulation can also affect smooth muscle contractility and hence affect transit (Kien, 1996). For example, butyrate produced by bacteria stimulates serotonin (5HT) release from enterochromaffin cells (Fukumoto et al., 2003). 5HT activates intrinsic primary afferent neurons (Fig 3) to initiate peristaltic reflexes (Hord, 2008) and has pro-inflammatory actions (Lakhan & Kirchgessner, 2010). 5HT receptor subtypes differ between animals and humans such that their function in peristalsis in humans is not fully determined (Wouters et al., 2007).

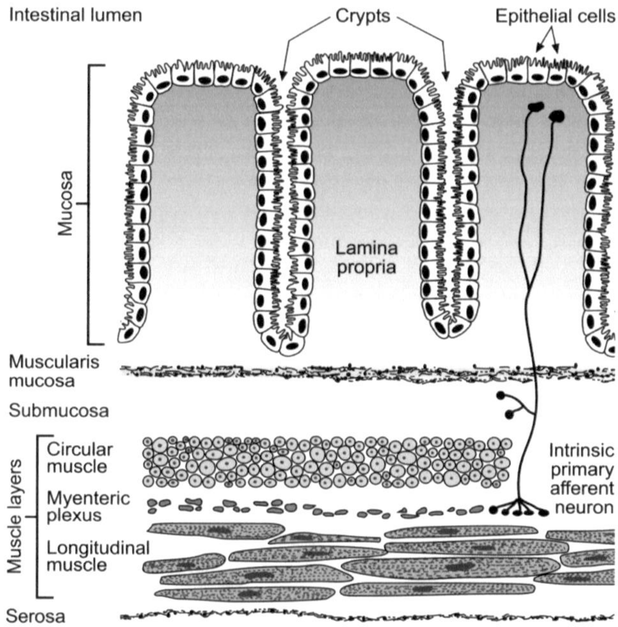

Fig. 3. Intestinal barrier and muscle layers in the colon.

Sympathetic nerves release norepinephrine which inhibits acetylcholine release from motor neurons and relaxes smooth muscle, decreasing gastrointestinal motility. Another enteric neurotransmitter is dopamine. Although the function of dopaminergic neurons is unclear, mice lacking the D_2 dopamine receptor subtype (present in smooth muscle from stomach to distal colon) have increased intestinal motility and stool water content and frequency (Zhi et al., 2006). Expression of most dopamine receptor subunits was detected in submucosal and myenteric neurons (Zhi et al., 2006). Since dopaminergic gene expression begins early at embryonic day 10 in the foetal intestines, prior to the appearance of neurons, it is possible that dopamine affects enteric nervous system development (Zhi et al., 2006).

3. Development and maturation of the intestinal barrier

The complexity of the intestinal barrier develops over time from early gestation through to childhood. The intestine undergoes incredible growth, elongating 1000-fold from 5-40 weeks gestation, to reach a mean length at birth of 275 cm (Neu, 2007). While growth occurs most rapidly during gestation, the intestine continues to lengthen until 3 to 4 years of age (Newell, 2000). The following sections describe the development and maturation of the intestinal barrier and the role of breast milk in these processes.

3.1 Maturation of the intestinal barrier in infants

The physical barrier begins developing from conception; its basic structure is formed by the end of the first trimester, and by week 22 of gestation the absorptive epithelial cells resemble those of the adult intestine (Montgomery et al., 1999). Initially, the absorptive lining of the intestine is stratified (Fig 4A) but soon becomes a single layer of columnar cells (Fig 4B). Simultaneously, structural differentiation begins with establishment of the crypt-villus axis.

Villi form by week 8 of gestation, beginning in the small intestine and progressing to the colon by week 10-12 with crypts developing throughout the intestine between weeks 12-19 (Fig 4C) (Maheshwari & Zemlin, 2009; Montgomery et al., 1999; Polak-Charcon et al., 1980). However, villi disappear from the colon at 30 weeks of gestation as the adult-type crypt epithelium is established (Fig 4D). Epithelial cells with microvilli, goblet and enteroendercrine cells, all derived from the same undifferentiated stem cells, appear by week 8 of gestation (Louis & Lin, 2009) and tight junctions are detected from week 10 (Fig 4B).

Many of the protective aspects of the foetal intestine are evident early in gestation and continue to mature throughout pregnancy (Louis & Lin, 2009). The goblet cells, responsible for producing the chemical barrier, start producing mucin by week 12 of gestation (Fig 4B)(Montgomery et al., 1999). The protective secretory cells of the innate immunological barrier are also formed early in gestation. For example, Paneth cells appear by the week 12 of gestation and begin to produce defensins by week 13 and lysozyme by week 20 with their number per crypt increasing with maturation until adulthood (Fig 4C-F) (Louis & Lin, 2009; Maheshwari & Zemlin, 2009; Rumbo & Schiffrin, 2005). M cells, specialised for antigen sampling, are first observed at week 17 of gestation, and distinct T cell zones and B cell follicles containing follicular dendritic cells, both associated with Peyer's patches, appear by week 19 (Fig 4C). All major components of the intestinal immune apparatus are identifiable by week 29 of gestation (Fig 4D) (Maheshwari & Zemlin, 2009).

Luminal factors play a crucial role in intestinal development. By week 16, the foetus begins to ingest amniotic fluid, which provides essential growth and trophic factors, such as epidermal growth factor and polyamines, that stimulate intestinal differentiation and growth (Pácha, 2000; Rumbo & Schiffrin, 2005). Other cytokines and growth factors necessary for maturation are provided by the systemic circulation and interstitial fluid (Harada et al., 1997; Hirai et al., 2002; Montgomery et al., 1999).

While the foetal intestinal mucosa is permeable to intact macromolecules allowing an exchange between amniotic fluid and foetal serum (Harada et al., 1997), "gut closure", or membrane closure, occurs during the first postnatal week. Any delay or change to these processes, particularly in pre-term or small-for-date infants, predisposes the infant to infection, inflammatory states and allergic sensitisation (Maheshwari & Zemlin, 2009). The gut closure process is mediated by human milk hormones and growth factors that play a crucial role in stimulating intestinal epithelial growth and maturation (Cummins & Thompson, 2002). These are described in more detail in section 3.2.

Formation of the microbial barrier is also crucial during this time. Unlike the adult intestinal tract, the newborn gastrointestinal tract was thought to be essentially sterile. However, recent discoveries point to pregnancy as the beginning of intestinal colonisation of the developing foetus (Jiménez et al., 2008) with a temporal progression towards an adult microbiota profile by the end of the first year of life (Fig 4E-F) (Palmer et al., 2007; Round & Mazmanian, 2009). Many factors contribute to the acquisition of intestinal microbiota including mode of delivery, gestational age, exposure to antibiotics (in either the mother or the infant), feeding (i.e. breast milk or formula, introduction of solids), and other environmental exposures. The first bacteria to colonise the intestine are facultative aerobes (such as *Staphylococcus, Streptococcus and Enterococcus*) while anaerobic bacteria such as eubacteria and clostridia appear later (Palmer et al., 2007).

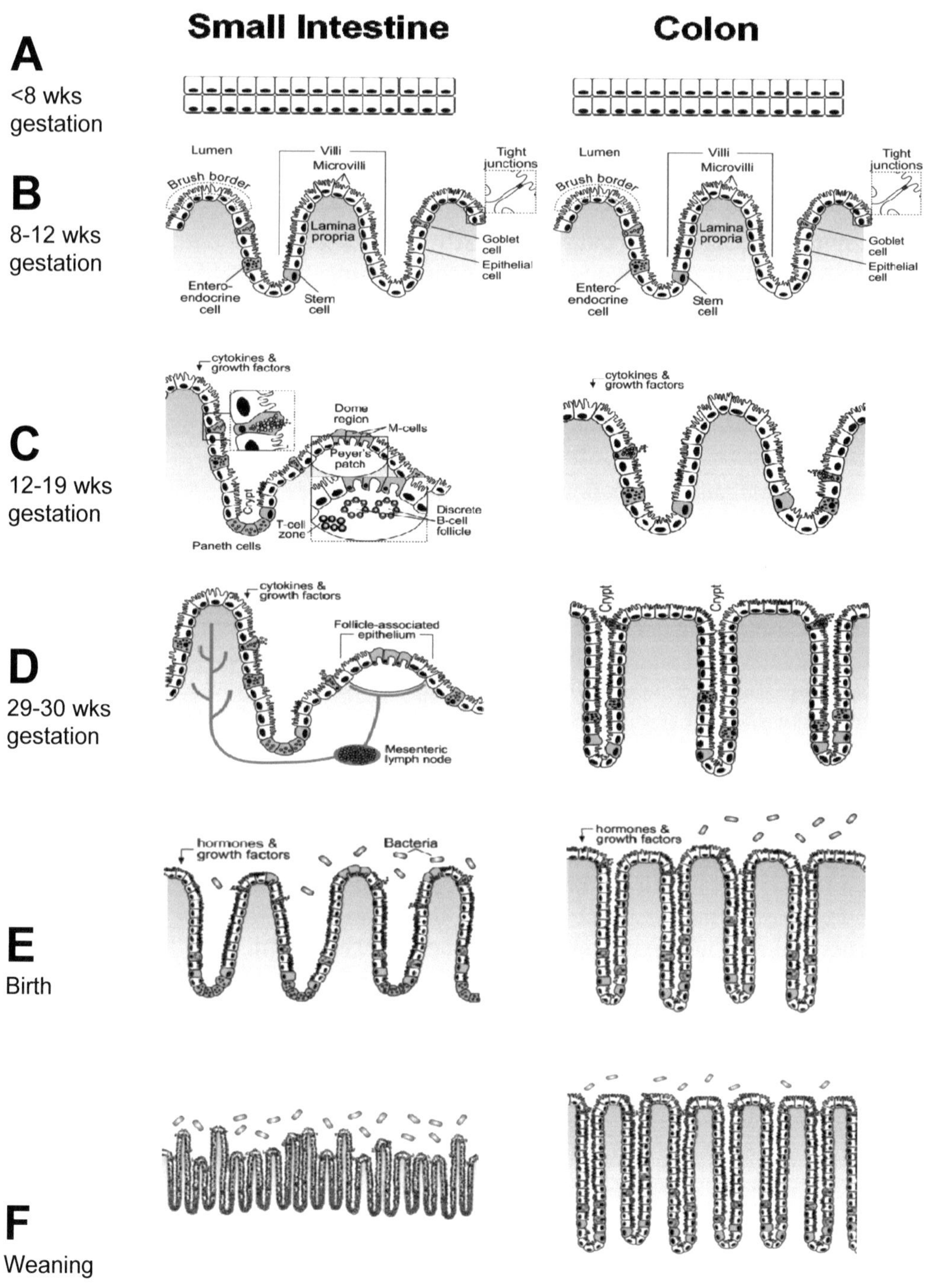

Fig. 4. Development and maturation of the intestinal barrier from conception to weaning.

Intestinal microbiota is necessary for both morphological and immunological maturation of the intestinal barrier (Hooper, 2004). For example, germ-free mice have hypoplastic villi that normalise when colonised with commensal bacteria (Louis & Lin, 2009). Other examples include bacterial-induced expression of the microbiocidal protein angiogenin-4 (Ang4) by paneth cells (Hooper et al., 2003), and induction of the development of networks of blood vessels in the villi (Stappenbeck et al., 2002).

The intestinal mucosal barrier continues to grow in a process that involves fission and deepening of crypts, increase in villus width and number, and appearance of submucosal folds (Cummins & Thompson, 2002). In the early postnatal period, development of intestinal mucosa is associated with profound tissue remodelling and modification of intestinal digestive and absorptive functions. An increase in the number of epithelial cells is also observed at the time of weaning; this involves a shift in the equilibrium between mitosis and apoptosis that is vital for maturation (Zabielski et al., 2008). Because the sIgA system is not fully mature until 4 years of age, it has been postulated that the intestinal barrier is in itself not fully mature until this time (Mayer, 2003).

3.2 Role of breast milk in intestinal barrier maturation

Human breast milk provides all the necessary ingredients for a newborn to make an optimal transition from intrauterine to extrauterine life. Breast milk contains numerous bioactive proteins, lipids and complex carbohydrates, including immune factors and growth factors that play roles in healthy structural and functional postnatal development of the intestinal barrier of the human infant. Although full-term infants are born with sufficiently developed absorptive and digestive function, the gastrointestinal tract undergoes significant postnatal development in the first year of life. The components in human breast milk that compensate for the developmental immaturity of the intestinal barrier include sIgA, lactoferrin, lysozyme, platelet activating factor-acetylhydrolase and cytokines.

Several studies have indicated that human breast milk decreases intestinal permeability and therefore enhances the physical barrier. Since the intestinal barrier is underdeveloped in pre-term babies, the influence of breast milk is particularly important. A study on pre-term infants in the first month post-birth found that those predominately fed human milk demonstrated lower intestinal permeability when compared with those fed minimal or no human milk (Taylor et al., 2009). A similar effect of breast feeding on intestinal permeability has also been reported for full-term babies (Catassi et al., 1995). The effect of formula-feeding on permeability appears to be related to the protein content: in a study using piglets, those fed a high-protein formula had increased intestinal permeability compared with those fed an adequate-protein formula (protein concentration the same as sows milk) and others fed by their mothers (Boudry et al., 2011). However, due to the complex composition of human breast milk and the interplay among its components, it has been difficult to delineate the roles of individual components on intestinal development.

4. Importance of the intestinal barrier in health and wellness

The controlled regulation of the intestinal barrier in the healthy intestine leads to antigenic tolerance. However, disruption of the intestinal barrier, in particular the tight junctions of the physical barrier, results in increased permeability (Fig 5). This allows direct access of antigens to the dendritic cells in the lamina propria, as opposed to the dendritic cells sampling the lumen, and results in an aberrant immune response that can target any organ or tissue in genetically predisposed individuals. As discussed in the following sections, this can lead to inflammatory and autoimmune diseases both during infancy and adulthood.

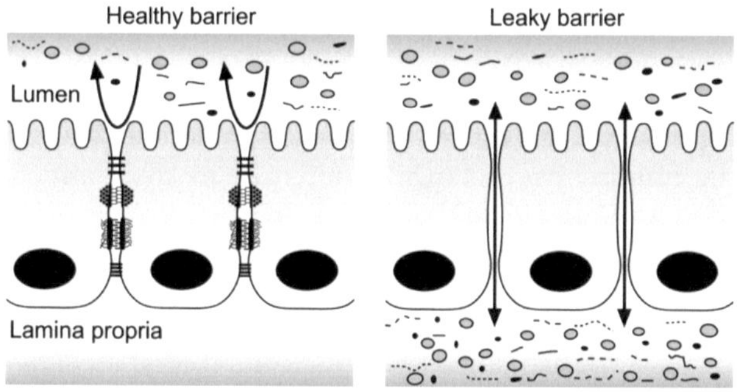

Fig. 5. When the intestinal barrier is functioning correctly, luminal bacteria and antigens are unlikely to pass across the epithelium into the lamina propria. In contrast, when the intestinal barrier is dysfunctional, paracellular permeability is increased.

4.1 Intestinal barrier dysfunction in infants

Dysfunction of intercellular junctions is a key factor in pathogenesis of several early infancy autoimmune diseases, including necrotising enterocolitis and allergic gastro-enteropathy, and may also a play a role in the pathogenesis of infectious diarrhoea. The following sections look at consequences of intestinal barrier dysfunction in the human infant.

4.1.1 Necrotising enterocolitis

Necrotising enterocolitis (NEC) is an inflammatory bowel necrosis that primarily afflicts the terminal ileum and proximal colon in pre-term infants (Caplan & MacKendrick, 1993). Although full-term infants can also develop NEC, there is usually an underlying cause such as birth asphyxia. Immaturity of intestinal barrier function may be a major risk factor for pre-term babies developing NEC. This includes: 1) an underdeveloped physical barrier with incomplete development of tight junctions; 2) a lack of proper chemical barrier due to lower gastric acid and mucin production, immature proteolytic enzyme activity (Udall, 1990), and deficiency of bacteriostatic proteins such as defensins (Salzman et al., 1998); and 3) a poor immunological barrier due to an under developed mucosal immune system.

In addition, the peristaltic muscle contractions can also be abnormal in pre-term infants, which can lead to increased bacterial adhesion, that in turn allows for bacterial overgrowth that could increase endotoxin exposure and predispose to NEC (Beeby & Jeffery, 1992). Pre-term infants have increased intestinal permeability and infants with NEC have even greater permeability (Neu, 2005). Thus any abnormality in maturation of the components of the intestinal barrier can predispose the neonatal intestine to insult by pathogenic or non-pathogenic invasion leading to tissue inflammation.

No case of NEC has been described *in utero,* supporting the importance of bacterial colonisation in the NEC pathophysiology. Most cases of NEC are sporadic, hence a specific infectious agent is not suspected. It is more likely that abnormal colonisation of the gastrointestinal tract with an unfavourable balance between desirable and undesirable microbes plays a significant role in the pathogenesis of NEC. In the case of a normal vaginal birth the infant first comes in contact with microbiota from the mother; whereas, in the case of caesarean birth it is the environment of the hospital or neonatal intensive care unit that provides the first bacterial exposure to the newborn. Indeed, there is evidence of abnormal colonisation in very low birth weight infants (Hoy et al., 2000).

Human breast milk contains a large amount of oligosaccharides that may promote growth of desirable bacteria. Studies have shown differences in the composition of microbiota between breast-fed and formula-fed babies (Rubaltelli et al., 1998; Wold & Adlerberth, 2000). This lack of human milk oligosaccharides in formula-fed pre-term babies may also contribute to NEC pathogenesis. Although the role of enteric bacteria is unclear, studies suggest that early colonisation with probiotics reduces the risk of NEC (Hoyos, 1999).

The likely common pathway in pathogenesis of NEC is the pro-inflammatory cascade initiated by bacteria, bacterial products and other antigens that gain access through a leaky intestinal barrier (Lin & Stoll, 2006). Inflammatory mediators implicated in NEC pathogenesis include platelet-activating factor (PAF), tumour necrosis factor (TNF-α) and pro-inflammatory cytokines such as IL-6, IL-8 and IL-12 (Edelson et al., 1999).

The definitive pathogenesis of NEC remains poorly understood. Hopefully, future research on the maturation of the intestinal barrier, role of probiotics and understanding of genetic predisposition will lead to better preventative and treatment strategies for this disease.

4.1.2 Infectious diarrhoea

Infectious diarrhoea is another disease where intestinal barrier dysfunction plays a role. It is defined as diarrhoea due to bacterial, viral or parasitic infection of the gastrointestinal tract that results in more than three bowel motions in a day with an excessive amount of watery stools. Diarrhoeal episodes are a major health problem in children worldwide and the global incidence of diarrhoeal disease has remained unchanged over the last decade; about 3.2 episodes per child per year (Kosek et al., 2003). In developing countries diarrhoeal illnesses are associated with a high risk of mortality and thus are a major concern.

Rotavirus infection is the single greatest cause of infectious diarrhoea in children worldwide (Dennehy, 2000). Rotavirus disrupts absorptive function by the selective invasion of mature enterocytes by the invading pathogen, resulting in osmolar diarrhoea. Rotavirus acts on epithelial cells by altering protein trafficking, disrupting cell-cell interactions, and damaging tight junctions, thereby increasing paracellular permeability (Obert et al., 2000). The toxic rotavirus unstructured protein-4 induces age- and calcium ion-dependent chloride secretion and disrupts sodium-dependent glucose transporter-1 mediated reabsorption of water (Ball et al., 2005).

There are a number of other pathogens that are responsible for infectious diarrhoea. The prevalence and type of individual pathogen varies widely between geographies and age groups. Common bacteria responsible for infectious diarrhoea include *Campylobacter, Salmonella, Clostridium, Shigella,* and *E. coli*; whereas *Giardia* and *Cryptosporidum* are among the most common parasites. The mechanisms by which these enteropathogens cause diarrhoea are highly variable, and include crypt cell proliferation, cellular invasion, production of enterotoxins or cytotoxins, and enteroadhesion. Infectious agents usually induce diarrhoea by directly damaging epithelial barrier function. For example, the *Viberio cholera* zonula occludens toxin acts by disrupting tight junctions leading to fluid secretion into the lumen (Fasano et al., 1991). Others affect ionic permeability, for example, enterotoxins produced by bacterial pathogens selectively and specifically increase either cyclic adenosine monophosphate (e.g., heat labile *E. coli* toxin) or cyclic guanosine monophosphate (e.g., enterotoxigenic *E. coli,* or *Klebsiella* heat stable toxin - Sta), resulting in the opening of Cl channels in the luminal membrane.

One of the most rapidly expanding areas in prevention and treatment of diarrhoeal diseases is the use of probiotics. A growing number of rigorous meta-analyses show the efficacy of probiotics in prevention of acute infectious diarrhoea in children (Guandalini 2006). Analysis shows that probiotics may shorten the duration and severity of diarrhoea, particularly in young children. Some evidence suggests that probiotics may improve intestinal barrier function (Anderson et al., 2010a; Anderson et al., 2010b). This will be discussed further in Section 5.1.

4.1.3 Allergic gastroenteropathy

Allergic gastroenteropathy is a term that describes an immune-mediated process that can affect any area of the gastrointestinal tract and may include classic allergic reaction, protein losing enteropathy, malabsorption syndrome and post-enteritis milk protein intolerance (Moon & Kleinman, 1995). The features of enteropathy may include lymphocyte and plasma cell infiltration, epithelial abnormality, or crypt hyperplastic villus atrophy and impaired absorption. Allergic gastroenteropathy is more common in infants, but may occur at any age.

The pathophysiologic basis of allergic gasteroenteropathy remains elusive and the primary treatment is the elimination of offending antigens. An elemental diet may prove beneficial in many patients, but the process of identifying causal allergens is time-consuming and often frustrating. The onset of symptoms after the addition of a problematic food may be delayed, adding to the diagnostic difficulties. Cows' milk-sensitive enteropathy is the most common food allergic gasteroenteropathy (Walker-Smith et al., 1978).

The most common type of eosinophilic gastroenteropathy, and most difficult to diagnose and manage, is allergic eosinophilic esophagitis. This disorder is particularly challenging to diagnose because the symptoms overlap those of gastroesophageal reflux (Sicherer, 2003).

4.2 Life-long impact of intestinal barrier dysfunction

Intestinal barrier dysfunction in infancy underlies predisposition to and exacerbation of various autoimmune and inflammatory diseases. In addition, compromised tight junctions are involved in cancer development, infections, and allergies (Fasano, 2011; Groschwitz & Hogan, 2009). The following sections highlight the life-long impact of intestinal barrier dysfunction.

4.2.1 Inflammatory bowel diseases

Inflammatory bowel disease (IBD) is a collection of conditions characterised by chronic and relapsing inflammation of the gastrointestinal tract, and includes Crohn's disease and ulcerative colitis. The exact etiology and pathogenesis of IBD is still unclear, although there is strong evidence for a genetic contribution to disease susceptibility, with more than 40 IBD loci identified (Frank et al., 2011). IBD is considered to involve overly aggressive acquired (T cell) responses to a subset of intestinal microbiotia that develop in genetically susceptible individuals where environmental factors precipitate the onset or reactivation of the disease (Sartor, 2006).

The immune-pathogenesis of IBD occurs in three distinct stages: 1) barrier defects allow luminal contents to penetrate the underlying tissues; 2) clearing of foreign material from the intestinal wall is impaired; and 3) a compensatory immune response, leading to the production of pro-inflammatory cytokines, perpetuates the increased intestinal permeability by re-organising the tight junction proteins (Fasano & Shea-Donohue, 2005; Matricon et al., 2010). This results in a vicious cycle in which barrier dysfunction allows further leakage of luminal contents, thereby triggering an immune response that in turn promotes further leakiness.

Although the intestinal microbiota has been shown to play a role in the development of IBD, specific contributions are undefined due to the complexity of this microbial community. *IL10*-gene-deficient mice that develop colitis in response to colonisation by enteric bacteria, but not under germ-free conditions, demonstrate that bacteria are required to initiate IBD (Hoffmann et al., 2011). However, studies of IBD patients have shown that while there are significant shifts in the composition of the microbiota, there is no consistent microbial profile associated with IBD (Frank et al., 2007; Frank et al., 2011), nor in chronic IBD (Nell et al., 2010). Toll-like receptors, which recognise conserved microbial molecules, and regulatory T cells have an important role in maintaining tolerance and immune homeostasis to prevent chronic inflammation (Levin & Shibolet, 2008; Nell et al., 2010). Likewise, NOD2, which plays an important part in the detection and elimination of intracellular pathogens, is also a recognised risk allele for Crohn's disease (Nell et al., 2010).

Receptors associated with colitis suggest targets for modulation by beneficial bacteria or functional foods to strengthen barrier integrity, immune tolerance and defence. An example is the intermediate conductance K^+ ion channel (IK, KCNN4) for which a gene variant has been implicated in Crohn's disease in an Australia/New Zealand cohort in which IK mRNA expression is significantly reduced (Simms et al., 2010). Decreased IK expression would limit its role in colonic anion secretion (Barmeyer et al., 2010) and positive modulation of motility (Wang et al., 2010), which would affect the microbiota environment. Since IK is also expressed in the colon and lamina propria and modulates T cell activation and cytokine production (Logsdon et al., 1997), reduced expression might impact immune function.

4.2.2 Celiac disease

Celiac disease is an autoimmune disorder of the small intestine that occurs in genetically predisposed individuals. It is caused by a reaction to gliadin, a prolamin component of gluten found in wheat, and similar proteins found in other cereals within the grass genus *Triticum*, such as barley and rye. Symptoms include chronic diarrhoea, failure to thrive and fatigue. Some patients also experience lactose intolerance due to the decrease in intestinal surface and reduced production of lactase but this is usually resolved once the condition is treated. Currently, the only known effective treatment for Celiac disease is a lifelong gluten-free diet. However, enhanced intestinal permeability persists even in asymptomatic patients while on a gluten-free diet (Chahine & Bahna, 2010; Schulzke et al., 1998).

Normally, gliadin is prevented from crossing the intestinal barrier by the intercellular tight junctions. However, in susceptible individuals, interplay between gliadin and the intestinal cells triggers tight junction disassembly. Gliadin causes a reorganisation of actin filaments and altered expression of the tight junction proteins occludin, claudin-3 and claudin-4, the tight junction-associated protein ZO-1 and the adherens junction protein E-cadherin resulting in increased intestinal permeability (Sander et al., 2005). This is thought to precede gliadin-induced immune events that eventually lead to Celiac disease (Schuppan, 2000).

Following tight junction disassembly, gliadin peptides can cross the epithelium and reach the lamina propria where they are recognised by antigen presenting cells. This triggers an inflammatory reaction; the body produces antibodies which damage the villi lining the small intestine and make it difficult for the body to absorb vitamins, minerals and other nutrients (Clemente et al., 2003; Fasano, 2011). Exercise can contribute to the disease by increasing intestinal permeability (Chahine & Bahna, 2010).

4.2.3 Irritable bowel syndrome

Irritable bowel syndrome (IBS) is characterised by abdominal pain and cramping, discomfort, bloating, and changes in bowel movements. Diarrhoea or constipation may predominate, or they may alternate, classified as IBS-D, IBS-C or IBS-A, respectively. While IBS is a common malady, the mechanisms by which the symptoms arise are poorly understood. IBS is associated with psychological disturbance (Drossman et al., 1999), food intolerance (Atkinson et al., 2004; Francis & Whorwell, 1994), and prior gastroenteritis (Dunlop et al., 2006; Spiller, 2003). The psychological aspect of this disease is not surprising given that stress is a well-documented inducer of intestinal permeability (Söderholm & Perdue, 2001).

Growing evidence suggests that patients with IBS have decreased intestinal barrier function and that some forms of IBS are associated with low-grade intestinal inflammation (Collins et al., 2001). Permeability of colonic biopsies is significantly higher in patients with IBS compared with healthy subjects (Piche et al., 2009). Furthermore, intestinal permeability profiles differ among IBS subtypes with increased small bowel permeability both in post infectious-IBS and IBS-D without an infectious onset when compared with both controls and IBS-C (Dunlop et al., 2006).

A number of other IBS-like intestinal disorders are associated with increased intestinal permeability. For instance, chronic alcohol consumption leads to enhanced translocation of endotoxins from the intestine to other organs resulting in inflammation and tissue damage (Groschwitz & Hogan, 2009). Non-steroidal anti-inflammatory drugs (NSAIDs), such as aspirin, also promote altered intestinal barrier dysfunction and hypermotility (Sigthorsson et al., 1998), as do the enterotoxins produced by bacterial pathogens such as *Vibrio cholerae,* and enteropathogenic *E. coli* (Fasano et al., 1991; Groschwitz & Hogan, 2009). The inflammatory responses elicited by bacteria and bacterial toxins due to changes in the integrity of the intestinal barrier have also been shown to enhance cancer progression (Fukata & Abreu, 2008). In some studies of IBD, the degree and prolongation of the duration of ulcerative colitis were recognised as factors leading to increased risk of gastrointestinal cancer development (McConnell & Yang, 2009; Tlaskalová-Hogenová et al., 2011), although the mechanisms involved are not fully understood.

Stress induced in early life by neonatal maternal separation may affect colonic permeability and motility (Bian et al., 2010; Coutinho et al., 2002; Gareau et al., 2007). When this condition is mimicked in a rat model of IBS, colonic smooth muscle contraction amplitude is increased and this is associated with an increased expression of L-type calcium ion channels in colonic smooth muscle, as the level of calcium in smooth muscle cells increased in response to L-type calcium ion channel activation (Zhang et al., 2010).

4.2.4 Non-intestinal disorders

There is increasing evidence to suggest intestinal barrier dysfunction results in immune responses that can target any organ or tissue in genetically predisposed individuals (Fasano & Shea-Donohue, 2005; Fasano, 2011), such as the skeletal system (ankylosing spondylitis, rheumatoid arthritis: Edwards, 2008), pancreas (type 1 diabetes: (Carratù et al., 1999), kidney (IgA nephropathy: Davin et al., 1988), liver (nonalcoholic steatohepatitis: Wigg et al., 2001), and brain (multiple sclerosis; Yacyshyn et al., 1996). Barrier dysfunction can also result in an aberrant or exaggerated inflammatory response to the intestinal microbiota. This has been implicated in a wide range of diseases such as cardiovascular disease, neoplastic diseases, diabetes and obesity (Chahine & Bahna, 2010). Intestinal microbiota and increased intestinal permeability have also been linked to atopic diseases such as eczema and dermatitis (Penna et al., 2008).

5. Improving intestinal barrier function

Ingestion of specific foods or bacteria to reverse barrier dysfunction has the potential to break the vicious cycle that occurs in colitis, that is, to improve physical barrier integrity and to maintain an immune homeostasis. Food and probiotics are intricately linked in their effects on colitis. In addition to the direct effects of food on intestinal barrier growth and survival, many food components are prebiotics, promoting the growth of beneficial bacteria. While effects of food components are generally studied in isolation it is the net effect of these interactions with the intestinal barrier that will determine their impact in colitis.

5.1 Probiotic bacteria that enhance intestinal barrier function

Probiotics are microorganisms that when ingested transiently occupy the gastrointestinal tract to confer health benefits (Saavedra, 2007). *Lactobacillus*, *Bifidobacterium* and *Streptococcus* species are widely used in foods for fermentation, and some strains are probiotic in that they help maintain intestinal barrier and immune functions (Saavedra, 2007). Multiple mechanisms have been implicated in beneficial probiotic modes of action. These include immune modulation of the host, production of substances that inhibit pathogens or toxins, competition with and therefore inhibition of pathogen growth, mucosal barrier repair (decrease permeability) (Penna et al., 2008), increased mucus secretion (Saavedra, 2007), and altered motility (Verdu, 2009). More specifically, probiotics have been reported to exert beneficial effects including altered cytokine secretion (particularly to down-regulate inflammation in infants), to affect T cell differentiation, and to increase macrophage activation (Saavedra, 2007).

Some probiotic bacteria, such as *Lactobacillus plantarum* (Anderson et al., 2010a; Anderson et al., 2010b), can improve tight junction integrity (physical barrier). For a recent review see Ulluwishewa et al. (2011). Probiotic bacteria may also enhance mucin production (chemical barrier). For example, a probiotic formula composed of *Lactobacillus, Bifidobacterium,* and *Streptococcus* species induces mucin gene expression and secretion in colonic epithelial cells (Caballero-Franco et al., 2007). Additionally, some probiotic bacteria can reduce the risk of infection (immunological barrier), for example, non-pathogenic *E. coli* have been shown to protect pre-term infants from infection (and reduce allergy) (Candy et al., 2008). Supplementation with probiotic bacteria can also alter the microbiota composition (microbial barrier). For example, when pre-term formula-fed infants are supplemented with bifidobacteria, their microbiota composition more closely resembles that of breast milk-fed infants (Saavedra, 2007).

Finally, probiotics can alter intestinal motility, which in turn can affect intestinal barrier function as discussed in Section 2.4. Probiotics that increase motility can also have the benefit of reducing constipation; whereas those that decrease motility may reduce diarrhoea (permeability changes are also relevant). Some *Lactobacillus, Bifidobacterium* and *Streptococcus* species increase intestinal motility *in vitro* (Massi et al., 2006; Wang et al., 2010) and *in vivo* (Ohashi et al., 2001) and reduce transit times from approximately 4 to 3 days in patients with chronic constipation (Krammer et al., 2011).

5.2 Foods that enhance intestinal barrier function

The most common way to alter intestinal barrier function using dietary intervention is via modification of the intestinal microbiota composition (microbial barrier). A prebiotic is a non-digestable ingredient that results in activity of the intestinal microbiota that is beneficial to the host (Roberfroid et al., 2010). The main substrates for bacterial growth are dietary non-digestible carbohydrates (e.g. pectins), non-digestible oligosaccharides (e.g. galactins), undigested disaccharide components (lactose), and sugar alcohols (Scheppach et al., 1996). Many of these are fermented by colonic bacteria to short chain fatty acids, which are also beneficial in that they acidify the lumen suppressing pathogen growth, and alter motility as described in Section 2.4 (Yajima, 1985). Short chain oligosaccharide fermentation increases bifidobacteria concentrations in adult faecal samples *in vitro* (Hernot et al., 2009). Although promotion of bifidobacteria concentration has been demonstrated in a number of infant studies (Rautava & Walker, 2008), few reports exist on the clinical benefits of dietary oligosaccharides in infants (Roberfroid et al., 2010). In pre-term infants, an oligosaccharide mix did not enhance the postnatal decrease in intestinal permeability (Westerbeek et al., 2010). However, treatment of healthy pre-term formula-fed infants with oligosaccharides has been shown to speed gastric emptying by 30% (Indrio et al., 2009). This is consistent with clinical studies on the effects of galacto-oligosaccharides reported for adults and the elderly that increase motility (Niittynen et al., 2007). The relatively slow mode of action of prebiotics in promoting bacterial growth is reflected in studies which demonstrate its effectiveness in prophylaxis rather than treatment (Roberfroid et al., 2010). Prebiotic supplementation to formula-fed infants increased bifidobacteria counts and reduced the occurrence of diarrhoea four-fold (Rao et al., 2009).

Some food components can improve tight junction integrity (physical barrier). For example: green pepper, nutmeg, and bay leaf extracts (Hashimoto et al., 1997), star anise, black tea (Konishi, 2003), and the flavonoid quercetin (Amasheh et al., 2008; Suzuki & Hara, 2009). Curcumin, a polyphenolic from turmeric, reduced inflammation in a mouse model of colonic inflammation (Nones et al., 2009). Black tea has multiple effects on physical aspects of the intestinal barrier in that it can improve tight junction integrity and speed gastrointestinal transit (Chaudhuri et al., 2000; Hashimoto et al., 1997). Some polyunsaturated fatty acids (PUFAs) are able to decrease intestinal permeability (Vine et al., 2002) and reduce intestinal inflammation (Knoch et al., 2009). Some dairy compounds can also enhance barrier function, for example, β-lactoglobulin (Hashimoto et al., 1995) and the casein peptide Asn-Pro-Trp-Asp-Gln (Yasumatsu & Tanabe, 2010) improve tight junction integrity. Bovine colostrum and goat milk powder were shown to reduce heat-induced intestinal hyperpermeability in a rat model (Prosser et al., 2004).

Additionally, food components can promote immune system development and homeostasis (immunological barrier). For example, lectin from kidney beans can accelerate the process of intestinal mucosa maturation in piglets (Zabielski et al., 2008). Bovine milk is a rich source of proteins and peptides that are important in immune system development and function. For example, glycomacropeptide derived from kappa casein, has anti-inflammatory activity in a rat model of colitis, suggesting potential for IBD treatment (Daddaoua et al., 2005). Oligosaccharides from goat milk have been shown to enhance recovery from colonic inflammatory damage in a rat model of colitis and may therefore also be useful for treatment of IBD (Daddaoua et al., 2006).

6. Delivering ingredients to infants

The delivery of required nutrients during the neonatal period is critical to later health outcomes. It is therefore essential that when breast feeding is not possible, steps are taken to incorporate functional ingredients suitable for infants into appropriate food systems, and deliver them to the required areas of the body. Infants can only ingest foods in liquid form until they are 4-6 months old, after which formulas and more structured food matrices, such as puréed/semi-solid foods can be introduced to their diet. The addition of functional ingredients can cause a range of adverse effects such as changes in stability, appearance and taste of the product. Additionally, the effects of processing, lack of bio-accessibility, or interaction with the food matrix may reduce the activity of the functional ingredient (Patel & Velikov, 2011).

6.1 Delivering probiotic bacteria to infants

Since probiotics do not colonise the intestines, they must be continually supplemented via food products to be of benefit. Probiotics are now added to many established infant formula ranges (e.g., Nestle-Nan Pro Gold, Danone-Aptamil and Nutirica-Karicare). The main difficulty associated with the incorporation of probiotics into foods is ensuring that the bacteria are both viable (at quantities sufficient enough to show an effect) and functional when they are delivered to the intestine. The three main obstacles to viability and functionality are the effects of processing, storage, and transition through the gastrointestinal tract. Industrial preparations of various probiotic strains can be bought in a number of forms (e.g. spray- and freeze-dried). A solution to delivering probiotic bacteria through the gastrointestinal tract is encapsulation. Matrices that can be used for probiotics have been comprehensively reviewed (Anal & Singh, 2007). It is important to understand the possible effects of the protective matrix on intestinal barrier function. For example, the food grade polymer chitosan, used in encapsulation matrices, can itself increase tight junction permeability (Sadeghi et al., 2008). Such particles are used in the drug/medical industry to help open tight junctions to allow particles through (targeted drug delivery).

The composition of the food matrix used to deliver the probiotic bacteria, including its pH, water activity, dissolved oxygen level and storage temperature, can affect viability. The pH of a fruit juice system for example will be low (3-4), and therefore this factor along with the organic acids present can cause a decrease in viability of most probiotic strains over storage time (Saarela et al., 2006). Researchers have found that milk-based systems perform well as delivery systems for probiotics due to the buffering capacity and pH of the milk, which can protect the bacterial strain from detrimental effects of gastric acid (Ranadheera et al., 2010). The amount and type of fat present in yoghurts can have an effect, with lower levels of fat showing greater probiotic viability for certain strains (Vinderola et al., 2000).

The delivery matrix can also have a significant effect on probiotic functionality due to positive or negative interactions. The response of probiotics to their surrounding environment could affect the level of organic acid produced, and therefore limit the extent of health benefit conferred. Interactions between probiotics and macromolecules in the matrix are also important. For example, a probiotic strain of *Lactobacillus reuteri* interacts preferentially with the fat globule membrane in dairy products (Brisson et al., 2010).

The survival of probiotics can also be enhanced by the addition of prebiotics, which are now added in varying quantities to food systems such as infant formulas (Boehmm G., 2007). For example, fructo and galacto-oligosaccharides have been found to promote the growth rate of bifidobacteria (Siggers et al., 2011).

6.2 Delivery of food components to infants

Peptides that play a role in promoting intestinal barrier function can be released from bovine milk proteins, casein (β- and α-) and whey (β-lactalbumin and α-lactoglobulin) (Yasumatsu & Tanabe, 2010), through commercial processing and gastric digestion. A number of factors can affect peptide activity, such as processing, shelf life of the product and the food system in which they are delivered to the body. An example of how both the intrinsic properties of the peptides and external factors can affect bioactivity was described in a recent study (Dupont et al., 2010). It was found that casein fractions (κ- and α_{s2}) were more resistant to infant digestion, due to both hydrophobic areas on the protein at pH 3 and heat processes during preparation of the product. This resistance to hydrolysis within the intestine may also be attributed partially to interactions with whey protein, which may protect the casein fractions to an extent. Conversely, a casein hydrolysate was found that can withstand manufacturing processes (atomisation, homogenisation, pasteurisation) and storage for a considerable time without any significant effect on its activity (Contreras et al., 2011). Recently a few studies have focused on assessing the effect of digestion on various peptides such as caseinophosphopeptides (García-Nebot et al., 2010). Further hydrolysis can occur as the peptides move through the stomach that may not always be desirable as it may reduce bioactivity within the body (Kamau et al., 2010). The effect of high temperatures on aminopeptides and lipids during processing in the presence of reducing sugars can lead to the formation of advanced glycation end products (AGEs). While these milk fractions may have been placed in the food system to potentially decrease intestinal permeability, the formation of AGEs can actually have the opposite effect (Rapin & Wiernsperger, 2010). Therefore it is of vital importance that the properties of the bioactive ingredients are considered, along with the composition of the food matrix and changes that occur to the product during processing and storage.

As with probiotics, there are many limitations that prevent the delivery of functional food components to the required site in the body. Encapsulation and protection have been identified as critical to the incorporation and delivery of biologically active ingredients to infants. The reasons are varied; from protection of the ingredient against processing conditions as discussed above, to masking of taste and also providing protection between the ingredient and the surrounding environment (gastric acid). The site of release is also important in order for these ingredients to confer a health benefit. Some peptides have been found to give a bitter taste, therefore effects on the organoleptic properties of food products are also a concern. This bitterness has been attributed to the hydrophobic nature of their amino acid side chains. Both the hydrophobicity and bitterness of milk peptides have lead to the use of encapsulation as a means to incorporate these ingredients into food systems. Methods such as spray drying have been recently used to try and reduce the extent of the bitterness of a casein hydrolysate (Favaro-Trindade et al., 2010). Mixtures of soy protein isolate and gelatin as carriers for the peptide helped to mask the adverse effects of the powdered samples.

7. Conclusions

It is well-established that intestinal barrier dysfunction can lead to gastrointestinal illness in infants and is a risk factor for inflammatory and autoimmune disease during adulthood. Since it is difficult to permanently alter intestinal barrier integrity in adults, greater success may be achieved by intervening in early-life to ensure the intestinal barrier matures appropriately, improving health both during infancy and adulthood.

Breast feeding is the most beneficial way to feed an infant and promote intestinal barrier maturation; however, this may not always be possible. Many infants, even while being breast-fed, also receive formula in order to meet their nutritional needs. Therefore, the optimisation of infant formulas and foods with ingredients that enhance intestinal barrier function is necessary to promote life-long wellness. However, more research is needed to fully understand how the intestinal barrier develops and the mechanisms by which food ingredients may enhance this process. In addition, there are still challenges in delivering ingredients to ensure that functional food ingredients maintain their activity throughout production, storage, and digestion.

8. Acknowledgments

This work was funded by the New Zealand Ministry of Science and Innovation (Contract C10X1003). The authors acknowledge Pauline Hunt, the AgResearch graphic designer, for drawing all of the figures included in this chapter, and Drs Tim Coolbear (Fonterra) and Rodrigo Bibiloni (AgResearch) for reviewing the manuscript.

9. References

Amasheh, M., Schlichter, S., Amasheh, S., Mankertz, J., Zeitz, M., Fromm, M. & Schulzke, J.D. (2008). Quercetin enhances epithelial barrier function and increases claudin-4 expression in caco-2 cells. *Journal of Nutrition,* 138, 6, 1067-1073

Anal, A.K. & Singh, H. (2007). Recent advances in microencapsulation of probiotics for industrial applications and targeted delivery. *Trends in Food Science and Technology,* 18, 5, 240-251

Anderson, R.C., Cookson, A.L., McNabb, W.C., Kelly, W.J. & Roy, N.C. (2010a). *Lactobacillus plantarum* dsm 2648 is a potential probiotic that enhances intestinal barrier function. *FEMS Microbiology Letters,* 309, 2, 184-192

Anderson, R.C., Cookson, A.L., McNabb, W.C., Park, Z., McCann, M.J., Kelly, W.J. & Roy, N.C. (2010b). *Lactobacillus plantarum* mb452 enhances the function of the intestinal barrier by increasing the expression levels of genes involved in tight junction formation. *BMC Microbiology,* 10, art. no. 316

Atkinson, W., Sheldon, T.A., Shaath, N. & Whorwell, P.J. (2004). Food elimination based on igg antibodies in irritable bowel syndrome: A randomised controlled trial. *Gut,* 53, 10, 1459-1464

Ball, J.M., Mitchell, D.M., Gibbons, T.F. & Parr, R.D. (2005). Rotavirus nsp4: A multifunctional viral enterotoxin. *Viral Immunology,* 18, 1, 27-40

Bar, F., Von Koschitzky, H., Roblick, U., Bruch, H.P., Schulze, L., Sonnenborn, U., Bottner, M. & Wedel, T. (2009). Cell-free supernatants of *escherichia coli* nissle 1917 modulate human colonic motility: Evidence from an in vitro organ bath study. *Neurogastroenterology and Motility,* 21, 5, 559-e517

Barmeyer, C., Rahner, C., Yang, Y., Sigworth, F.J., Binder, H.J. & Rajendran, V.M. (2010). Cloning and identification of tissue-specific expression of kcnn4 splice variants in rat colon. *American Journal of Physiology - Cell Physiology,* 299, 2, C251-C263

Beeby, P.J. & Jeffery, H. (1992). Risk factors for necrotising enterocolitis: The influence of gestational age. *Archives of Disease in Childhood,* 67, 4 SUPPL., 432-435

Bian, Z.X., Zhang, M., Han, Q.B., Xu, H.X. & Sung, J.J.Y. (2010). Analgesic effects of jcm-16021 on neonatal maternal separation-induced visceral pain in rats. *World Journal of Gastroenterology,* 16, 7, 837-845

Bibiloni, R. & Schiffrin, E.J. (2010). Intestinal host-microbe interactions under physiological and pathological conditions. *International Journal of Inflammation,* 2010, 1-8

Bienenstock, J., Forsythe, P., Karimi, K. & Kunze, W. (2010). Neuroimmune aspects of food intake. *International Dairy Journal,* 20, 4, 253-258

Boudry, G., Morise, A., Seve, B. & Huërou-Luron, I. (2011). Effect of milk formula protein content on intestinal barrier function in a porcine model of lbw neonates. *Pediatric Research,* 69, 1, 4-9

Brisson, G., Payken, H.F., Sharpe, J.P. & Jimenez-Flores, R. (2010). Characterization of lactobacillus reuteri interaction with milk fat globule membrane components in dairy products. *Journal of Agricultural and Food Chemistry,* 58, 9, 5612-5619

Caballero-Franco, C., Keller, K., De Simone, C. & Chadee, K. (2007). The vsl#3 probiotic formula induces mucin gene expression and secretion in colonic epithelial cells. *American Journal of Physiology - Gastrointestinal and Liver Physiology,* 292, 1, G315-G322

Candy, D.C., Heath, S.J., Lewis, J.D. & Thomas, L.V. (2008). Probiotics for the young and the not so young. *International Journal of Dairy Technology,* 61, 3, 215-221

Caplan, M.S. & MacKendrick, W. (1993). Necrotizing enterocolitis: A review of pathogenetic mechanisms and implications for prevention. *Pediatric Pathology,* 13, 3, 357-369

Carratù, R., Secondulfo, M., De Magistris, L., Iafusco, D., Urio, A., Carbone, M.G., Pontoni, G., Cartenì, M. & Prisco, F. (1999). Altered intestinal permeability to mannitol in diabetes mellitus type i. *Journal of Pediatric Gastroenterology and Nutrition,* 28, 3, 264-269

Catassi, C., Bonucci, A., Coppa, G.V., Carlucci, A. & Giorgi, P.L. (1995). Intestinal permeability changes during the first month: Effect of natural versus artificial feeding. *Journal of Pediatric Gastroenterology and Nutrition,* 21, 4, 383-386

Cereijido, M., Contreras, R.G., Flores-Benítez, D., Flores-Maldonado, C., Larre, I., Ruiz, A. & Shoshani, L. (2007). New diseases derived or associated with the tight junction. *Archives of Medical Research,* 38, 5, 465-478

Chahine, B.G. & Bahna, S.L. (2010). The role of the gut mucosal immunity in the development of tolerance versus development of allergy to food. *Current Opinion in Allergy and Clinical Immunology,* 10, 4, 394-399

Chaudhuri, L., Basu, S., Seth, P., Chaudhuri, T., Besra, S.E., Vedasiromoni, J.R. & Ganguly, D.K. (2000). Prokinetic effect of black tea on gastrointestinal motility. *Life Sciences,* 66, 9, 847-854

Clemente, M.G., De Virgiliis, S., Kang, J.S., Macatagney, R., Musu, M.P., Di Pierro, M.R., Drago, S., Congia, M. & Fasano, A. (2003). Early effects of gliadin on enterocyte intracellular signalling involved in intestinal barrier function. *Gut,* 52, 2, 218-223

Collins, S.M., Piche, T. & Rampal, P. (2001). The putative role of inflammation in the irritable bowel syndrome. *Gut,* 49, 6, 743-745

Contreras, M.d.M., Sevilla, M.A., Monroy-Ruiz, J., Amigo, L., Gómez-Sala, B., Molina, E., Ramos, M. & Recio, I. (2011). Food-grade production of an antihypertensive casein hydrolysate and resistance of active peptides to drying and storage. *International Dairy Journal,* 21, 7, 470-476

Coutinho, S.V., Plotsky, P.M., Sablad, M., Miller, J.C., Zhou, H., Bayati, A.I., McRoberts, J.A. & Mayer, E.A. (2002). Neonatal maternal separation alters stress-induced responses to viscerosomatic nociceptive stimuli in rat. *American Journal of Physiology - Gastrointestinal and Liver Physiology,* 282, 2 45-2, G307-G316

Cummins, A.G. & Thompson, F.M. (2002). Effect of breast milk and weaning on epithelial growth of the small intestine in humans. *Gut,* 51, 5, 748-754

Daddaoua, A., Puerta, V., Zarzuelo, A., Suárez, M.D., Sánchez De Medina, F. & Martínez-Augustin, O. (2005). Bovine glycomacropeptide is anti-inflammatory in rats with hapten-induced colitis. *Journal of Nutrition,* 135, 5, 1164-1170

Daddaoua, A., Puerta, V., Requena, P., Martínez-Férez, A., Guadix, E., Sánchez De Medina, F., Zarzuelo, A., Suárez, M.D., Boza, J.J. & Martínez-Augustin, O. (2006). Goat milk oligosaccharides are anti-inflammatory in rats with hapten-induced colitis. *Journal of Nutrition,* 136, 3, 672-676

Davin, J.C., Forget, P. & Mahieu, P.R. (1988). Increased intestinal permeability to (51 cr) edta is correlated with iga immune complex-plasma levels in children with iga-associated nephropathies. *Acta Paediatrica Scandinavica,* 77, 1, 118-124

DeMeo, M.T., Mutlu, E.A., Keshavarzian, A. & Tobin, M.C. (2002). The small intestine and nutrition: Intestinal permeation and gastrointestinal disease. *Journal of Clinical Gastroenterology,* 34, 4, 385-396

Dennehy, P.H. (2000). Transmission of rotavirus and other enteric pathogens in the home. *Pediatric Infectious Disease Journal,* 19, 10 SUPPL., S103-S105

Deplancke, B. & Gaskins, H.R. (2001). Microbial modulation of innate defense: Goblet cells and the intestinal mucus layer. *American Journal of Clinical Nutrition,* 73, 6, 1131S-1141S

Drossman, D.A., Creed, F.H., Olden, K.W., Svedlund, J., Toner, B.B. & Whitehead, W.E. (1999). Psychosocial aspects of the functional gastrointestinal disorders. *Gut,* 45, SUPPL. 2, II25-II30

Dunlop, S.P., Hebden, J., Campbell, E., Naesdal, J., Olbe, L., Perkins, A.C. & Spiller, R.C. (2006). Abnormal intestinal permeability in subgroups of diarrhea-predominant irritable bowel syndromes. *American Journal of Gastroenterology,* 101, 6, 1288-1294

Dupont, D., Mandalari, G., Mollé, D., Jardin, J., Rolet-Répécaud, O., Duboz, G., Léonil, J., Mills, C.E.N. & Mackie, A.R. (2010). Food processing increases casein resistance to simulated infant digestion. *Molecular Nutrition and Food Research,* 54, 11, 1677-1689

Eckburg, P.B., Bik, E.M., Bernstein, C.N., Purdom, E., Dethlefsen, L., Sargent, M., Gill, S.R., Nelson, K.E. & Relman, D.A. (2005). Diversity of the human intestinal microbial flora. *Science,* 308, 5728, 1635-1638

Edelson, M.B., Bagwell, C.E. & Rozycki, H.J. (1999). Circulating pro- and counterinflammatory cytokine levels and severity in necrotizing enterocolitis. *Pediatrics,* 103, 4 I, 766-771

Farquhar, M.G. & Palade, G.E. (1963). Junctional complexes in various epithelia. *The Journal of cell biology,* 17, 375-412

Fasano, A., Baudry, B., Pumplin, D.W., Wasserman, S.S., Tall, B.D., Ketley, J.M. & Kaper, J.B. (1991). *Vibrio cholerae* produces a second enterotoxin, which affects intestinal tight junctions. *Proceedings of the National Academy of Sciences of the United States of America,* 88, 12, 5242-5246

Fasano, A. & Shea-Donohue, T. (2005). Mechanisms of disease: The role of intestinal barrier function in the pathogenesis of gastrointestinal autoimmune diseases. *Nature Clinical Practice Gastroenterology and Hepatology,* 2, 9, 416-422

Fasano, A. (2011). Zonulin and its regulation of intestinal barrier function: The biological door to inflammation, autoimmunity, and cancer. *Physiological Reviews,* 91, 1, 151-175

Favaro-Trindade, C.S., Santana, A.S., Monterrey-Quintero, E.S., Trindade, M.A. & Netto, F.M. (2010). The use of spray drying technology to reduce bitter taste of casein hydrolysate. *Food Hydrocolloids,* 24, 4, 336-340

Francis, C.Y. & Whorwell, P.J. (1994). Bran and irritable bowel syndrome: Time for reappraisal. *Lancet,* 344, 8914, 39-40

Frank, D.N., St. Amand, A.L., Feldman, R.A., Boedeker, E.C., Harpaz, N. & Pace, N.R. (2007). Molecular-phylogenetic characterization of microbial community imbalances in human inflammatory bowel diseases. *Proceedings of the National Academy of Sciences of the United States of America,* 104, 34, 13780-13785

Frank, D.N., Robertson, C.E., Hamm, C.M., Kpadeh, Z., Zhang, T., Chen, H., Zhu, W., Sartor, R.B., Boedeker, E.C., Harpaz, N., Pace, N.R. & Li, E. (2011). Disease phenotype and genotype are associated with shifts in intestinal-associated microbiota in inflammatory bowel diseases. *Inflammatory Bowel Diseases,* 17, 1, 179-184

Fukata, M. & Abreu, M.T. (2008). Role of toll-like receptors in gastrointestinal malignancies. *Oncogene,* 27, 2, 234-243

Fukumoto, S., Tatewaki, M., Yamada, T., Fujimiya, M., Mantyh, C., Voss, M., Eubanks, S., Harris, M., Pappas, T.N. & Takahashi, T. (2003). Short-chain fatty acids stimulate colonic transit via intraluminal 5-ht release in rats. *American Journal of Physiology - Regulatory Integrative and Comparative Physiology,* 284, 5 53-5, R1269-R1276

García-Nebot, M.J., Alegría, A., Barberá, R., Contreras, M.d.M. & Recio, I. (2010). Milk versus caseinophosphopeptides added to fruit beverage: Resistance and release from simulated gastrointestinal digestion. *Peptides,* 31, 4, 555-561

Gareau, M.G., Jury, J. & Perdue, M.H. (2007). Neonatal maternal separation of rat pups results in abnormal cholinergic regulation of epithelial permeability. *American Journal of Physiology - Gastrointestinal and Liver Physiology,* 293, 1, G198-G203

Groschwitz, K.R. & Hogan, S.P. (2009). Intestinal barrier function: Molecular regulation and disease pathogenesis. *Journal of Allergy and Clinical Immunology,* 124, 1, 3-20; quiz 21-22

Harada, I., Tsutsumi, O., Momoeda, M., Horikawa, R., Yasunaga, T., Tanaka, T. & Taketani, Y. (1997). Comparative concentrations of growth hormone-binding protein in maternal circulation, fetal circulation, and amniotic fluid. *Endocrine Journal,* 44, 1, 111-116

Hashimoto, K., Takeda, K., Nakayama, T. & Shimizu, M. (1995). Stabilization of the tight junction of the intestinal caco-2 cell monolayer by milk whey proteins. *Bioscience, Biotechnology, and Biochemistry,* 59, 10, 1951-1952

Hashimoto, K., Kawagishi, H., Nakayama, T. & Shimizu, M. (1997). Effect of capsianoside, a diterpene glycoside, on tight-junctional permeability. *Biochimica et Biophysica Acta - Biomembranes,* 1323, 2, 281-290

Hernot, D.C., Boileau, T.W., Bauer, L.L., Middelbos, I.S., Murphy, M.R., Swanson, K.S. & Fahey Jr, G.C. (2009). *In vitro* fermentation profiles, gas production rates, and microbiota modulation as affected by certain fructans, galactooligosaccharides, and polydextrose. *Journal of Agricultural and Food Chemistry,* 57, 4, 1354-1361

Hirai, C., Ichiba, H., Saito, M., Shintaku, H., Yamano, T. & Kusuda, S. (2002). Trophic effect of multiple growth factors in amniotic fluid or human milk on cultured human fetal small intestinal cells. *Journal of Pediatric Gastroenterology and Nutrition,* 34, 5, 524-528

Hoffmann, M., Messlik, A., Kim, S.C., Sartor, R.B. & Haller, D. (2011). Impact of a probiotic enterococcus faecalis in a gnotobiotic mouse model of experimental colitis. *Molecular Nutrition and Food Research,* 55, 5, 703-713

Hooper, L.V., Stappenbeck, T.S., Hong, C.V. & Gordon, J.I. (2003). Angiogenins: A new class of microbicidal proteins involved in innate immunity. *Nature Immunology,* 4, 3, 269-273

Hooper, L.V. (2004). Bacterial contributions to mammalian gut development. *Trends in Microbiology,* 12, 3, 129-134

Hord, N.G. (2008). Eukaryotic-microbiota crosstalk: Potential mechanisms for health benefits of prebiotics and probiotics. *Annual Review of Nutrition,* 28, 215-231

Hoy, C.M., Wood, C.M., Hawkey, P.M. & Puntis, J.W.L. (2000). Duodenal microflora in very-low-birth-weight neonates and relation to necrotizing enterocolitis. *Journal of Clinical Microbiology,* 38, 12, 4539-4547

Hoyos, A.B. (1999). Reduced incidence of necrotizing enterocolitis associated with enteral administration of lactobacillus acidophilus and bifidobacterium infantis to neonates in an intensive care unit. *International Journal of Infectious Diseases,* 3, 4, 197-202

Indrio, F., Riezzo, G., Raimondi, F., Francavilla, R., Montagna, O., Valenzano, M.L., Cavallo, L. & Boehm, G. (2009). Prebiotics improve gastric motility and gastric electrical activity in preterm newborns. *Journal of Pediatric Gastroenterology and Nutrition,* 49, 2, 258-261

Jiménez, E., Marín, M.L., Martín, R., Odriozola, J.M., Olivares, M., Xaus, J., Fernández, L. & Rodríguez, J.M. (2008). Is meconium from healthy newborns actually sterile? *Research in Microbiology,* 159, 3, 187-193

Kamau, S.M., Lu, R.R., Chen, W., Liu, X.M., Tian, F.W., Shen, Y. & Gao, T. (2010). Functional significance of bioactive peptides derived from milk proteins. *Food Reviews International,* 26, 4, 386-401

Kelly, D., King, T. & Aminov, R. (2007). Importance of microbial colonization of the gut in early life to the development of immunity. *Mutation Research - Fundamental and Molecular Mechanisms of Mutagenesis,* 622, 1-2, 58-69

Kien, C.L. (1996). Digestion, absorption, and fermentation of carbohydrates in the newborn. *Clinics in Perinatology,* 23, 2, 211-228

Kim, J.W. & Lin, H.C. (2007). Contribution of gut microbes to gastrointestinal motility disorders. *Practical Gastroenterology,* 31, 4, 51-60

Knoch, B., Barnett, M.P.G., Zhu, S., Park, Z.A., Nones, K., Dommels, Y.E.M., Knowles, S.O., McNabb, W.C. & Roy, N.C. (2009). Genome-wide analysis of dietary eicosapentaenoic acid- and oleic acid-induced modulation of colon inflammation in interleukin-10 gene-deficient mice. *Journal of Nutrigenetics and Nutrigenomics,* 2, 1, 9-28

Konishi, Y. (2003). Modulations of food-derived substances on intestinal permeability and caco-2 cell monolayers. *Bioscience, Biotechnology, and Biochemistry,* 67, 10, 2297-2299

Kosek, M., Bern, C. & Guerrant, R.L. (2003). The global burden of diarrhoeal disease, as estimated from studies published between 1992 and 2000. *Bulletin of The World Health Organization,* 81, 3, 197-204

Krammer, H.J., von Seggern, H., Schaumburg, J. & Neumer, F. (2011). Effect of *lactobacillus casei* shirota on colonic transit time in patients with chronic constipation. *Coloproctology,* 1-5

Lakhan, S.E. & Kirchgessner, A. (2010). Neuroinflammation in inflammatory bowel disease. *Journal of Neuroinflammation,* 7, art. no. 37,

Levin, A. & Shibolet, O. (2008). Toll-like receptors in inflammatory bowel disease-stepping into uncharted territory. *World Journal of Gastroenterology,* 14, 33, 5149-5153

Lin, P.W. & Stoll, B.J. (2006). Necrotising enterocolitis. *Lancet,* 368, 9543, 1271-1283

Logsdon, N.J., Kang, J., Togo, J.A., Christian, E.P. & Aiyar, J. (1997). A novel gene, hkca4, encodes the calcium-activated potassium channel in human t lymphocytes. *Journal of Biological Chemistry,* 272, 52, 32723-32726

Louis, N.A. & Lin, P.W. (2009). The intestinal immune barrier. *NeoReviews,* 10, 4, e180-e190

Maheshwari, A. & Zemlin, M. (2009). Ontogeny of the intestinal immune system. *h [Haematologica Reports]*, 2, 10, 18-26

Massi, M., Ioan, P., Budriesi, R., Chiarini, A., Vitali, B., Lammers, K.M., Gionchetti, P., Campieri, M., Lembo, A. & Brigidi, P. (2006). Effects of probiotic bacteria on gastrointestinal motility in guinea-pig isolated tissue. *World Journal of Gastroenterology*, 12, 37, 5987-5994

Matricon, J., Barnich, N. & Ardid, D. (2010). Immunopathogenesis of inflammatory bowel disease. *Self/Nonself - Immune Recognition and Signaling*, 1, 4, 299-309

Mayer, L. (2003). Mucosal immunity. *Pediatrics*, 111, 6 III, 1595-1600

McConnell, B.B. & Yang, V.W. (2009). The role of inflammation in the pathogenesis of colorectal cancer. *Current Colorectal Cancer Reports*, 5, 2, 69-74

Montgomery, R.K., Mulberg, A.E. & Grand, R.J. (1999). Development of the human gastrointestinal tract: Twenty years of progress. *Gastroenterology*, 116, 3, 702-731

Moon, A. & Kleinman, R.E. (1995). Allergic gastroenteropathy in children. *Annals of Allergy*, 74, 1, 5-12

Neish, A.S. (2009). Microbes in gastrointestinal health and disease. *Gastroenterology*, 136, 1, 65-80

Nell, S., Suerbaum, S. & Josenhans, C. (2010). The impact of the microbiota on the pathogenesis of ibd: Lessons from mouse infection models. *Nature Reviews Microbiology*, 8, 8, 564-577

Neu, J. (2005). Neonatal necrotizing enterocolitis: An update. *Acta Paediatrica, International Journal of Paediatrics, Supplement*, 94, 449, 100-105

Neu, J. (2007). Gastrointestinal maturation and implications for infant feeding. *Early Human Development*, 83, 12, 767-775

Newell, S.J. (2000). Enteral feeding of the micropremie. *Clinics in Perinatology*, 27, 1, 221-234

Niittynen, L., Kajander, K. & Korpela, R. (2007). Galacto-oligosaccharides and bowel function. *Scandinavian Journal of Food and Nutrition*, 51, 2, 62-66

Nones, K., Dommels, Y.E.M., Martell, S., Butts, C., McNabb, W.C., Park, Z.A., Zhu, S., Hedderley, D., Barnett, M.P.G. & Roy, N.C. (2009). The effects of dietary curcumin and rutin on colonic inflammation and gene expression in multidrug resistance gene-deficient (mdr1a-/-) mice, a model of inflammatory bowel diseases. *British Journal of Nutrition*, 101, 2, 169-181

Obert, G., Peiffer, I. & Servin, A.L. (2000). Rotavirus-induced structural and functional alterations in tight junctions of polarized intestinal caco-2 cell monolayers. *Journal of Virology*, 74, 10, 4645-4651

Ohashi, Y., Inoue, R., Tanaka, K., Umesaki, Y. & Ushida, K. (2001). Strain gauge force transducer and its application in a pig model to evaluate the effect of probiotic on colonic motility. *Journal of Nutritional Science and Vitaminology*, 47, 5, 351-356

Pácha, J. (2000). Development of intestinal transport function in mammals. *Physiological Reviews*, 80, 4, 1633-1667

Palmer, C., Bik, E.M., DiGiulio, D.B., Relman, D.A. & Brown, P.O. (2007). Development of the human infant intestinal microbiota. *PLoS Biology*, 5, 7, 1556-1573

Park, H.K., Shim, S.S., Kim, S.Y., Park, J.H., Park, S.E., Kim, H.J., Kang, B.C. & Kim, C.M. (2005). Molecular analysis of colonized bacteria in a human newborn infant gut. *Journal of Microbiology*, 43, 4, 345-353

Patel, A.R. & Velikov, K.P. (2011). Colloidal delivery systems in foods: A general comparison with oral drug delivery. *LWT - Food Science and Technology,* In Press, Corrected Proof, In press,

Penna, F.J., Péret, L.A., Vieira, L.Q. & Nicoli, J.R. (2008). Probiotics and mucosal barrier in children. *Current Opinion in Clinical Nutrition and Metabolic Care,* 11, 5, 640-644

Piche, T., Barbara, G., Aubert, P., Des Varannes, S.B., Dainese, R., Nano, J.L., Cremon, C., Stanghellini, V., De Giorgio, R., Galmiche, J.P. & Neunlist, M. (2009). Impaired intestinal barrier integrity in the colon of patients with irritable bowel syndrome: Involvement of soluble mediators. *Gut,* 58, 2, 196-201

Polak-Charcon, S., Shoham, J. & Ben-Shaul, Y. (1980). Tight junctions in epithelial cells of human fetal hindgut, normal colon, and colon adenocarcinoma. *Journal of the National Cancer Institute,* 65, 1, 53-62

Prosser, C., Stelwagen, K., Cummins, R., Guerin, P., Gill, N. & Milne, C. (2004). Reduction in heat-induced gastrointestinal hyperpermeability in rats by bovine colostrum and goat milk powders. *Journal of Applied Physiology,* 96, 2, 650-654

Ranadheera, R.D.C.S., Baines, S.K. & Adams, M.C. (2010). Importance of food in probiotic efficacy. *Food Research International,* 43, 1, 1-7

Rao, S., Srinivasjois, R. & Patole, S. (2009). Prebiotic supplementation in full-term neonates: A systematic review of randomized controlled trials. *Archives of Pediatrics and Adolescent Medicine,* 163, 8, 755-764

Rapin, J. & Wiernsperger, N. (2010). Possible links between intestinal permeablity and food processing: A potential therapeutic niche for glutamine. *Clinics [online],* 65, 6, 635-643

Roberfroid, M., Gibson, G.R., Hoyles, L., McCartney, A.L., Rastall, R., Rowland, I., Wolvers, D., Watzl, B., Szajewska, H., Stahl, B., Guarner, F., Respondek, F., Whelan, K., Coxam, V., Davicco, M.J., Léotoing, L., Wittrant, Y., Delzenne, N.M., Cani, P.D., Neyrinck, A.M. & Meheust, A. (2010). Prebiotic effects: Metabolic and health benefits. *British Journal of Nutrition,* 104, SUPPL.2, S1-S63

Round, J.L. & Mazmanian, S.K. (2009). The gut microbiota shapes intestinal immune responses during health and disease. *Nature Reviews Immunology,* 9, 5, 313-323

Rubaltelli, F.F., Biadaioli, R., Pecile, P. & Nicoletti, P. (1998). Intestinal flora in breast- and bottle-fed infants. *Journal of Perinatal Medicine,* 26, 3, 186-191

Rumbo, M. & Schiffrin, E.J. (2005). Ontogeny of intestinal epithelium immune functions: Developmental and environmental regulation. *Cellular and Molecular Life Sciences,* 62, 12, 1288-1296

Saarela, M., Virkajärvi, I., Alakomi, H.-L., Sigvart-Mattila, P. & Mättö, J. (2006). Stability and functionality of freeze-dried probiotic bifidobacterium cells during storage in juice and milk. *International Dairy Journal,* 16, 12, 1477-1482

Saavedra, J.M. (2007). Use of probiotics in pediatrics: Rationale, mechanisms of action, and practical aspects. *Nutrition in Clinical Practice,* 22, 3, 351-365

Sadeghi, A.M.M., Dorkoosh, F.A., Avadi, M.R., Weinhold, M., Bayat, A., Delie, F., Gurny, R., Larijani, B., Rafiee-Tehrani, M. & Junginger, H.E. (2008). Permeation enhancer effect of chitosan and chitosan derivatives: Comparison of formulations as soluble polymers and nanoparticulate systems on insulin absorption in caco-2 cells. *European Journal of Pharmaceutics and Biopharmaceutics,* 70, 1, 270-278

Salzman, N.H., Polin, R.A., Harris, M.C., Ruchelli, E., Hebra, A., Zirin-Butler, S., Jawad, A., Porter, E.M. & Bevins, C.L. (1998). Enteric defensin expression in necrotizing enterocolitis. *Pediatric Research,* 44, 1, 20-26

Sander, G.R., Cummins, A.G. & Powell, B.C. (2005). Rapid disruption of intestinal barrier function by gliadin involves altered expression of apical junctional proteins. *FEBS Letters,* 579, 21, 4851-4855

Sanderson, I.R. (2004). Short chain fatty acid regulation of signaling genes expressed by the intestinal epithelium. *Journal of Nutrition,* 134, 9, 2450S-2454S

Scheppach, W., Bartram, H.P., Richter, F., Müller, J.G., Greinwald, K., Tauschel, H.D., Gierend, M., Weber, A., Hegemann, D., Kubetzko, W., Rabast, U., Schütz, E., Raedsch, R., Britsch, R., Rehmann, I.H., Otto, P., Judmaier, G., Press, A.G., Wördehoff, D., Mlitz, H., Stein, J. & Schmidt, C. (1996). Treatment of distal ulcerative colitis with short-chain fatty acid enemas. A placebo-controlled trial. *Digestive Diseases and Sciences,* 41, 11, 2254-2259

Schreiber, R.A. & Walker, W.A. (1988). The gastrointestinal barrier: Antigen uptake and perinatal immunity. *Annals of Allergy,* 61, 6 Pt 2, 3-12

Schulzke, J.D., Bentzel, C.J., Schulzke, I., Riecken, E.O. & Fromm, M. (1998). Epithelial tight junction structure in the jejunum of children with acute and treated celiac sprue. *Pediatric Research,* 43, 4 I, 435-441

Schuppan, D. (2000). Current concepts of celiac disease pathogenesis. *Gastroenterology,* 119, 1, 234-242

Sicherer, S.H. (2003). Clinical aspects of gastrointestinal food allergy in childhood. *Pediatrics,* 111, 6 III, 1609-1616

Siggers, R.H., Siggers, J., Thymann, T., Boye, M. & Sangild, P.T. (2011). Nutritional modulation of the gut microbiota and immune system in preterm neonates susceptible to necrotizing enterocolitis. *The Journal of Nutritional Biochemistry,* 22, 6, 511-521

Sigthorsson, G., Tibble, J., Hayllar, J., Menzies, I., Macpherson, A., Moots, R., Scott, D., Gumpel, M.J. & Bjarnason, I. (1998). Intestinal permeability and inflammation in patients on nsaids. *Gut,* 43, 4, 506-511

Simms, L.A., Doecke, J.D., Roberts, R.L., Fowler, E.V., Zhao, Z.Z., McGuckin, M.A., Huang, N., Hayward, N.K., Webb, P.M., Whiteman, D.C., Cavanaugh, J.A., McCallum, R., Florin, T.H.J., Barclay, M.L., Gearry, R.B., Merriman, T.R., Montgomery, G.W. & Radford-Smith, G.L. (2010). Kcnn4 gene variant is associated with ileal crohn's disease in the australian and new zealand population. *American Journal of Gastroenterology,* 105, 10, 2209-2217

Söderholm, J.D. & Perdue, M.H. (2001). Stress and the gastrointestinal tract ii. Stress and intestinal barrier function. *American Journal of Physiology - Gastrointestinal and Liver Physiology,* 280, 1 43-1, G7-G13

Spiller, R.C. (2003). Postinfectious irritable bowel syndrome. *Gastroenterology,* 124, 6, 1662-1671

Stappenbeck, T.S., Hooper, L.V. & Gordon, J.I. (2002). Developmental regulation of intestinal angiogenesis by indigenous microbes via paneth cells. *Proceedings of the National Academy of Sciences of the United States of America,* 99, 24, 15451-15455

Suzuki, T. & Hara, H. (2009). Quercetin enhances intestinal barrier function through the assembly of zonula [corrected] occludens-2, occludin, and claudin-1 and the expression of claudin-4 in caco-2 cells. *Journal of Nutrition,* 139, 5, 965-974

Taylor, S.N., Basile, L.A., Ebeling, M. & Wagner, C.L. (2009). Intestinal permeability in preterm infants by feeding type: Mother's milk versus formula. *Breastfeeding Medicine,* 4, 1, 11-15

Tlaskalová-Hogenová, H., Tpánková, R., Kozáková, H., Hudcovic, T., Vannucci, L., Tuková, L., Rossmann, P., Hrní, T., Kverka, M., Zákostelská, Z., Klimeová, K., Pibylová, J., Bártová, J., Sanchez, D., Fundová, P., Borovská, D., Rtková, D., Zídek, Z., Schwarzer, M., Drastich, P. & Funda, D.P. (2011). The role of gut microbiota (commensal bacteria) and the mucosal barrier in the pathogenesis of inflammatory and autoimmune diseases and cancer: Contribution of germ-free and gnotobiotic animal models of human diseases. *Cellular and Molecular Immunology,* 8, 2, 110-120

Udall, J.N. (1990). Gasterointestinal host defense and necrotising enterocolitis. *Journal of Pediatrics,* 117, S33-S43,

Ulluwishewa, D., Anderson, R.C., McNabb, W.C., Moughan, P.J., Wells, J.M. & Roy, N.C. (2011). Regulation of tight junction permeability by intestinal bacteria and dietary components. *Journal of Nutrition,* 141, 5, 769-776

Van Der Flier, L.G. & Clevers, H. (2009). Stem cells, self-renewal, and differentiation in the intestinal epithelium. *Annual Review of Physiology,* 71, 241-260

Verdu, E.F. (2009). Probiotics effects on gastrointestinal function: Beyond the gut? *Neurogastroenterology and Motility,* 21, 5, 477-480

Verhasselt, V. (2010). Neonatal tolerance under breastfeeding influence. *Current Opinion in Immunology,* 22, 5, 623-630

Vinderola, C.G., Bailo, N. & Reinheimer, J.A. (2000). Survival of probiotic microflora in argentinian yoghurts during refrigerated storage. *Food Research International,* 33, 2, 97-102

Vine, D.F., Charman, S.A., Gibson, P.R., Sinclair, A.J. & Porter, C.J.H. (2002). Effect of dietary fatty acids on the intestinal permeability of marker drug compounds in excised rat jejunum. *Journal of Pharmacy and Pharmacology,* 54, 6, 809-819

Walker-Smith, J., Harrison, M. & Kilby, A. (1978). Cow's milk-sensitive enteropathy. *Archives of Disease in Childhood,* 53, 5, 375-380

Wang, B., Mao, Y.K., Diorio, C., Wang, L., Huizinga, J.D., Bienenstock, J. & Kunze, W. (2010). *Lactobacillus reuteri* ingestion and ikca channel blockade have similar effects on rat colon motility and myenteric neurones. *Neurogastroenterology and Motility,* 22, 1, 98-107+e133

Westerbeek, E.A.M., Van Den Berg, A., Lafeber, H.N., Fetter, W.P.F. & Van Elburg, R.M. (2010). The effect of enteral supplementation of a prebiotic mixture of non-human milk galacto-, fructo- and acidic oligosaccharides on intestinal permeability in preterm infants. *British Journal of Nutrition,* 105, 2, 268-274

Wigg, A.J., Roberts-Thomson, I.C., Grose, R.H., Cummins, A.G., Dymock, R.B. & McCarthy, P.J. (2001). The role of small intestinal bacterial overgrowth, intestinal permeability, endotoxaemia, and tumour necrosis factor α in the pathogenesis of non-alcoholic steatohepatitis. *Gut,* 48, 2, 206-211

Wold, A. & Adlerberth, I. (2000). Breast feeding and intestinal microbiota of the infant - implications for protection against infectious diseases. *Advances in Experimental Medicine and Biology,* 478, 77-93

Wouters, M.M., Farrugia, G. & Schemann, M. (2007). 5-ht receptors on interstitial cells of cajal, smooth muscle and enteric nerves. *Neurogastroenterology and Motility,* 19, SUPPL.2, 5-12

Yacyshyn, B., Meddings, J., Sadowski, D. & Bowen-Yacyshyn, M.B. (1996). Multiple sclerosis patients have peripheral blood cd45ro+ b cells and increased intestinal permeability. *Digestive Diseases and Sciences,* 41, 12, 2493-2498

Yajima, T. (1985). Contractile effect of short-chain fatty acids on the isolated colon of the rat. *Journal of Physiology,* 368, 667-678

Yasumatsu, H. & Tanabe, S. (2010). The casein peptide asn-pro-trp-asp-gln enforces the intestinal tight junction partly by increasing occludin expression in caco-2 cells. *British Journal of Nutrition,* 104, 7, 951-956

Zabielski, R., Godlewski, M.M. & Guilloteau, P. (2008). Control of development of gastrointestinal system in neonates. *Journal of Physiology and Pharmacology,* 59, SUPPL.1, 35-54

Zhang, M., Leung, F.P., Huang, Y. & Bian, Z.X. (2010). Increased colonic motility in a rat model of irritable bowel syndrome is associated with up-regulation of l-type calcium channels in colonic smooth muscle cells. *Neurogastroenterology and Motility,* 22, 5, e162-e170

Zhi, S.L., Schmauss, C., Cuenca, A., Ratcliffe, E. & Gershon, M.D. (2006). Physiological modulation of intestinal motility by enteric dopaminergic neurons and the d2 receptor: Analysis of dopamine receptor expression, location, development, and function in wild-type and knock-out mice. *Journal of Neuroscience,* 26, 10, 2798-2807

2

Resolution of Colitis-Associated Inflammation

Hennebert Olivier, Pelissier Marie-Agnès and Morfin Robert
Biotechnologie, CNAM, Paris, France

1. Introduction

Ulcerative colitis (UC) is an inflammatory bowel disease related to chronic relapsing inflammation of the intestinal tract of unknown aetiology (Podolsky, 2003). Maintenance of colonic inflammation involves a network of inflammatory mediators resulting in a dramatic increase in the production of reactive oxygen species that contribute to the functional change characteristic of UC (Pavlick et al, 2002). Animal models provide evidence that altered cytokine (IL-1β) and eicosanoid secretion patterns may play a role in UC (Blumberg et al, 1999; Stenson, 2007). Eicosanoids, including leukotrienes generated by the 5-lipoxygenase pathway (Murthy et al, 1997) and prostaglandins (PGs) produced by the cyclooxygenases COX-1 or COX-2, are lipid mediators implicated in the pathophysiology of UC (Funk, 2001).

Inflammation in experimentally induced colitis is characterized by increased PGs such as PGE_2 and PGD_2. PGD_2 (Ajuebor et al, 2000; Melgar et al, 2006) is further converted by dehydratation to 15-deoxy-$\Delta^{12,14}$-PGJ_2 (15d- PGJ_2) (Monneret et al, 2002), a stable PG and putative endogenous PPARγ ligand with cytoprotective and anti-inflammatory properties, and hence a new potential therapeutic target in inflammatory bowel diseases (Dubuquoy et al, 2006).

7α-Hydroxy-DHEA, the innate metabolite of dehydroepiandrosterone (DHEA), is normally produced in the colon and many other tissues (Doostzadeh & Morfin, 1996; Morfin & Courchay, 1994) but overproduced by IL-1β during the inflammatory process as shown in mice and humans (Dulos et al, 2004; Dulos et al, 2005). We have previously shown that pre-treatment with DHEA and 7α-hydroxy-DHEA resulted in protective anti-oxidant effects in the colon of healthy and colitis rats (Pelissier et al, 2004; Pelissier et al, 2006). 7α-Hydroxy-DHEA is converted by NADP(H)-dependent 11β-hydroxysteroid dehydrogenase type 1 (11β-HSD1) to 7β-hydroxy-DHEA through an oxido-reductive process via 7-oxo-DHEA (Muller et al, 2006b). Through this mechanism, 7α-hydroxy-DHEA may inhibit 11β-HSD1-dependent production of inactive cortisone from active cortisol (Hennebert et al, 2007a).

Epiandrosterone (EpiA), which is derived from DHEA, is also converted into 7-hydroxylated metabolites (Kim et al, 2004). We have recently shown that 11β-HSD1 is responsible for converting 7α-hydroxy-EpiA into 7β-hydroxy-EpiA (Chalbot & Morfin, 2005; Hennebert et al, 2007b), which is readily produced in small quantities in human tissues (Jacolot et al, 1981; Kim et al, 2004).

7β-Hydroxy-EpiA has been shown to exert neuroprotective effects *in vivo* at remarkably low doses in animal models of cerebral ischemia (Pringle et al, 2003) and Alzheimer's disease (Dudas et al, 2004). However, dose levels needed to demonstrate these effects are far below the concentrations necessary to inhibit the 11β-HSD1-dependent-cortisol transformation indicating that other mechanisms may be involved.

Finally, studies in rheumatoid arthritis and brain injury models have shown that DHEA can modulate the expression of COX-2 mRNA or PGE_2 synthesis (Malik et al, 2003; Sun et al, 2006).

Taken together, these finding suggest that certain 7-hydroxysteroids may play a role in the modulation of PGs production in inflammation. This role may permit to resolve inflammation in inflammatory bowel diseases.

2. The resolution of inflammation

Inflammatory resolution occurs after the sharp PGE_2-driven inflammation process and is thought to result from cytoprotective PGD_2 and 15d-PGJ_2 action. A shift from arachidonic acid-derived PGE_2 to PGD_2 production occurs to these ends (Haworth & Buckley, 2007; Rajakariar et al, 2007) and is illustrated in Figure 1.

Figure 1 outlines the native inflammation process and its relations to immunity onset and circulating steroid metabolism. Inflammation-triggered increase in cellular cytochrome P450-7B1 which results in augmented 7α-hydroxy-steroid production was shown both in a

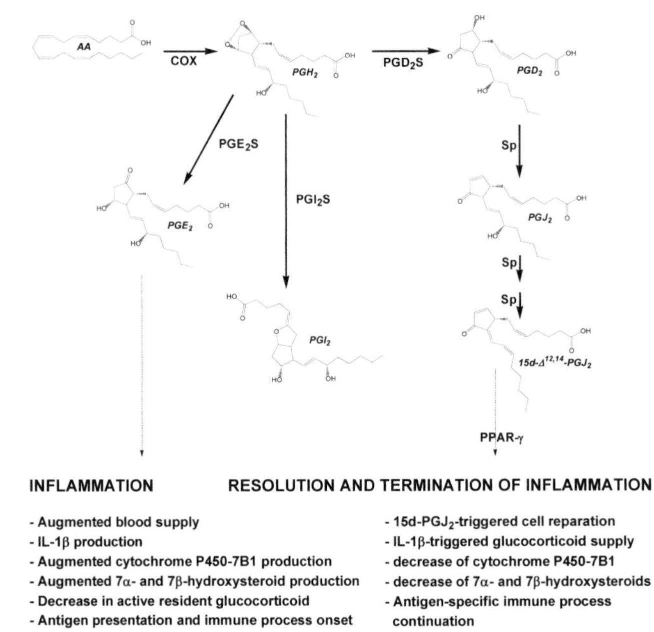

Fig. 1. At the onset of inflammatory response, arachidonic acid (AA) is converted to PGH_2 via COX. In turn, PGE_2, PGI_2 and PGD_2 are produced from PGH_2 by synthases (PGE_2S, PGI_2S, PGD_2S). PGD_2 is transformed non-enzymatically (Sp) to 15d-PGJ_2 which interacts with PPAR-γ. Non PPAR-γ-mediated action of 15d-PGJ_2 are not shown.

mouse model of rheumatoid arthritis and in humans with rheumatoid arthritis (Dulos et al, 2004; Dulos et al, 2005). Due to this increase, competitive inhibition of the cellular 11β-HSD1 may occur (Muller et al, 2006a) through use of the enzyme for transformation of 7α-hydroxysteroid into 7β-hydroxysteroids (Hennebert et al, 2007a; Muller et al, 2006b). Thus, the circulating inactive cortisone made available to the inflamed cells is not activated into cortisol which would quench the onset of immune processes. Our finding of a 7α-hydroxy-dehydroepiandrosterone-triggered increase of immune response in mice supports this relation to immunity onset (Morfin & Courchay, 1994).

These basic facts led to questions relative to the effect of 7β-hydroxysteroids on inflammation, PG metabolism, cell protection and related mechanisms of action. Answers were found through investigations using several models of inflammation in rats and humans.

3. Choice in the 7β-Hydroxysteroid used in treatments

Among 7β-hydroxysteroids, 7β-hydroxy-epiandrosterone (7β-hydroxy-EpiA) was selected because of its reported effects as a neuroprotector (Pringle et al, 2003). 7β-Hydroxy-EpiA is a native steroid which derives from testosterone and dehydroepiandrosterone as reported (Niro et al, 2010) and illustrated in Figure 2. The chemical synthesis of 7β-hydroxy-EpiA was carried out (Ricco et al, 2011) and provided 400 mg of the steroid which is available now for investigations in our group and abroad. Several doses of 7β-hydroxy-EpiA (0.01, 0.1 and 1 mg/kg) were used for the treatments.

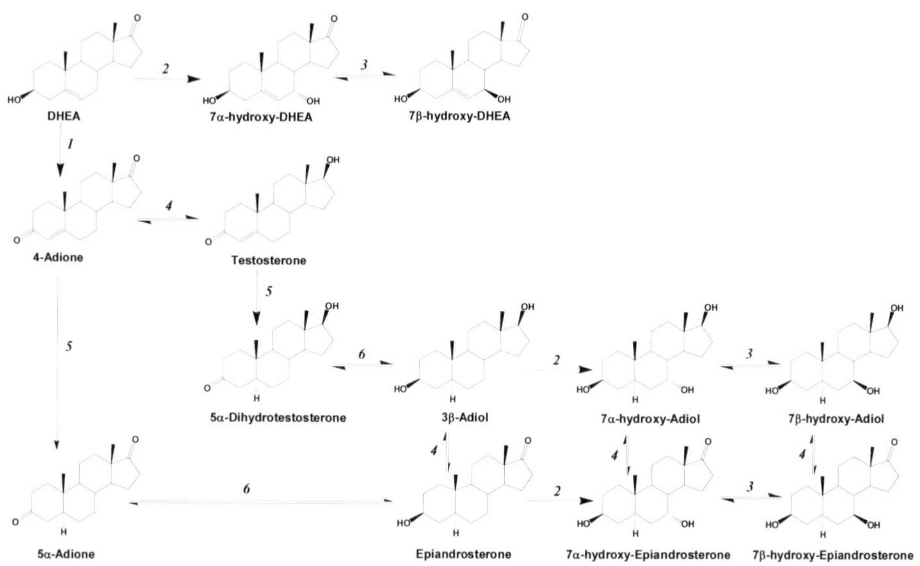

Fig. 2. Epiandrosterone derives from testosterone and dehydroepiandrosterone (DHEA) and is a substrate for cytochrome P450-7B1 (**2** EC 1.14.13.100) producing 7α-hydroxy-epiandrosterone which is inter-converted then into 7β-hydroxy-epiandrosterone by 11β-hydroxysteroid dehydrogenase type 1 (**3** EC 1.1.1.148). Other enzymes are **1**. 3β-hydroxy-5-ene steroid dehydrogenase (EC 1.1.1.145, EC 5.3.3.1) **4.** 17β-hydroxysteroid dehydrogenase (EC 1.1.1.51) **5.** Steroid Δ4-5α-reductase (EC 1.3.99.5) **6.** 3β-hydroxysteroid dehydrogenase (EC 1.1.1.51).

4. Investigations in rats with dextran sodium sulphate-induced colitis

4.1 Colitis induction and experimental design

Male Wistar rats (180-200g) were acclimated for 7 days and were divided into 2 controls groups (one sham-treated and one treated) and 2 colitis groups (one sham-treated and one treated). Treatments with 7β-hydroxy-EpiA were carried out for 7 days prior to colitis induction (Figure 3). Doses (0.01, 0.1 and 1 mg/kg) were dissolved in dimethyl sulfoxide and injected *i.p.* daily for 7 days. Dimethyl sulfoxide alone was injected to the sham-treated animals. Colitis was then induced by addition of 5% dextran sodium sulphate (DSS) to drinking water for 7 days. Plain water was given to the control groups. Clinical and histological signs of colitis occurred in all the DSS-treated rats. Typically, all the rats exhibited symptoms of colitis and severe diarrhea 5 days after the onset of DSS treatment followed by rectal bleeding and shortening of the colon after 7 days. Increase in colonic myeloperoxidase activity indicated an invasion of the colonic mucosa by neutrophils (Hennebert et al, 2008).

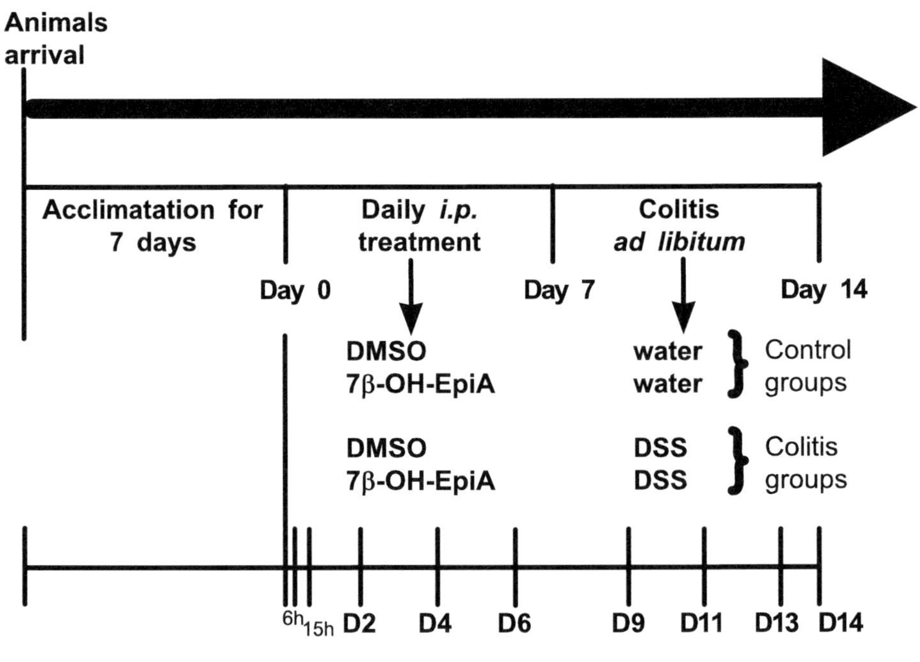

Fig. 3. Experimental design. DSS: 5% DSS in drinking water; DMSO: dimethyl sufoxide; 7β-OH-EpiA: 7β-hydroxy-EpiA in DMSO.

4.2 Histological examinations

A portion (1 cm) of the proximal colon was fixed in 4% formaldehyde and embedded in paraffin. Tissue sections (5 μm) were stained either with hematoxylin/eosin or Alcian blue for evaluation of colonic damage and mucus goblet cells content, respectively.

Major hallmarks of colonic inflammation, namely cryptic distorsion, neutrophil infiltration in the mucosal tissue (Figure 4B1), and loss of goblet cells which contained less mucins

(Figure 4B2) were apparent in the colitis group at day 13 and were more pronounced at day 14 (Figure 4D1-4D2) when compared with sham-control group (Figure 4A1,A2 and C1,C2).

The two low doses of 7β-hydroxy-EpiA (0.01, 0.1 mg/kg) prevented the DSS-induced colonic damages as indicated by the suppression of diarrhea and rectal bleeding. The colon length reduction was less pronounced in the groups treated by the low steroid doses (0.01, 0.1 mg/kg) than in the colitis group. All 7β-hydroxy-EpiA doses (0.01, 0.1 and 1 mg/kg) antagonized mucus depletion in goblet cells (Figure 4E2,F2,G2) and improved histological changes such as the abnormality of crypts and neutrophil infiltration (Figure 4E1,F1,G1) (Hennebert et al, 2008).

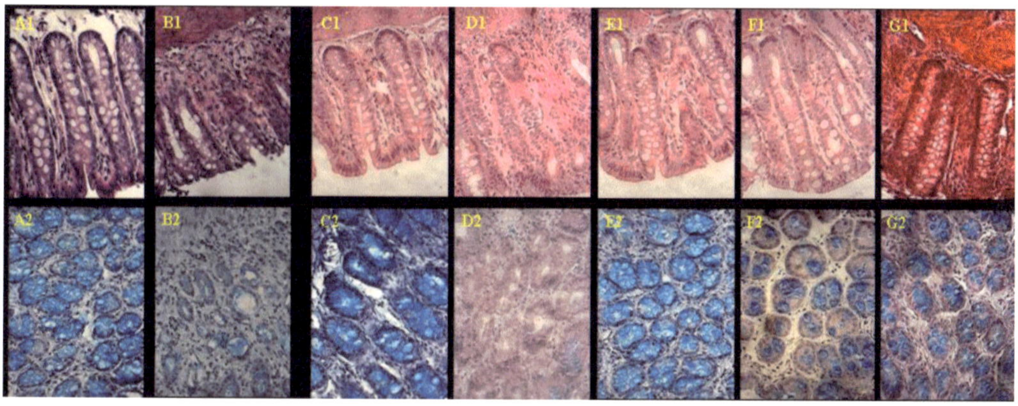

Fig. 4. Acute colitis induced by DSS: effect of 7β-hydroxy-EpiA on colon injury. Histological appearance of rat colonic mucosa after hematoxylin/eosin (A1-G1) or alcian blue stain (A2-G2) at days 13 and 14: sham (A1,A2) and DSS-treated (B1,B2) at day 13; sham (C1,C2) and DSS-treated (D1,D2) at day 14; and 0.01 mg/kg 7β-hydroxy-EpiA (E1,E2), 0.1 mg/kg (F1,F2) and 1 mg/kg (G1,G2) at day 14. No histological modification was present in sham animals (A and C) at days 13 and 14. Mucosal injury in DSS-induced colitis rats starting at day 13 and being more pronounced at day 14 (D) was characterized by necrosis of the epithelium, focal ulceration, infiltration of inflammatory cells and mucin goblet cell depletion. Treatment with 7β-hydroxy-EpiA (E-G) reduced the morphological alteration associated with DSS administration protecting the mucosal architecture. Magnification was 40x for all slices.

4.3 7β-Hydroxy-EpiA-induced changes in PG colonic tissue levels

7β-Hydroxy-EpiA treatments did not alter PGE_2 and PGD_2 colonic tissue levels in control rats without colitis (data not shown). DSS administration resulted into a marked increase of PGE_2, PGD_2 and 15d-PGJ_2 colonic synthesis at day 13 (Figure 5). At day 14, PGE_2 levels whereas PGD_2 synthesis was increased and 15d-PGJ_2 levels were reduced (Figure 5).

7β-Hydroxy-EpiA treatment in rats with DSS-induced colitis significantly decreased the colonic PGE_2 synthesis at days 13 and 14 when compared with untreated colitis rats. The greatest decrease was observed with the lowest dose (0.01 mg/kg) which led to a return towards basal values (Figure 5A). PGD_2 levels remained unchanged with the highest steroid-doses whereas the low doses (0.01 and 0.1mg/kg) caused a small but significant decrease (Figure 5B). Following the treatment with 7β-hydroxy-EpiA and throughout colitis induction, 15d-PGJ_2 levels were maintained above control levels ranging from 5 to 14-fold increase (Figure 5C). Since 15d-PGJ_2 results from the produced PGD_2, addition of both PG levels may reflect the total production of PGD_2. This leads to observations identical with those derived from 15d-PGJ_2 measurements alone (Figure 4D). The decrease in 15d-PGJ_2 observed at the end of colitis induction underlies that 7β-hydroxy-EpiA treatment produced large amounts of 15d-PGJ_2 prior to colitis induction. This was confirmed after measurement of colonic 15d-PGJ_2 during 7β-hydroxy-EpiA treatment (Figure 5). Thus, a 51-fold increase was obtained with the 0.1 mg/kg dose at day 2 (D2) and decreased progressively from D4 to D6 (increments ranging from of 44-fold to 5-fold) (Figures 5C and 6). Conclusion of these findings is that 7β-hydroxy-EpiA treatments induced a shift from PGE_2 to 15d-PGJ_2 production (Hennebert et al, 2008).

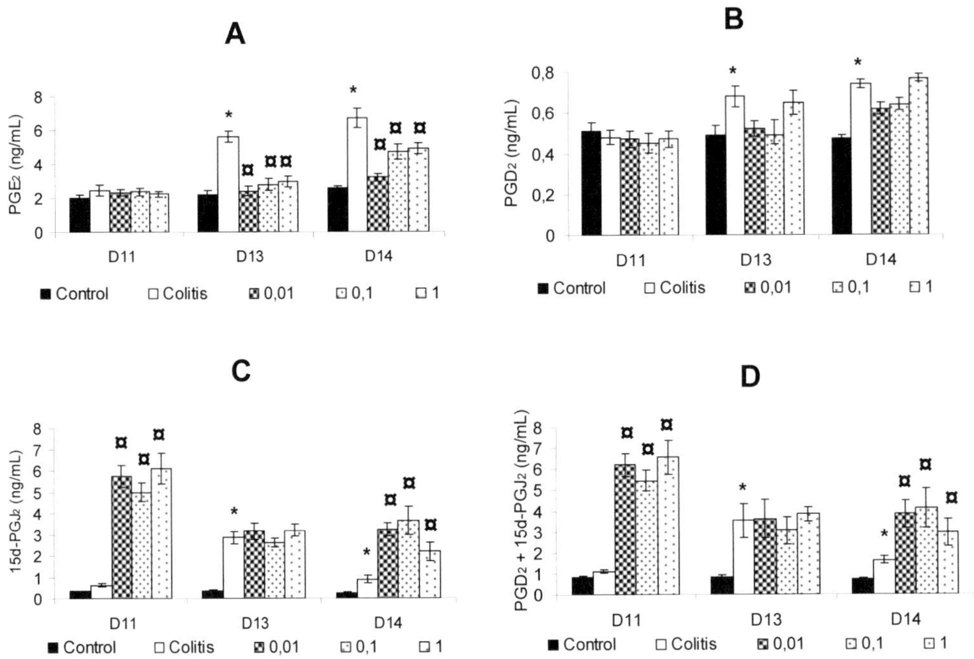

Fig. 5. Effect of 7β-hydroxy-EpiA on colonic synthesis of PGE2 (A), PGD2 (B), 15d-PGJ2 (C) and PGD2+15d-PGJ2 (D). Measurements were carried out in triplicate during DSS administration at days D11, D13 and D14. Data are expressed as mean ± S.E.M. with n=3-15 (*) Dextran sodium sulphate-induced colitis group versus Sham-control group; (¤) 7β-hydroxy-EpiA treated group versus Dextran sodium sulphate-induced colitis group ($p < 0.05$).

4.4 7β-Hydroxy-EpiA-induced changes in PG-producing enzymes

Because significant modifications in prostaglandin levels were observed with DSS administration and 7β-hydroxy-EpiA treatments, we tested whether the expression of COX-2, mPGES-1 and H-PGDS was altered by quantifying specific mRNA by real-time RT-PCR. Transcription of these genes was examined and related to that of the HPRT1 house-keeping gene (Hennebert et al, 2008).

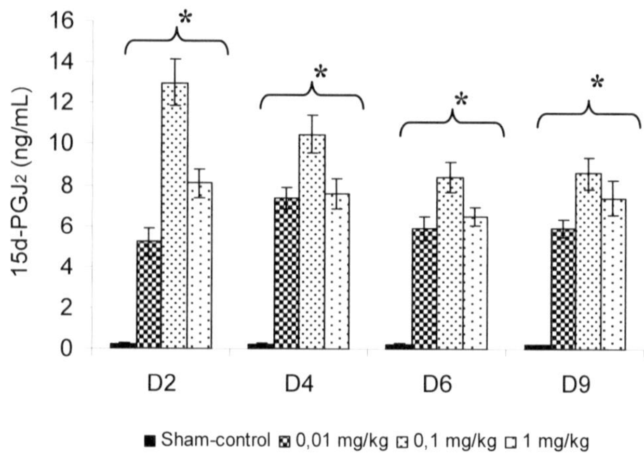

Fig. 6. Colonic 15d-PGJ2 levels at various times during and after 7β-hydroxy-EpiA treatment (D2-D9). Values are mean ± S.E.M. (n= 3-15) . (*) comparison to the sham-control group (p<0.05).

In control rats without colitis, the daily 7β-hydroxy-EpiA treatment (0.1 mg/kg) induced a significant 1.5 fold increase in COX-2 mRNA levels at 15h followed by a decrease up to day 4 and thereafter returned to basal values (Figure 7A). mPGES-1 mRNA expression increased transiently between 6h to 15h returning towards basal levels at day 2. H-PGDS mRNA expression remained similar to that in sham-control rats throughout the time course.

After colitis induction, a 2.5 fold increase in COX-2 mRNA expression was observed at days 13 and 14 of DSS administration (Figure 7B) while mPGES-1 mRNA was significantly augmented at day 13 only (Figure 7C). H-PGDS was not altered by colitis (Figure 7D). In conclusion, 7β-hydroxy-EpiA treatment (all doses) suppressed the increase in both COX-2 and mPGES-1 mRNA synthesis in the colitis group from day 13 to day 14 (Figure 7).

4.5 7β-Hydroxy-EpiA overall effects on colitis

Colitis was fully induced in untreated rats after DSS administration for 7 days. Treatment for 7 days with several doses of 7β-hydroxy-EpiA prior to colitis induction led to a prevention of colitis onset. Examination of myeloperoxidase activity and oxidative stress markers such as carbonylated proteins and Tbars provided evidence of their decrease after steroid treatment (Hennebert et al, 2008). The preventive effects of 7β-hydroxy-EpiA could result in part from the early increase of the prostaglandin 15d-PGJ_2 that might contribute to down regulate the inflammatory response. 7β-Hydroxy-EpiA triggered an increase in COX-2 and m-PGES1 expression but depressed the elevation of colonic PGE_2 synthesis in dextran sodium sulphate-treated rats. Thus, 7β-hydroxy-EpiA triggered a shift from the PGE pathway towards the PGD pathway, causing increased production of 15d-PGJ_2, the dehydrated stable metabolite of PGD_2 (Scher & Pillinger, 2005). Our finding that small doses of 7β-hydroxy-EpiA, an endogenous steroid produced in colon, can prevent colonic damage through a shift from PGE_2 to PGD_2 production via changes in COX-2 expression, followed by an increase of 15d-PGJ_2 levels in the colon result from investigations carried out on a rat

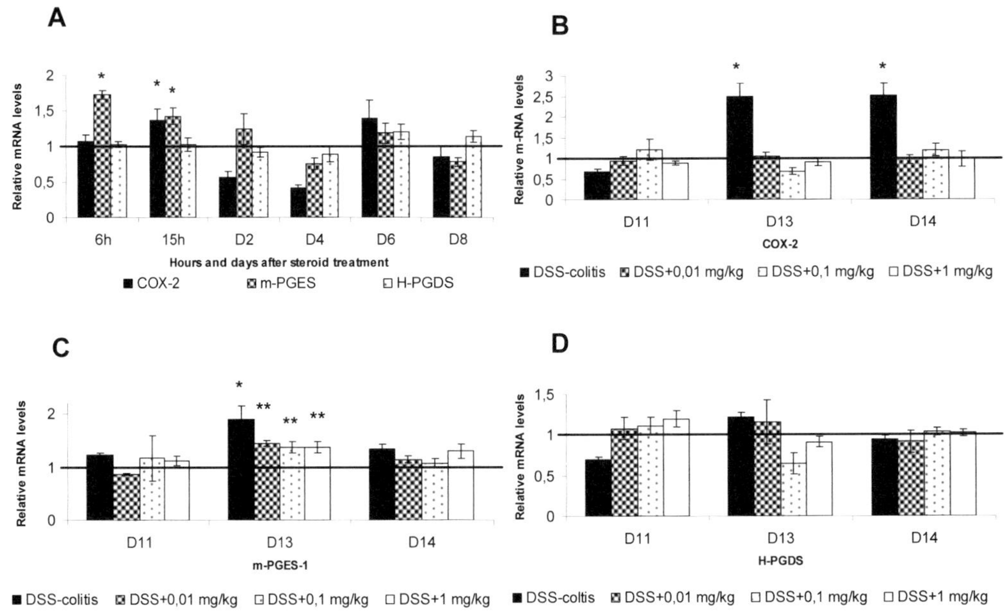

Fig. 7. Colonic expression of COX-2, m-PGES1 and H-PGDS mRNA after 0.1 mg/kg 7β-hydroxy-EpiA treatment and before colitis induction (A). During colitis induction, mRNA levels for COX-2 (B), m-PGES-1 (C) and H-PGDS (C) were measured at days 11, 13 and 14. mRNA levels are expressed relative to that of HPRT1 standing at a basal level of 1 shown as a continuous line. (*) DSS-colitis versus basal level ($p < 0.05$). (**) DSS + 0.01, 0.1 and 1 mg/kg 7β-hydroxy-EpiA-treated group versus DSS-colitis group ($p < 0.05$).

model where inflammation and colitis were obtained by dextran sodium sulphate administration. Two immediate questions arise from these findings: i) does this process, leading to the resolution of inflammation, occur in any inflammation? ii) is 7β-hydroxy-EpiA as efficient in humans as in rats when faced with inflammation? Answers to these questions were seek in human cell cultures.

5. A model for inflammation studies in humans

Addition of TNF-α to cultures of human peripheral blood monocytes (PBMC) results into the cellular stress found in inflammatory conditions through production of mediators released from the eicosanoid pathway. These mediators include PGE_2 that is associated with inflammation, and PGD_2 and 15d-PGJ_2 which are associated with the resolution of inflammation (Haworth & Buckley, 2007). Therefore, we used human PBMC cultured in the presence or absence of 0.01 μg/mL TNF-α in order to test the effects of 7β-hydroxy-EpiA on PG production (Le Mee et al, 2008). PBMC were cultivated either for 4 or 24 hours. RIA measurements were carried out for the PG levels released in the medium, and mRNA of the eicosanoid pathway were measured in cell extracts by quantitative PCR. All mRNA measurements were made relative to the expression of house-keeping gene HPRT1 (Le Mee et al, 2008).

5.1 7β-Hydroxy-EpiA-induced a shift in PG production

7β-Hydroxy-EpiA addition to the medium induced no significant change in PG levels in PBMC cultured for 4 h. In marked contrast, significantly increased 15d-PGJ_2 levels were obtained after cultivation for 24 h (Figure 8). This increment occurred both in the presence and in the absence of TNF-α. A significant decrease in PGE_2 levels was also obtained in the presence of TNF-α only (Figure 8B). These findings indicated that 7β-hydroxy-EpiA treatment of TNF-α-associated inflammation patterns were causative of a shift from PGE_2 to 15d-PGJ_2 production. Since 15d-PGJ_2 is a spontaneous dehydrated derivative of PGD_2, production of PGD_2 must have been increased along with the inflammation-related conditions for its conversion to 15d-PGJ_2 (Le Mee et al, 2008). 7β-Hydroxy-EpiA-triggered changes in the expression of the enzymes producing PGE_2 and PGD_2 had to be examined then.

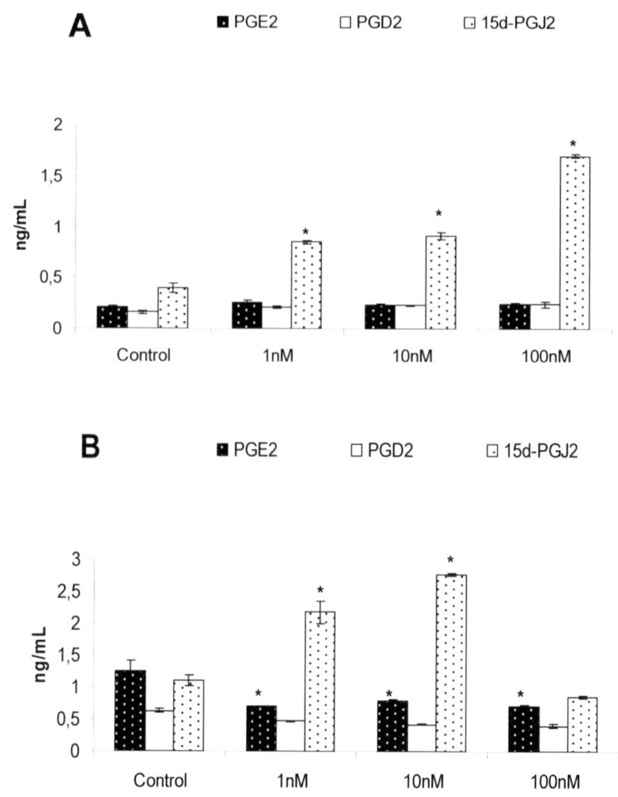

Fig. 8. PG levels released in the medium of human PBMC cultured for 24 h fortified with 1-100 nM 7β-hydroxy-EpiA. Cultures were carried out in the absence (A) or in the presence of TNF-α (B). (*) significantly different from controls ($p < 0.05$).

5.2 7β-Hydroxy-EpiA-induced changes in eicosanoid pathway enzyme expression

In addition to COX-2 and m-PGES1 which are responsible for arachidonic acid conversion to PGH2 and PGE2, respectively, we measured the mRNA levels of the known two enzymes responsible for PGD2 production, namely H-PGDS and L-PGDS. No significant change in enzyme mRNA levels was found in cells culture with 7β-hydroxy-EpiA for 4 h. In marked contrast, cultivation for 24 h led to significant differences in enzyme expression. Cultures without addition of TNF-α showed that 7β-hydroxy-EpiA significantly increased m-PGES1 and decreased H-PGDS mRNA levels (Figure 9A). The findings were opposite in the presence of TNF-α, with significant decrease in m-PGES1 and no change in H-PGDS mRNA levels (Figure 9B). No significant effect of 7β-hydroxy-EpiA was found for COX-2 and L-PGDS. These findings parallel well with PG levels measurements, and imply that the 7β-hydroxy-EpiA-triggered shift from PGE_2 to 15d-PGJ_2 production is mainly due to a lower expression of the m-PGES1 enzyme responsible for PGE2 production (Le Mee et al, 2008).

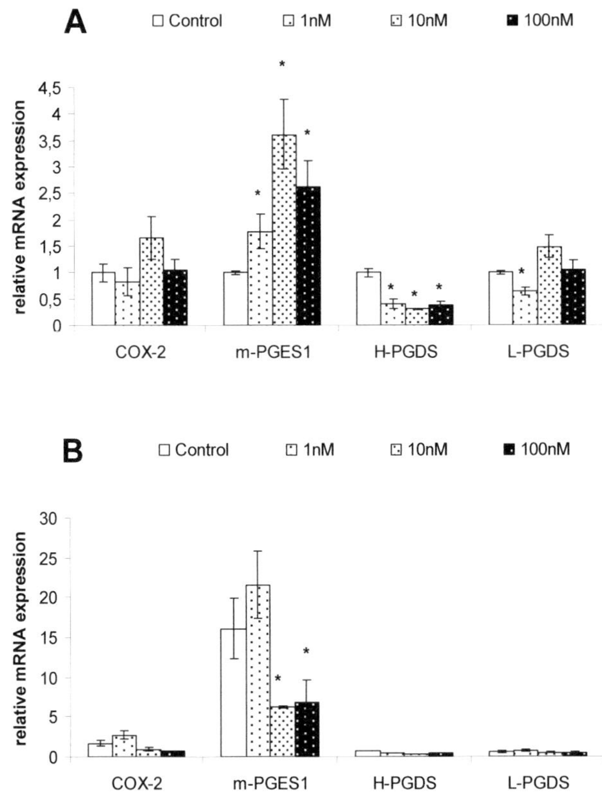

Fig. 9. Measurement of COX-2, m-PGES1, H-PGDS and L-PGDS mRNA levels relative to the expression of house-keeping gene HPRT1. The human PBMC were cultured for 24 h without or with 1-100 nM 7β-hydroxy-EpiA. Cultures were carried out in the absence (A) or the presence of TNF-α. (*) significantly different from control group ($p < 0.05$).

5.3 A putative specific receptor for 7β-Hydroxy-EpiA

Our findings that a 10^{-9} M dose of 7β-hydroxy-EpiA was a trigger for the resolution of inflammation and for cellular protection led us to consider this steroid as a possible candidate for interference with a putative nuclear receptor. A precursor for 7β-hydroxy-

EpiA, namely 5α-androstane-3β,17β-diol, was shown to bind preferentially to the estrogen receptor-β (ER-β) with agonistic activity and a K_d of 2 nM (20 times larger than for estradiol) (Kuiper et al, 1997). Several reports inferred that ER-β was involved in the protection against breast and prostate cancer (Dondi et al, 2010; Nilsson et al, 2001), and this led us to test this hypothesis on three breast cancer cell lines, namely, MCF-7, MDA-231 and SKBR-3 (Niro et al, 2011).

6. Tamoxifen-like effect of 7β-Hydroxy-EpiA on breast cancer cell proliferation

Among ERs, MCF-7 cells are known to express ER-α, ER-β and GPR30. MCF-7 cells proliferate in the presence of 10^{-8} M estradiol, and their proliferation is markedly inhibited by 10^{-6} M tamoxifen (TAM), even in the presence of estradiol. Cultivations in the presence of 10^{-7}-10^{-9} M 7β-hydroxy-EpiA without TAM or estradiol inhibited MCF-7 cell proliferation to TAM levels, whereas use of both TAM and 7β-hydroxy-EpiA, or estradiol + 7β-hydroxy-EpiA, decreased the proliferation below TAM levels (Figure 10A). These results indicated that 7β-hydroxy-EpiA doses 10-10^3 lower than the TAM dose produced TAM-like effects on MCF-7 growth. In contrast, the MDA-231 cell receptor status is ER-β+, GPR30+. Their proliferation was not increased by estradiol, and TAM effects were not as strikingly important as in MCF-7 cells (Niro et al, 2011).

Cultivations of the MDA-231 cells in the presence of 10^{-7}-10^{-9} M 7β-hydroxy-EpiA without TAM or estradiol did not significantly change the proliferation patterns, whereas use of either estradiol + TAM or estradiol + 7β-hydroxy-EpiA, decreased the proliferation much below TAM or estradiol levels (Figure 10B). In the case of SKBR-3 cells, le receptor status is GPR30+. SKBR-3 cell line proliferation was not significantly changed by estradiol, TAM or 10^{-7}-10^{-9} M 7β-hydroxy-EpiA. Cultivations of SKBR-3 cells in the presence of estradiol + 7β-hydroxy-EpiA significantly decreased cell proliferation (Figure 10C) (Niro et al, 2011).

The conclusions drawn from these studies imply the native 7β-hydroxy-EpiA in the regulation of ER-mediated estrogen effects. As for TAM, the responsiveness of MCF-7 cells to 7β-hydroxy-EpiA was better than for MDA-231 and SKBR-3 cells, and this implied that the antiproliferative and cytoprotective effects can be mediated by a receptor linked to one or several ERs. In any case, the receptor responsible for 7β-hydroxy-EpiA effects needs to be identified and whether and how ERs are involved in the mechanism leading to cell protection require further examination.

7. Pathophysiological significance of 7β-Hydroxy-EpiA levels

The first requirement for the production of native 7β-hydroxy-EpiA is the presence of the steroid hormone substrate testosterone for generation of epiandrosterone by the classical steroid metabolism (Figure 2). Scarce studies were addressed to the levels of circulating epiandrosterone in humans. This may be due to ignorance of its fate in hormonal and physiological processes. Two key enzymes are required then for 7β-hydroxy-EpiA production. One is CYP7B1 which provides a hydroxyl at the 7α- position on epiandrosterone, and the second is 11β-HSD1 which converts 7α-hydroxy-EpiA into 7β-hydroxy-EpiA. Both enzymes

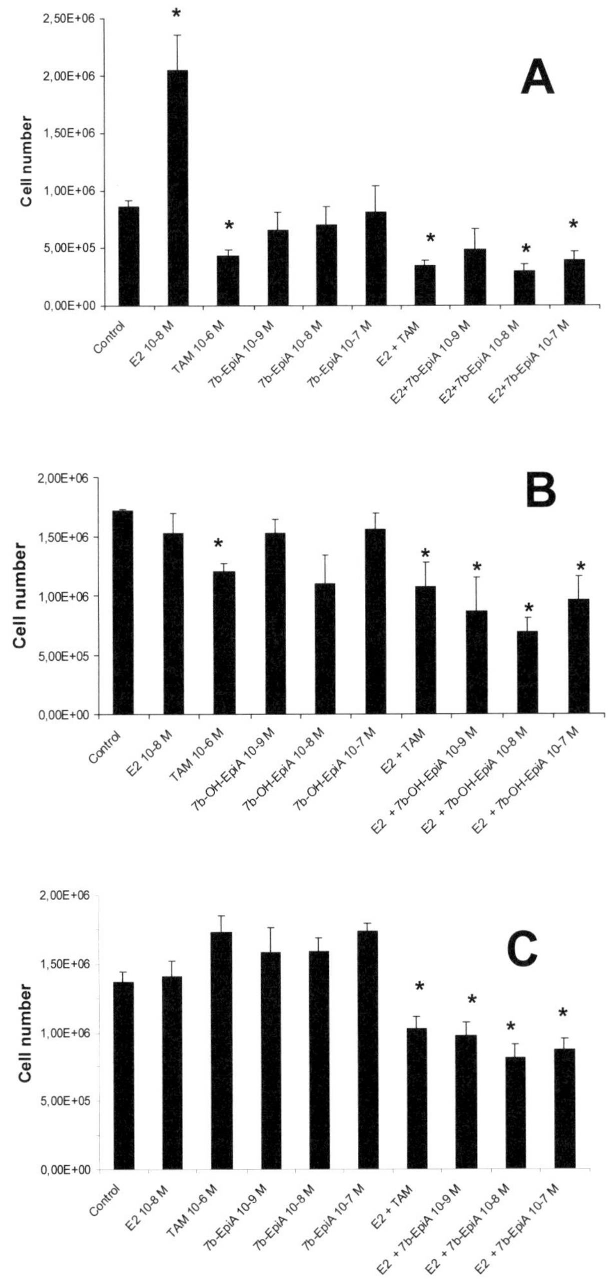

Fig. 10. Tamoxifen-like effects of 7β-hydroxy-EpiA on the proliferation of MCF-7 (A), MDA-231 (B) and SKBR-3 cell lines. Cells (10^5) were seeded in triplicate in 24-well plates, and adherent cells were cultivated in 1 mL growth medium at 37°C, 95% humidity and in the presence of 5% CO_2 for 72h. Estradiol (E2), 7β-hydroxy-EpiA (7β-EpiA) and tamoxifen (TAM) were administered in 5μL ethanol at the beginning of assays. Controls contained 5μL ethanol only. * Indicates a significant difference with controls ($p < 0.05$).

are ubiquitous in human tissues, and any deficit in their expression may lead to related pathologies. Their outcome may also be related to aging since the production and levels of steroid precursors such as DHEA and testosterone are known to be significantly decreased after the fifth decade in humans. These considerations would be strongly supported by precise measurements of the 7β-hydroxy-EpiA circulating levels in humans.

Finally, variations in the susceptibility for the development of diseases may depend on 7β-hydroxy-EpiA receptor availability and function (Nilsson & Gustafsson, 2002). The precise mechanism of action and the Ers involvement are to be deciphered in order to give a full support to 7β-hydroxy-EpiA beneficial effects.

8. Concluding remarks

DHEA and testosterone-derived metabolites, namely epiandrosterone and 5α-androstane-3β,17β-diol, are substrates for the CYP7B1 and their 7α-hydroxylated products are also converted into 7β epimer by the 11β-HSD1. When assayed in rat colitis and inflamed human PBMC at doses 10^4 lower than circulating free DHEA or testosterone, 7β-hydroxy-EpiA was shown to shift the PG metabolism from PGE_2 to 15d-PGJ_2 production, thus triggering the resolution of inflammation. In addition, 7β-hydroxy-EpiA (1 nM) exerted the same effects as TAM (1 μM) on the proliferation of MCF-7, MDA-231 and SKBR-3 human beast cancer cell lines. These findings suggest that the observed effects of 7β-hydroxy-EpiA could be mediated in part by ERs.

This overview of recent studies implies that DHEA and/or testosterone are precursors for 7β-hydroxy-EpiA acting on inflamed tissues for the resolution of inflammation through a putative receptor. CYP7B1 and 11β-HSD1 are two key enzymes involved in 7β-hydroxy-EpiA production, and their expression in colitis and other inflammatory diseases could be a rewarding target in further studies.

9. References

Ajuebor, Singh, & Wallace (2000). Cyclooxygenase-2-derived prostaglandin D(2) is an early anti-inflammatory signal in experimental colitis. *Am. J. Physiol Gastrointest. Liver Physiol.* 279, G238-G244.

Blumberg, Saubermann, & Strober (1999). Animal models of mucosal inflammation and their relation to human inflammatory bowel disease. *Curr. Opin. Immunol.* 11, 648-656.

Chalbot & Morfin (2005). Neurosteroids: metabolism in human intestine microsomes. *Steroids* 70, 319-326.

Dondi, Piccolella, Biserni, Della, Ramachandran, Locatelli, Rusmini, Sau, Caruso, Maggi, Ciana, & Poletti (2010). Estrogen receptor beta and the progression of prostate cancer: role of 5alpha-androstane-3beta,17beta-diol. *Endocr. Relat Cancer* 17, 731-742.

Doostzadeh & Morfin (1996). Studies of the enzyme complex responsible for pregnenolone and dehydroepiandrosterone 7 alpha-hydroxylation in mouse tissues. *Steroids* 61, 613-620.

Dubuquoy, Rousseaux, Thuru, Peyrin-Biroulet, Romano, Chavatte, Chamaillard, & Desreumaux (2006). PPARgamma as a new therapeutic target in inflammatory bowel diseases. *Gut* 55, 1341-1349.

Dudas, Hanin, Rose, & Wulfert (2004). Protection against inflammatory neurodegeneration and glial cell death by 7beta-hydroxy epiandrosterone, a novel neurosteroid. *Neurobiol. Dis.* 15, 262-268.

Dulos, van der Vleuten, Kavelaars, Heijnen, & Boots (2005). CYP7B expression and activity in fibroblast-like synoviocytes from patients with rheumatoid arthritis: regulation by proinflammatory cytokines. *Arthritis Rheum.* 52, 770-778.

Dulos, Verbraak, Bagchus, Boots, & Kaptein (2004). Severity of murine collagen-induced arthritis correlates with increased CYP7B activity: enhancement of dehydroepiandrosterone metabolism by interleukin-1beta. *Arthritis Rheum.* 50, 3346-3353.

Funk (2001). Prostaglandins and leukotrienes: advances in eicosanoid biology. *Science* 294, 1871-1875.

Haworth & Buckley (2007). Resolving the problem of persistence in the switch from acute to chronic inflammation. *Proc. Natl. Acad. Sci. U. S. A.* 104, 20647-20648.

Hennebert, Chalbot, Alran, & Morfin (2007a). Dehydroepiandrosterone 7alpha-hydroxylation in human tissues: possible interference with type 1 11beta-hydroxysteroid dehydrogenase-mediated processes. *J. Steroid Biochem. Mol. Biol.* 104, 326-333.

Hennebert, Pelissier, Le Mee, Wulfert, & Morfin (2008). Anti-inflammatory effects and changes in prostaglandin patterns induced by 7beta-hydroxy-epiandrosterone in rats with colitis. *J. Steroid Biochem. Mol. Biol.* 110, 255-262.

Hennebert, Pernelle, Ferroud, & Morfin (2007b). 7alpha- and 7beta-hydroxy-epiandrosterone as substrates and inhibitors for the human 11beta-hydroxysteroid dehydrogenase type 1. *J. Steroid Biochem. Mol. Biol.* 105, 159-165.

Jacolot, Berthou, Dreano, Bercovici, & Floch (1981). In vivo metabolism of ^{14}C-labelled 5α-androstane-3β,17β-diol. *J. Steroid Biochem.* 14, 663-669.

Kim, Chalbot, Pompon, Jo, & Morfin (2004). The human cytochrome P4507B1: catalytic activity studies. *J. Steroid Biochem. Mol. Biol.* 92, 383-389.

Kuiper, Carlsson, Grandien, Enmark, Haggblad, Nilsson, & Gustafsson (1997). Comparison of the ligand binding specificity and transcript tissue distribution of estrogen receptors alpha and beta. *Endocrinology* 138, 863-870.

Le Mee, Hennebert, Ferrec, Wulfert, & Morfin (2008). 7beta-Hydroxy-epiandrosterone-mediated regulation of the prostaglandin synthesis pathway in human peripheral blood monocytes. *Steroids* 73, 1148-1159.

Malik, Narayan, Wendling, Cole, Pashko, Schwartz, & Strauss (2003). A novel dehydroepiandrosterone analog improves functional recovery in a rat traumatic brain injury model. *J. Neurotrauma* 20, 463-476.

Melgar, Drmotova, Rehnstrom, Jansson, & Michaelsson (2006). Local production of chemokines and prostaglandin E2 in the acute, chronic and recovery phase of murine experimental colitis. *Cytokine* 35, 275-283.

Monneret, Li, Vasilescu, Rokach, & Powell (2002). 15-Deoxy-delta 12,14-prostaglandins D2 and J2 are potent activators of human eosinophils. *J. Immunol.* 168, 3563-3569.

Morfin & Courchay (1994). Pregnenolone and dehydroepiandrosterone as precursors of native 7-hydroxylated metabolites which increase the immune response in mice. *J. Steroid Biochem. Mol. Biol.* 50, 91-100.

Muller, Hennebert, & Morfin (2006a). The native antiglucocorticoid paradigm. *J. Steroid Biochem. Mol. Biol.* 100, 95-105.

Muller, Pompon, Urban, & Morfin (2006b). Inter-conversion of 7alpha- and 7beta-hydroxy-dehydroepiandrosterone by the human 11beta-hydroxysteroid dehydrogenase type 1. *J. Steroid Biochem. Mol. Biol.* 99, 215-222.

Murthy, Murthy, Coppola, & Wood (1997). The efficacy of BAY y 1015 in dextran sulfate model of mouse colitis. *Inflamm. Res.* 46, 224-233.

Nilsson & Gustafsson (2002). Biological role of estrogen and estrogen receptors. *Crit. Rev. Biochem. Molec. Biol.* 37, 1-28.

Nilsson, Makela, Treuter, Tujague, Thomsen, Andersson, Enmark, Pettersson, Warner, & Gustafsson (2001). Mechanisms of estrogen action. *Physiol. Rev.* 81, 1535-1565.

Niro, Hennebert, & Morfin (2010). A native steroid hormone derivative triggers the resolution of inflammation. *Hormone Molecular Biology and Clinical Investigation* 1, 11-19.

Niro, Hennebert, & Morfin (2011). New insights into the protective effects of DHEA. *Hormone Molecular Biology and Clinical Investigation* 4, 489-498.

Pavlick, Laroux, Fuseler, Wolf, Gray, Hoffman, & Grisham (2002). Role of reactive metabolites of oxygen and nitrogen in inflammatory bowel disease. *Free Radic. Biol. Med.* 33, 311-322.

Pelissier, Muller, Hill, & Morfin (2006). Protection against dextran sodium sulfate-induced colitis by dehydroepiandrosterone and 7alpha-hydroxy-dehydroepiandrosterone in the rat. *Steroids* 71, 240-248.

Pelissier, Trap, Malewiak, & Morfin (2004). Antioxidant effects of dehydroepiandrosterone and 7a-hydroxy-dehydroepiandrosterone in the rat colon, intestine and liver. *Steroids* 69, 137-144.

Podolsky (2003). The future of IBD treatment. *J. Gastroenterol.* 38 Suppl 15, 63-66.

Pringle, Schmidt, Deans, Wulfert, Reymann, & Sundstrom (2003). 7-Hydroxylated epiandrosterone (7-OH-EPIA) reduces ischaemia-induced neuronal damage both in vivo and in vitro. *Eur. J. Neurosci.* 18, 117-124.

Rajakariar, Hilliard, Lawrence, Trivedi, Colville-Nash, Bellingan, Fitzgerald, Yaqoob, & Gilroy (2007). Hematopoietic prostaglandin D2 synthase controls the onset and resolution of acute inflammation through PGD2 and 15-deoxyDelta12 14 PGJ2. *Proc. Natl. Acad. Sci. U. S. A.* 104, 20979-20984.

Ricco, Revial, Ferroud, Hennebert, & Morfin (2011). Synthesis of 7beta-hydroxy-epiandrosterone. *Steroids* 76, 28-30.

Scher & Pillinger (2005). 15d-PGJ2: the anti-inflammatory prostaglandin? *Clin. Immunol.* 114, 100-109.

Stenson (2007). Prostaglandins and epithelial response to injury. *Curr. Opin. Gastroenterol.* 23, 107-110.

Sun, Wu, Tsuang, Chen, & Sheu (2006). The in vitro effects of dehydroepiandrosterone on chondrocyte metabolism. *Osteoarthritis. Cartilage.* 14, 238-249.

Part 2

Infectious Colitis

3

Amebic Colitis

María Carolina Isea[1], Andrés Escudero-Sepulveda[2] and Alfonso J. Rodriguez-Morales[3]

[1]*Fundación Jiménez Díaz-UTE, Madrid*
[2]*Faculty of Health Sciences, Universidad Autónoma de Bucaramanga, Bucaramanga*
[3]*Faculty of Medicine, Universidad Central de Venezuela, Caracas*
[1]*Spain*
[2]*Colombia*
[3]*Venezuela*

1. Introduction

Gastrointestinal pathologies constitute among the most frequent form of disease in the World, especially enteric infections represent a significant burden of morbidity and mortality particularly in developing countries, where barriers between human feces and food and water supplies are inadequate. Enteric infections can be produce by a varied type of organisms, including bacteria, fungi, viruses and parasites. Among the parasites, two different types of them can produce gastrointestinal infections: helminths and protozoans. Inside the protozoans, these would be classified as flagellates (eg. *Giardia intestinalis*), spore-forming or coccidia (eg. *Cyclospora cayetanensis*), ciliates (eg. *Balantidium coli*) and amebas (eg. *Entamoeba histolytica*).

Amebas parasites include a large number of genuses and species among three subphyla of the phylum *Amoebozoa*: *Conosa, Lobosa* and *Protamoebae*. Pathogenic species are included in the families *Achanthamoebidae* (eg. *Acanthamoeba*), *Vahlkampfia* (eg. *Naegleria*), *Balamuthiidae* (eg. *Balamuthia*) and *Entamoebidae* (eg. *Entamoeba histolytica*). *Entamoeba histolytica* is the only recognized intestinal pathogenic ameba. Other species in the genus can be present in the human intestinal tract but are non-pathogenic (eg. *E. dispar*).

Over the past decade, since it was formally recognized, through molecular biology and phylogenetic analyses, that *Entamoeba histolytica* and *Entamoeba dispar* were two distinct species, studies in this field have made dramatic in-roads into the understanding of *E. histolytica* and the pathogenesis of invasive amebiasis (Adams & MacLeod, 1977), which in fact represent a low proportion of the cases of amebiasis; most of then are asymptomatic. Given this knowledge an extensive understanding of the epidemiology, pathophysiology, and the molecular and genetic biology of the organism has been reached, improving not just the diagnosis, medical and surgical treatment options but, ultimately, the development of a safe and efficacious vaccine, which is actually in process (Bercu, et al 2007 ; Blessmann & Tannich, 2002 ; Gonzales, et al 2009).

2. Epidemiology

In the last two decades too, it has also become clear that the true incidence of *E. histolytica* infection, particularly in vulnerable populations such as low socioeconomic children, is exceedingly high. Even more, in deprived areas of the World, especially in suburban and rural areas of the developing countries, particularly in tropical areas, amebiasis is a disease with a high burden of morbidity and mortality, with nations where prevalence estimates reach as high as 50% or more (eg. in Central and South America, Asia and Africa). However, this disease can be found worldwide and has been estimated that around 10% of the World's population is infected.

Morbidity from amebiasis represent around 40-50 million estimated cases per year in the World (World Health Organization, WHO). Although most cases are asymptomatic, dysentery and invasive extraintestinal disease can occur (Lysy, et al 1991). Amebic liver abscess is the most common manifestation of invasive amebiasis, but other organs can also be involved, including pleuropulmonary, cardiac, cerebral, renal, genitourinary, and cutaneous sites (Kenner & Rosen, 2006). Mortality due to amebiasis is estimated in 40,000-100,000 deaths per year (WHO). Its lethality or case fatality ratio in amebic colitis is estimated in 2-10%, however would be increased up to 40% when amebic colitis evolves to fulminant necrotizing colitis or rupture (Aristizabal, et al 1991).

Actually, amebiasis is the second leading cause of death from parasitic diseases worldwide. In many countries, the epidemiology of amebiasis has been recognized as a significant public health problem, even in many countries, before the 1990s, being overestimated and overdiagnosed due to the confusion between *E. histolytica* and *E. dispar* that many times generated a false positive diagnosis of amebiasis when incorrectly *E. dispar* infection was diagnosed as amebiasis due to *E. histolytica*. This happened because these species cannot be differentiated by direct examination, mainly by molecular techniques more often used these days.

Although that today is still controversial of the role of *E. histolytica* in certain type of patients (eg. immunocompromised hosts, particularly in Human Immunodeficiency Virus, HIV infection/Acquired Immunodeficiency Syndrome, AIDS, but additionally in cancer and pregnant women). Additionally to this, has been stated that are certain groups of patients predisposed to amebic colitis: very young patients, malnourished subjects and recipients of corticosteroids, men who have sex with men and institutionalized individuals. Otherwise, race, sex and age, in general, do not affect significantly the epidemiology of disease.

New contexts of disease include today the infection impact in transplant recipients (Franco-Paredes, et al 2010). Infection due to *Entamoeba histolytica* can occur in transplant recipients leading to severe colitis and liver abscesses.

Even more, in the context of globalization and migration, relevance of many gastrointestinal infections have been emphasised. Traveller's diarrhoea represents 20-60% of the estimated incidence of illness during travel to developing countries, being 5-10% of its etiology due to protozoan agents. In this context, travel and migration from those countries with high prevalence of amebiasis have been also considered of risk for infection. Amebic liver abscesses have been reported in travel exposures as short as 4 days, with a median of 3 months. Whereas amebic colitis is not common in short-term travellers (Cascio, et al 2011).

3. Pathology

The causative protozoan parasite, *E. histolytica* (Figure 1), is a potent pathogen, transmitted via ingestion of the cystic mature form (Figure 2), the infective stage of this protozoan parasite (Dickson-Gonzalez, et al 2009).

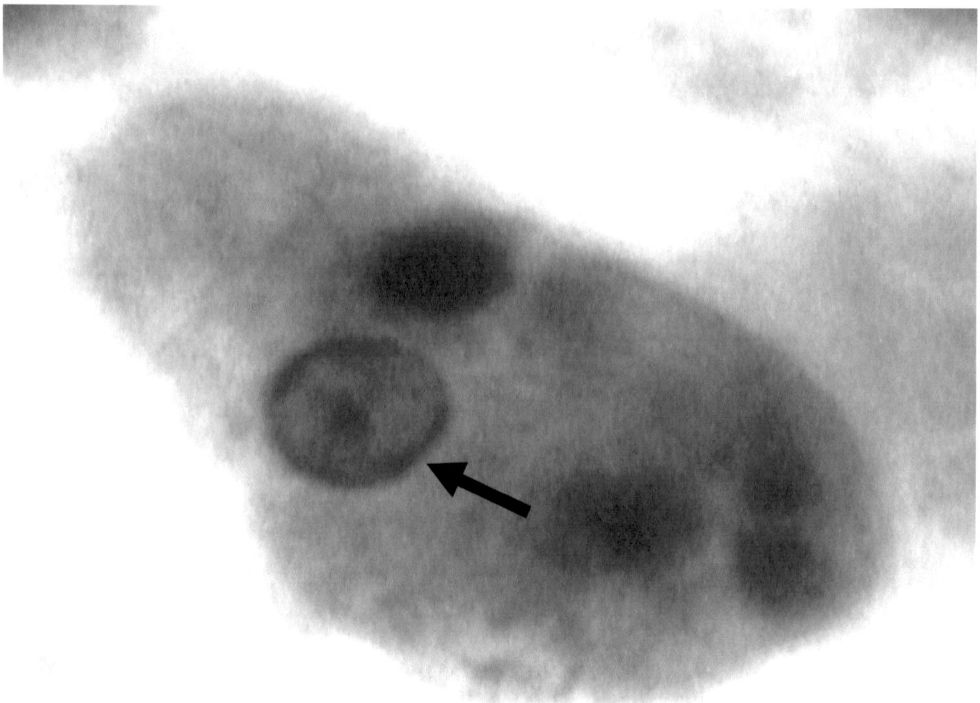

Fig. 1. *Entamoeba histolytica* throphozoites, showing nucleus and karyosoma (arrow) (HF, 1000X) (Dickson-Gonzalez et al., 2009)

Viable in the environment for weeks to even months, cysts can be found in fecally contaminated soil, fertilizer, or water or on the contaminated hands of food handlers and contaminated elements that can be used during food preparation or ingestion (Dickson-Gonzalez, et al 2009).

Fecal-oral transmission can also occur in the setting of anal sexual practices, for which some series have been found a higher incidence in men who have sex with men (MSM), or in the context of direct rectal inoculation through colonic irrigation devices.

Excystation (Figure 2) occurs in the terminal ileum or colon (Figure 3), resulting in trophozoites, the invasive form.

The trophozoites can penetrate and invade the colonic mucosal barrier, leading to tissue destruction, secretory bloody diarrhea, and colitis resembling inflammatory bowel disease. In addition, the trophozoites can spread hematogenously via the portal circulation to the liver or even to more distant organs, which would include lungs, brain, kidneys and skin, among others (extraintestinal disease) (Figure 2) (Dickson-Gonzalez, et al 2009).

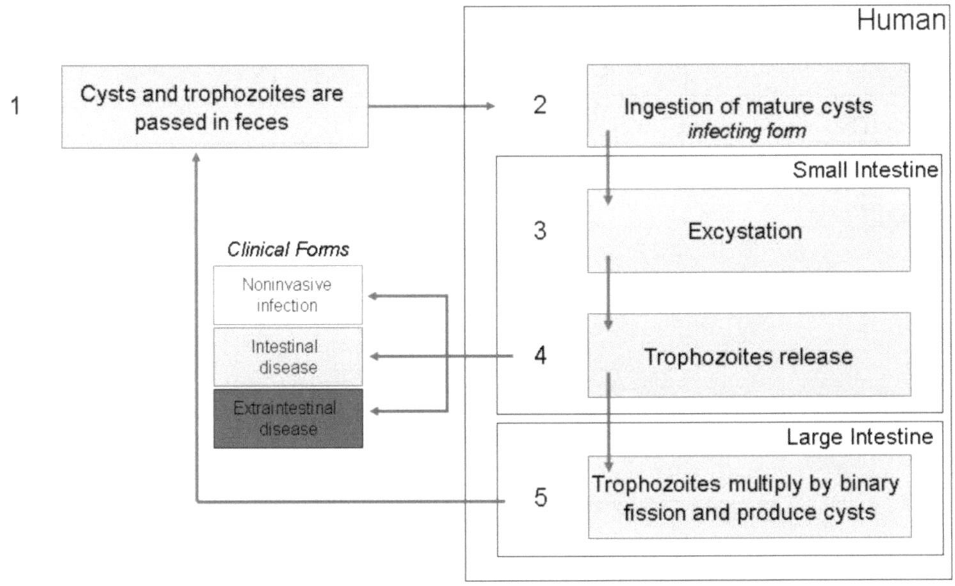

Fig. 2. Life cycle of *Entamoeba histolytica* infection

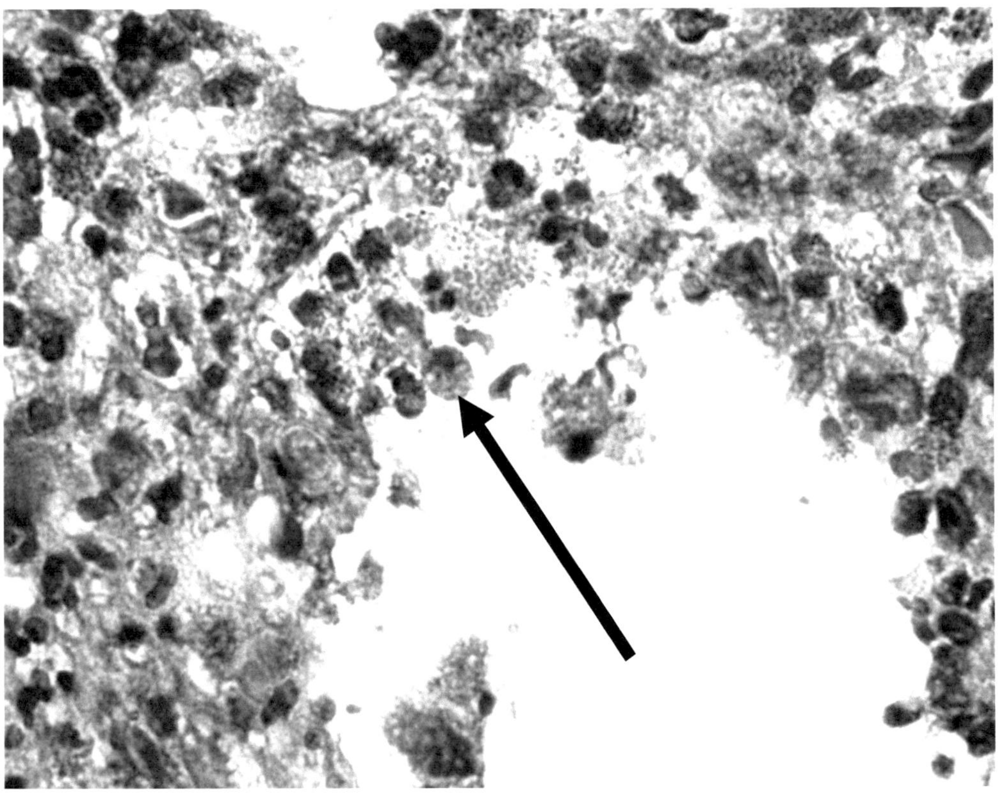

Fig. 3. *Entamoeba histolytica* throphozoites with a granulose cytoplasm (arrow), in the ileum producing an ulceration of the mucosa (HE, 200X) (Dickson-Gonzalez et al., 2009)

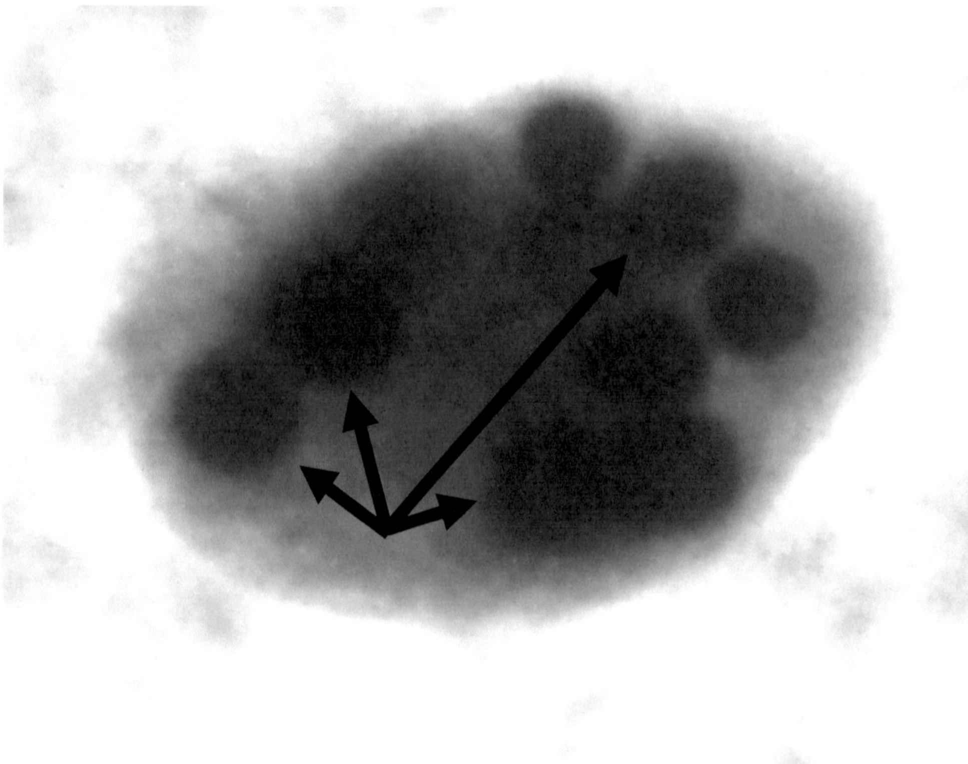

Fig. 4. *Entamoeba histolytica* throphozoites with abundant erythrophagia (arrows) (HF, 1000X) (Dickson-Gonzalez et al., 2009)

Today is well known that many pathogenic mechanisms are involved in the disease produced by this parasite, such as secreting proteinases that dissolve host tissues, killing host cells on contact, and engulfing red blood cells (Figure 4), leading to trophozoites to invade the intestinal mucosa, causing amebic colitis. Classically, the triad of Gal-lectin, cysteine proteinases and amoebapores of the parasite were thought to be the major proteins involved in the pathogenesis of amoebiasis (Accolla, 2006).

Regard to the pathophysiology, new evidences regard the interaction between *E. histolytica* and human polymorphonuclear neutrophils (PMN) has been investigated, based on *in vitro* and *in vivo* animal studies, which have found that PMN actively migrate toward amebae trophozoite cells (Al-Mofleh, et al 1989; Arbo, et al 1993 ; Guerrant, et al 1981). Later studies in tissue culture systems demonstrated that PMN were confirmed to play a vital role in amebic tissue invasion mechanisms (Accolla, 2006; Arbo, et al 1993).

Even more, at least axenic *E. histolytica* trophozoites and amebic protein preparations have been able to stimulate chemotaxis of human PMN *in vitro*. Additionally, *E. histolytica* inhibits the respiratory burst of PMN which represents a unique survival tactic and may contribute also to the pathogenesis of amebiasis (Dickson-Gonzalez, et al 2009).

More recently, some evidence has being reported on the findings regard to this interaction *in vivo* on human beings. In a study on biopsy samples taken by endoscopic surgical procedures from individuals with amebic colitis assessed histopathologically the relation between inflammatory infiltrating cells populations and the *E. histolytica* density in the intestinal lesions. PMN and lymphocytes are significantly associated with the extent of parasite presence (more significantly for PMN). Such findings support the theory that PMN interaction with *E. histolytica* contribute to the pathogenesis of lesions (Accolla, 2006).

However, further studies are necessary in order to improve the knowledge of pathophysiology as well the systemic and local immune response of this worldwide public health problem which may cause potentially life-threatening diseases (Accolla, 2006 ; Adams, et al 1993 ; Jhingran, et al 2008).

4. Gastrointestinal manifestations

The most common presentation of amebic colitis is gradual onset of bloody diarrhea, abdominal pain, and tenderness spanning several weeks' duration. Besides that, rectal bleeding without diarrhea can occur, especially in children. Other manifestations include heme-positive stools (seen in approximately 70-100%), diffuse abdominal tenderness (12-85%), weight loss (40%), fever (10-30%) and anorexia.

In the case of fulminant or necrotizing colitis, severe bloody diarrhea and widespread abdominal pain with evidence of peritonitis and fever are usually observed. Predisposing factors for this form of colitis include pregnancy, malnutrition, corticosteroid use and very young age (Hsu, et al 1995).

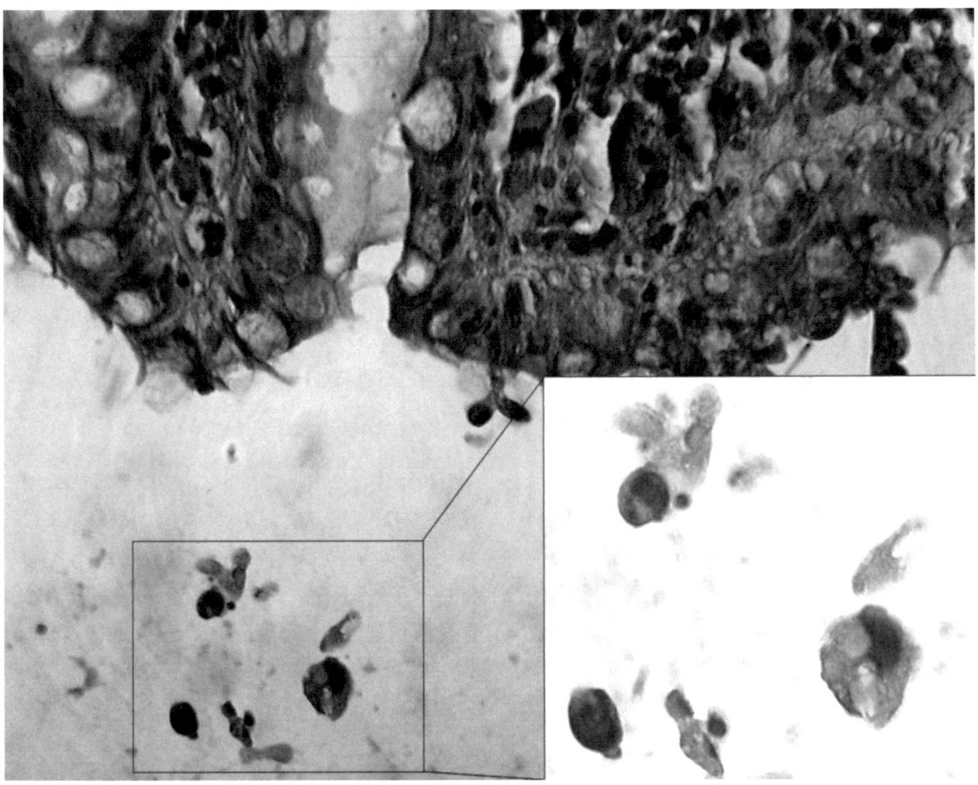

Fig. 5. Colon mucosa with mixed inflammatory infiltrate and congestion with presence of *E. histolytica* (HE, 400X, in the zooming, 1000X) (Dickson-Gonzalez et al., 2009)

Colonic findings in amebiasis have varied from thickening of the mucosa to flask-shaped ulceration, mostly in the cecum or appendix or near the ascending colon, but rarely in the sigmoidorectal area. These intestinal lesions can include: a colonic mucosa with mixed inflammatory infiltrate and congestion with presence of *E. histolytica* (Figure 5), inflammatory infiltrate in the superficial epithelium of the colon, with absortive cells denudated (Figure 6), interglandular corion with abundant inflammatory infiltrate rich in PMN and eosinophils (Figure 7), erosions of colonic mucosa with fibrinousleucocitary exudate in the surface (Figure 8), necrotic material and fibrinousleucocitary exudate (Figure 9) and the presence abundant eosinophils and edema in the interglandular corion (Figure 10).

The development of fulminant colitis, ameboma, cutaneous amebiasis and rectovaginal fistulas can occur as medical and surgical complications of intestinal amebiasis (Kenner & Rosen, 2006 ; Lejeune, et al, 2009).

5. Diagnosis

Diferential diagnosis of amebiasis include a large list of infectious and non-infectious causes (Table 1). Then multiple studies can be performed to confirm or rule-out the diagnosis, including stools microscopy, cultures, antigen detection, histopathology, serology and molecular biology techniques (Dickson-Gonzalez, et al 2009).

Microscopic evaluation using trichrome stain of stools is able to detect trophozoites in amebic colitis in 33-50%. Then serial stool samples (≥3) over no more than 10 days increase the sensitivity to 85-95%. Besides the trophozoite ingesting red blood cells, mostly happening in *E. histolytica* infection, leukocytes may be found (Burchard, et al 1993).

At cultures infection diagnosis can be achieved in 50% to 70%. Culture is not a routine process and is less sensitive than microscopy in detection. Then, it should be understood that cultures of *Entamoeba* are primarily research tools rather than diagnostic ones.

Differential diagnoses of amebiasis	
Infectious	**Non-infectious**
Abdominal Abscess	Arteriovenous Malformations
Campylobacter Infections	Diverticulitis
Cholecystitis	Hepatocellular Adenoma
Echinococcosis	Inflammatory Bowel Disease
Escherichia coli Infections	Ischemic Colitis
Hepatitis A	Perforated abdominal viscus
Other Viral Hepatitis	
Pericarditis	
Peritonitis	
Pyogenic Hepatic Abscesses	
Right lower lobe pneumonia	
Salmonellosis	
Shigellosis	

Table 1. Differential diagnoses of amebiasis

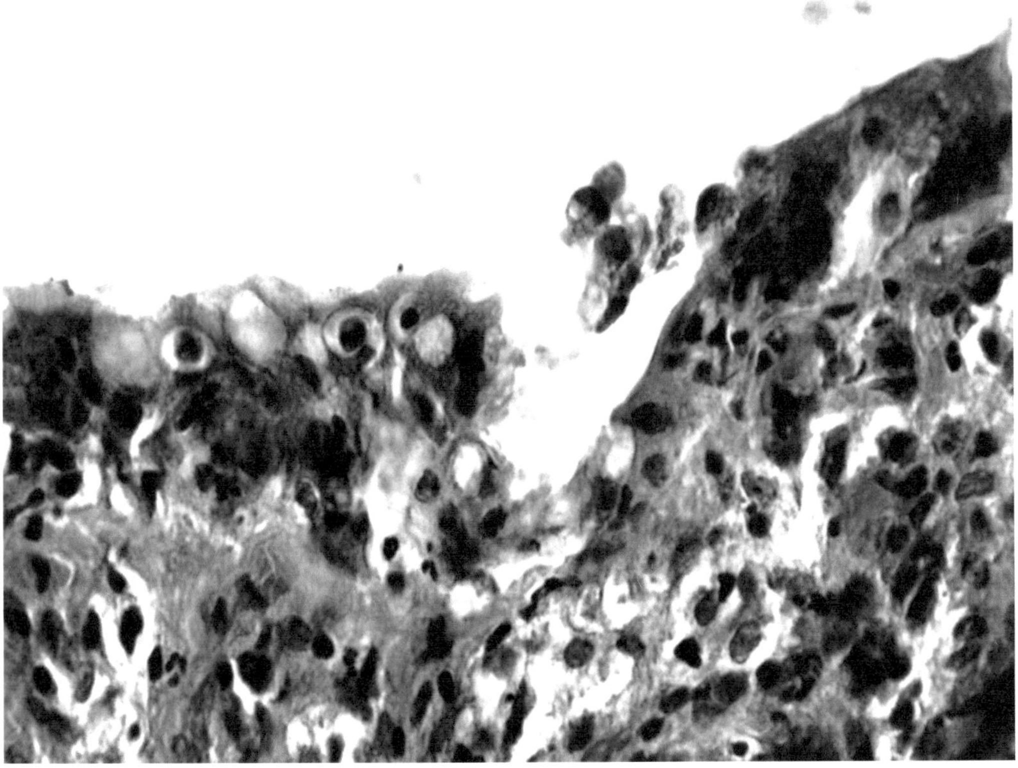

Fig. 6. Inflammatory infiltrate in the superficial epithelium of the colon, absorptive cells are denudated (HE, 1000X) (Dickson-Gonzalez et al., 2009)

Antigen detection through enzyme-linked immunosorbent assay (ELISA) is another test currently more available with multiple kits commercially available. In addition to it, kits using monoclonal antibodies against the GAL/GalNAc–specific lectin and the serine-rich antigen of *E. histolytica* yield an overall sensitivity up to 71%-100% and specificity up to 93%-100% (Dickson-Gonzalez, et al 2009).

Histopathological diagnosis of amebic colitis has been, until now, based on the demonstration of the amebic throphozoites in the histological sections, mostly without considering the environment of the parasite. However, cell populations such as PMN and eosinophils (Figure 6) would be predictive of the parasitic infection, which would change the diagnostic approach and criteria in the future.

Serology is also another form of diagnosis for amebiasis. Multiple serologic assays are currently available, being the ELISA the most used of them. This, measures the presence of serum IgG antibodies antilectin. Its sensitivity is high for extraintestinal disease up to 98%, but very low for active amebic colitis particularly in endemic areas due repeated exposure and development of some immunity, limiting antibody-based testing for diagnosing currently active disease, since antibodies can persist for years after infection. Other techniques for extraintestinal disease available include immunofluorescent assay (IFA), indirect hemagglutination (IHA) immunoelectrophoresis, counter-immunoelectrophoresis (CIE), immunodiffusion tests and complement fixation (CF) is less sensitive than other techniques.

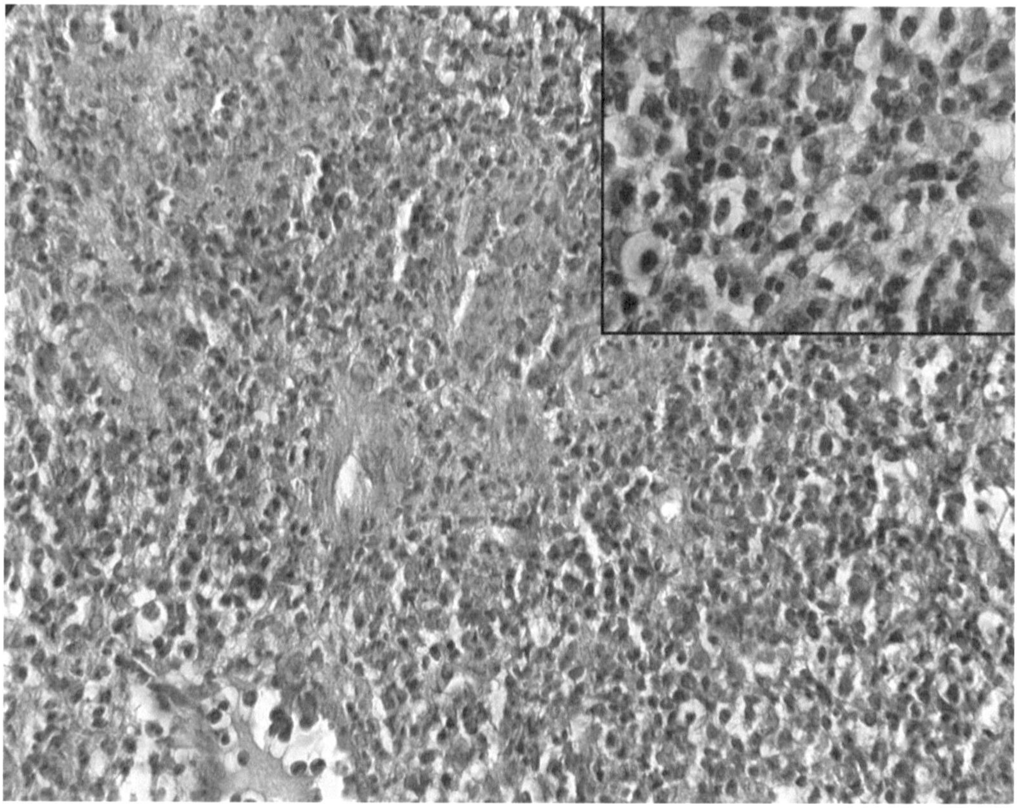

Fig. 7. Interglandular corion with abundant inflammatory infiltrate rich in PMN and eosinophils (HE, 400X, in the zooming 1000X) (Dickson-Gonzalez et al., 2009)

Molecular biology techniques can directly identify RNA and DNA of the parasite, being specific for the species. Right now using multiple targeting genes, including a small-subunit rRNA gene (18S rDNA), serine-rich protein gene, chitinase gene, 30-kDa antigen gene, hemolysin gene, and extrachromosomal circular DNA, among others, *E. histolytica* can be differentiated from other species. Although that, its wide application is still very limited for the routine diagnosis given the cost as well the availability of facilities for these technologies.

6. Treatment and prospects for a vaccine

Additionally to the clinical, epidemiological and diagnostic issues, therapeutic management of amebiasis is currently showing new options. For amebic colitis the main choice drug is still metronidazole (given for 5 to 10 days). Treatment requires the use of two groups of antiparasitic drugs: luminal and tissue agents. Asymptomatic intestinal colonization with *E. histolytica* can be treated with luminal agents alone. Drugs used for the treatment of luminal infections and generally prescribed for asymptomatic cyst passers include iodoquinol, diloxanide furoate, and paromomycin (5 to 20 days to eradicate colonization). Secnidazole has been used in some countries, but most studies coincide in that metronidazole, although more side effects such as headaches, anorexia, nausea, metallic taste, a disulfiram-like reaction to alcohol, and vomiting, is more effective than secnidazole. Recently some studies have also indicated a potential use of ivermectin for amebiasis (González-Salazar, et al 2009). In a systematic review published recently, information relating to the effectiveness and safety of the following interventions was described: diiodohydroxyquinoline (iodoquinol), diloxanide, emetine, metronidazole, nitazoxanide, ornidazole, paromomycin, secnidazole, and tinidazole.

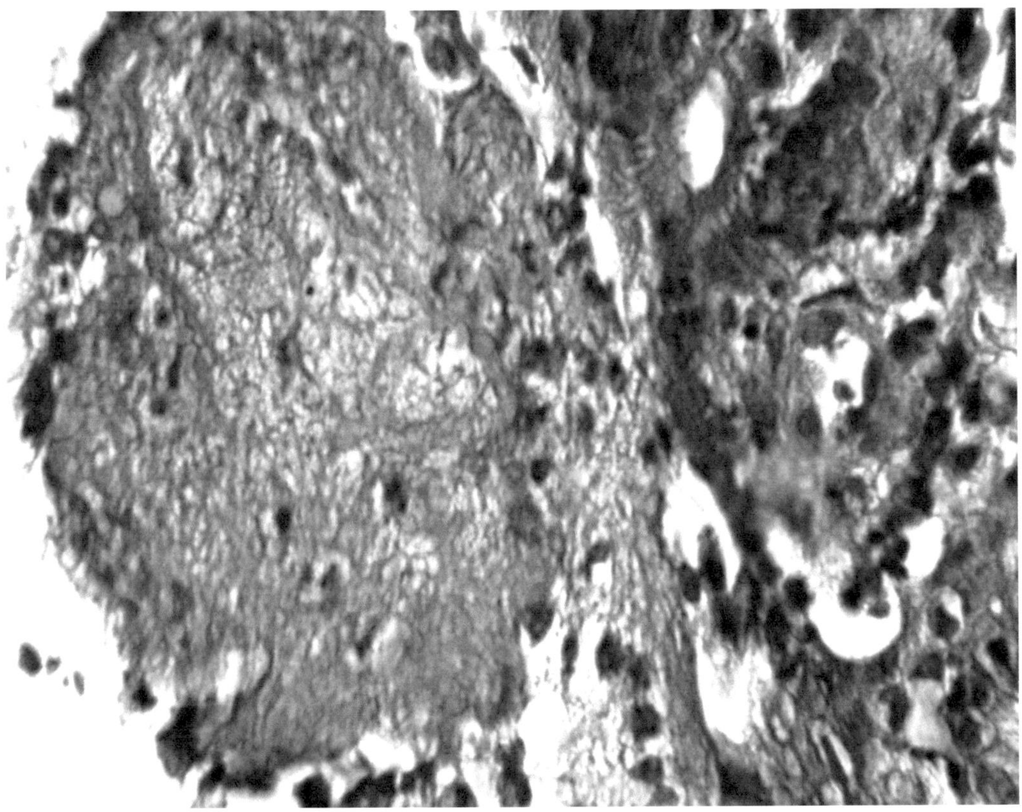

Fig. 8. Erosions of colonic mucosa with fibrinousleucocitary exudate in the surface (HE, 400X) (Dickson-Gonzalez et al., 2009)

Even more, in a recent review of the Cochrane Database Systematic Reviews, tinidazole was found as more effective in reducing clinical failure compared with metronidazole and has fewer associated adverse events. Combination drug therapy was found to be more effective in reducing parasitological failure compared with metronidazole alone. However, these results were based on trials with poor methodological quality so there is uncertainty in these conclusions. Further trials of the efficacy of antiamoebic drugs, with better methodological quality, are recommended.

The addition of broad-spectrum antibiotics to the treatment of acute amebic colitis may be appropriate if perforation is suspected. The possibility of coexisting bacteria causing dysentery must always be considered (Mackey-Lawrence & Petri 2011). Amebic colitis and some of its complications, such as ameboma, generally respond to medical treatment without surgical intervention, but for acute necrotizing colitis with toxic megacolon, partial or complete colectomy may be necessary.

Although not currently a significant problem, is expected that in the future antiparasitic drug resistance can emerge as a threat in the therapeutic management of amebiasis.

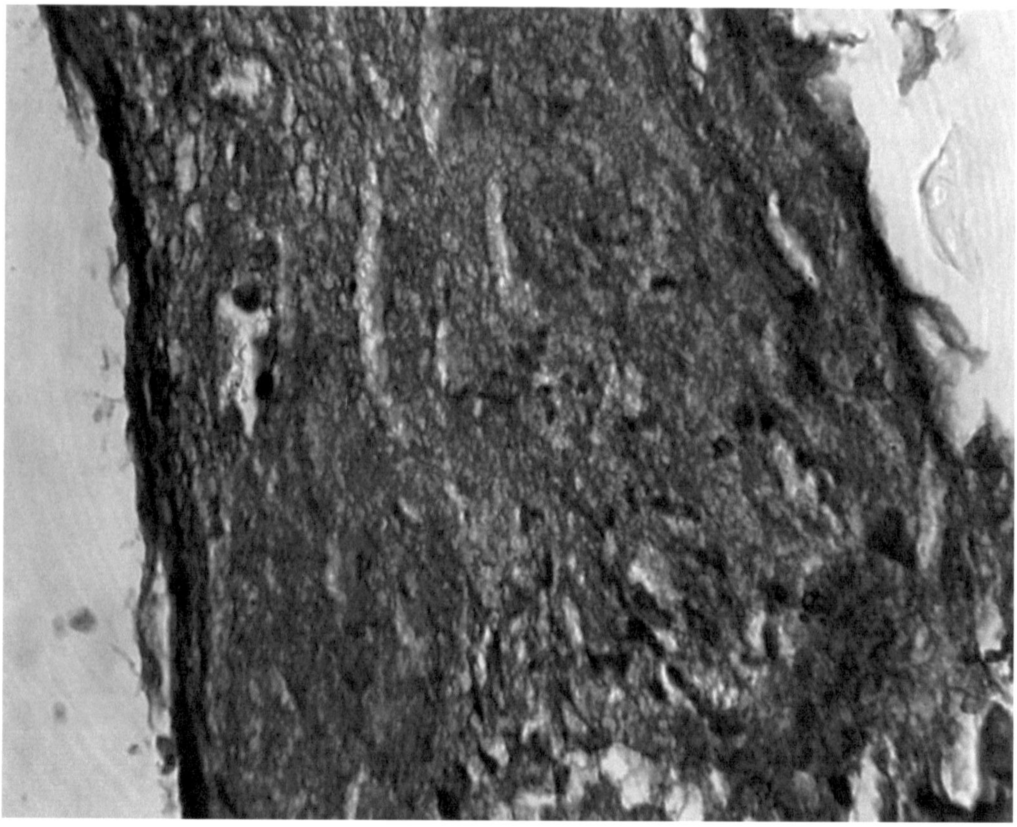

Fig. 9. Necrotic material and fibrinousleucocitary exudate (HE, 200X) (Dickson-Gonzalez et al., 2009)

Recently, the genome of *E. histolytica* has been sequenced, which has widened the scope to study additional virulence factors. *E. histolytica* genome-based approaches have now confirmed the presence of Golgi apparatus-like vesicles and the machinery for glycosylation, thus improving the chances of identifying potential drug targets for chemotherapeutic intervention. Gal-lectin-based vaccines are under development, but additionally, promising vaccine targets such as serine-rich *E. histolytica* protein have yielded encouraging results. Considerable efforts have also been made to skew vaccination responses towards appropriate T-helper cell immunity that could augment the efficacy of vaccine candidates under study. Thus, ongoing efforts mining the information made available with the sequencing of the *E. histolytica* genome will no doubt identify and characterize other important potential vaccine and drug targets and lead to effective immunologic strategies for the control of amebiasis.

Over the past decade, progress in vaccine development has been facilitated by new animal models that allow better testing of potential vaccine candidates and the application of recombinant technology to vaccine design. Oral vaccines and DNA-based vaccines have been successfully tested in animals models for immunogenicity and efficacy.

There has been significant progress on a number of fronts, but there are unanswered questions regarding the effectiveness of immune responses in preventing disease in man and, as yet, no testing of any of these vaccines in humans has been performed. In addition, there are strong economic barriers to developing an amebiasis vaccine and questions about how and where an effective vaccine would be utilized.

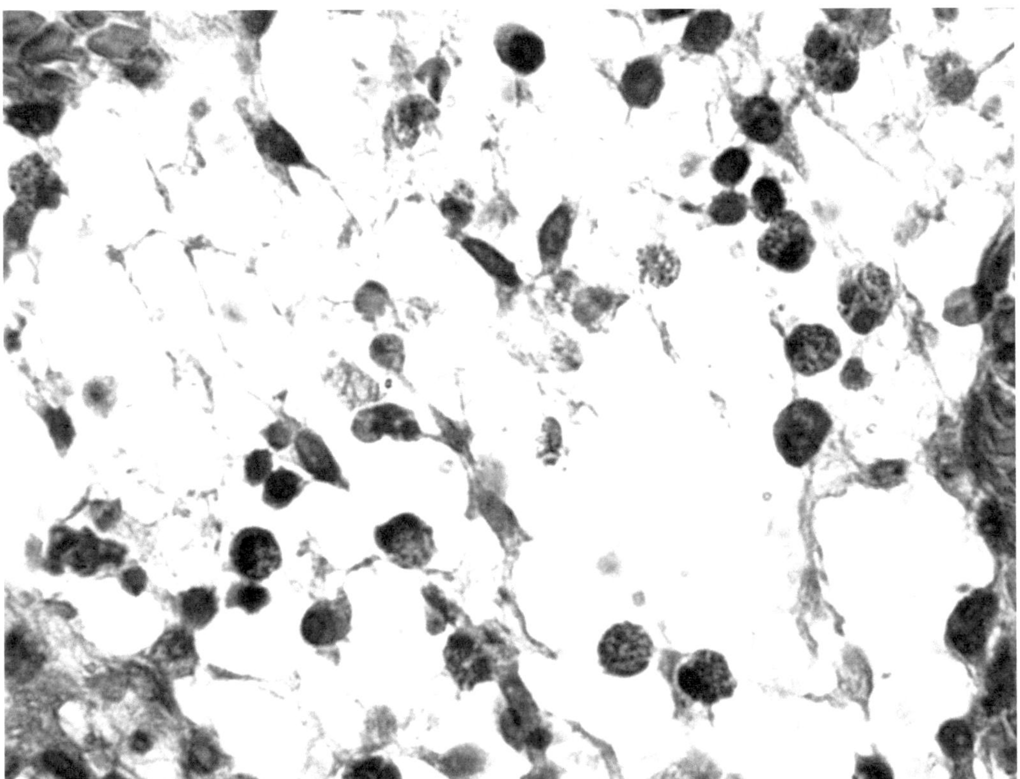

Fig. 10. Abundant eosinophils and edema in the interglandular corion (HE, 1000X) (Dickson-Gonzalez et al., 2009)

7. Conclusions

Amebiasis has been recently suggested as one of the new proposed neglected tropical diseases (NTDs), beyond the original list. Neglected tropical diseases include in order of decreasing prevalence: soil transmitted helminths (these include roundworms such as *Ascaris lumbricoides* which causes ascariasis, whipworm which causes trichuriasis, hookworms which, depending on the species, cause necatoriasis and ancylostomiasis), snail fever (schistosomiasis), lymphatic filariasis, trachoma, kala-azar black fever (and other clinical forms of leishmaniasis), Chagas disease (american trypanosomiasis), leprosy, African sleeping sickness (human African trypanosomiasis), Guinea-worm (dracunculiasis), and Buruli ulcer. The World Health Organization (WHO) list of neglected tropical diseases is including the following additional diseases: cysticercosis, dengue and dengue haemorrhagic fever, echinococcosis, fascioliasis, onchocerciasis, rabies, yaws, podoconiosis and snakebites.

Although its distribution is cosmopolitan, highest burden of amebiasis occurs in developing tropical countries, then, adding the low interest in research and in developing new drugs for its treatment, this pathology would be considered as neglected.

Additionally to these considerations, right now is not just important in endemic countries, but also in and non-endemic ones, due to international migration, which makes now that amebiasis would represents a global phenomenon with a changing geography of its epidemiology.

For all these reasons a high level of suspicion should be established into the medical practice not just in endemic countries in symptomatic and asymptomatic patients with epidemiological risk factors, but also in non-endemic countries in travellers and migrants from endemic countries.

Early diagnosis and prompt treatment is highly important in an adequate resolution of disease and avoidance of extraintestinal pathology. More on, deep research is needed in different clinical and epidemiological settings such as in immunosupressed individuals.

Fortunately recent insights into vaccine development promise potential candidates that would be effectively used in human beings in the next following years or decades, making a significant intervention into reduction of its high burden of morbidity and mortality especially in developing countries.

8. Acknowledgements

We would like to thank S. Dickson-Gonzalez for her review on the manuscript.

9. References

Accolla, R.S. (2006). Host defense mechanisms against pathogens. *Surgical infections,* Vol.7 Suppl 2, pp. S5-7.

Adams, E.B., MacLeod, I.N. (1977). Invasive amebiasis. I. Amebic dysentery and its complications. *Medicine,* Vol.56, pp.315-323.

Adams SA, Robson SC, Gathiram V, et al. (1993). Immunological similarity between the 170 kD amoebic adherence glycoprotein and human beta 2 integrins. *Lancet,* Vol.341, pp.17-19.

Al-Mofleh, I.A., Al-Tuwaijri, A.S., Mahmoud, A.A., Alam, M. (1989). *Entamoeba histolytica* depresses chemiluminescence in stimulated human polymorphonuclear leukocytes. *International journal of immunopharmacology,* Vol.11, No.1, pp. 529-536.

Arbo, A., Hoefsloot, M., Ramirez, A., Ignacio Santos J. (1993) *Entamoeba histolytica* inhibits the respiratory burst of polymorphonuclear leukocytes. *Archivos de investigacion medica* Vol.21, Suppl 1, pp.57-61.

Aristizabal H, Acevedo J, Botero M. (1991). Fulminant amebic colitis. *World journal of surgery,* Vol.15, pp.216-221.

Bercu TE, Petri WA, Behm JW. (2007). Amebic colitis: new insights into pathogenesis and treatment. *Curr Gastroenterol Rep.;* Vol. 9, pp.429-33.

Blessmann, J., Tannich, E. (2002). Treatment of asymptomatic intestinal *Entamoeba histolytica* infection. *N Engl J Med,* Vol.347, No.17, pp.1384.

Burchard GD, Prange G, Mirelman D. (1993) Interaction between trophozoites of *Entamoeba histolytica* and the human intestinal cell line HT-29 in the presence or absence of leukocytes. *Parasitology research;* Vol. 79, pp.140-145.

Cascio A, Bosilkovski M, Rodriguez-Morales AJ, Pappas G. (2011). The socio-ecology of zoonotic infections. *Clin Microbiol Infect;* Vol.17, pp.336-42.

Dickson-Gonzalez SM, de Uribe ML, Rodriguez-Morales AJ (2009). Polymorphonuclear neutrophil infiltration intensity as consequence of *Entamoeba histolytica* density in amebic colitis. *Surg Infect (Larchmt);* Vol. 10, pp.91-7.

Franco-Paredes C, Jacob JT, Hidron A, Rodriguez-Morales AJ, Kuhar D, Caliendo AM. (2010). Transplantation and tropical infectious diseases. *Int J Infect Dis;* Vol. 14, pp.e189-96.

Gonzales ML, Dans LF, Martinez EG. (2009). Antiamoebic drugs for treating amoebic colitis. *Cochrane Database Syst Rev;* Vol. 2, pp.CD006085.

González-Salazar F, Mata-Cárdenas BD, Vargas-Villareal J. (2009). Sensibility of *Entamoeba histolytica* trophozoites to ivermectin. *Medicina (B Aires)*;69(3):318-20.

Guerrant, R.L., Brush, J., Ravdin, J.I., et al. (1981). Interaction between *Entamoeba histolytica* and human polymorphonuclear neutrophils. *The Journal of infectious diseases,* Vol.143, No.2, (March 1981), pp. 83-93.

Hsu YB, Chen FM, Lee PH, et al. (1995). Fulminant amebiasis: a clinical evaluation. *Hepato-gastroenterology;* 42, pp.109-112.

Jhingran A, Padmanabhan PK, Singh S, et al. (2008). Characterization of the *Entamoeba histolytica* Ornithine Decarboxylase-Like Enzyme. *PLoS neglected tropical diseases*;2: , pp.e115.

Kenner BM, Rosen T. Cutaneous amebiasis in a child and review of the literature. *Pediatric dermatology* 2006;23: , pp.231-234.

Lejeune M, Rybicka JM, Chadee K. Recent discoveries in the pathogenesis and immune response toward *Entamoeba histolytica*. *Future Microbiol.* 2009 Feb;4(1):105-18.

Lysy J, Zimmerman J, Sherman Y, et al. Crohn's colitis complicated by superimposed invasive amebic colitis. *The American journal of gastroenterology*. 1991;86: , pp.1063-1065.

Mackey-Lawrence NM, Petri WA Jr. Amoebic dysentery. *Clin Evid (Online)*. 2011 Jan 13;2011. pii: 0918.

Mann BJ, Torian BE, Vedvick TS, Petri WA, Jr. Sequence of a cysteine-rich galactose-specific lectin of *Entamoeba histolytica*. Proceedings of the National Academy of Sciences of the United States of America 1991;88: , pp.3248-3252.

Pudifin DJ, Duursma J, Gathiram V, Jackson TF. Invasive amoebiasis is associated with the development of anti-neutrophil cytoplasmic antibody. Clinical and experimental immunology 1994;97: , pp.48-51.

Rodríguez-Morales AJ, Barbella RA, Case C, Arria M, Ravelo M, Perez H, Urdaneta O, Gervasio G, Rubio N, Maldonado A, Aguilera Y, Viloria A, Blanco JJ, Colina M, Hernández E, Araujo E, Cabaniel G, Benitez J, Rifakis P. Intestinal parasitic infections among pregnant women in Venezuela. *Infect Dis Obstet Gynecol*. 2006;2006:23125.

Salata, R.A., Ahmed, P., Ravdin, J.I. (1989). Chemoattractant activity of *Entamoeba histolytica* for human polymorphonuclear neutrophils. *The Journal of parasitology*, Vol.75, pp. 644-646.

Salata RA, Martinez-Palomo A, Murray HW, et al. Patients treated for amebic liver abscess develop cell-mediated immune responses effective in vitro against *Entamoeba histolytica*. *J Immunol*. 1986;136: , pp.2633-2639.

Salata RA, Ravdin JI. The interaction of human neutrophils and *Entamoeba histolytica* increases cytopathogenicity for liver cell monolayers. The Journal of infectious diseases 1986;154: , pp.19-26.

Seydel KB, Li E, Swanson PE, Stanley SL, Jr. Human intestinal epithelial cells produce proinflammatory cytokines in response to infection in a SCID mouse-human intestinal xenograft model of amebiasis. Infection and immunity 1997;65: , pp.1631-1639.

Stanley, S.L., Jr. (2003) Amoebiasis. *Lancet*, Vol.361, No.1, (May 2003), pp. 1025-1034.

Stanley SL Jr. Vaccines for amoebiasis: barriers and opportunities. Parasitology. 2006;133 Suppl:S81-6.

Stauffer, W., Ravdin. J.I. (2003). *Entamoeba histolytica*: an update. *Current Opinion In Infectious Diseases*, Vol.16, No.1, pp. 479-485.

Tanyuksel M, Petri WA, Jr. Laboratory diagnosis of amebiasis. Clinical microbiology reviews 2003;16: , pp.713-729.

Tsutsumi V, Mena-Lopez R, Anaya-Velazquez F, Martinez-Palomo A. Cellular bases of experimental amebic liver abscess formation. The American journal of pathology 1984;117: , pp.81-91.

Vega-Robledo GB, Leandro E, Silva R, et al. Effect of zinc-treated *Entamoeba histolytica* on the human polymorphonuclear respiratory burst. Archives of medical research 2005;36: , pp.75-79.

Yu Y, Chadee K. *Entamoeba histolytica* stimulates interleukin 8 from human colonic epithelial cells without parasite-enterocyte contact. Gastroenterology 1997;112: , pp.1536-1547.

4

Clostridium difficile-Associated Colitis: Role of the Immune Response and Approach to Treatment

Katie Solomon[1] and Lorraine Kyne[2,3]
[1]*School of Public Health, Physiotherapy and Population Science, University College Dublin,*
[2]*School of Medicine and Health Sciences, University College Dublin,*
[3]*Mater Misericordiae University Hospital, Dublin, Ireland*

1. Introduction

Clostridium difficile infection (CDI) is the most common infectious cause of healthcare-acquired diarrhoea. Approximately 15%–25% of all cases of antibiotic-associated colitis (AAC) are caused by *C. difficile* and this likelihood increases with the severity of disease, reaching 95%–100% among patients with documented antibiotic-associated pseudomembraneous colitis (PMC) (Bartlett, 1994). Since the initial report of *C. difficile* as the cause of AAC in 1978 (Larson *et al.*, 1978), subsequent work has provided important information regarding risk factors, diagnosis and effective therapy. More recently, significant challenges have arisen due to increases in frequency and severity of disease, limitations of standard therapy and propensity for recurrence of infection. There has been an unanticipated increase in morbidity and mortality attributed to this disease, linked in part to the emergence of antimicrobial-resistance and the epidemic bacterial strain, BI/NAP-1/ribotype 027 leading to a resurgence of CDI as a major cause of hospital-acquired infection.

2. Clinical presentation of CDI

Infection with *C. difficile* can result in clinical manifestations ranging from asymptomatic carriage to fulminant colitis and death (Bartlett, 1994). The pathogenesis of symptomatic CDI is characterised by an acute intestinal inflammatory response, prominent neutrophil infiltration and associated tissue injury (Savidge *et al.*, 2003). Features of severe CDI include pseudomembranes visible on endoscopy, abdominal cramps, fever, marked increase in white cell count, rise in serum creatinine level and hypoalbuminemia (Cloud *et al.*, 2009; Pepin *et al.*, 2009). Systemic symptoms may be absent in mild disease but are common in moderate or severe disease. Accurate diagnosis early in the disease course is important for the successful management of CDI.

2.2 Elevated white cell count and hypoalbuminemia

The increase in white cell count associated with CDI is mainly a result of a marked increase in peripheral blood neutrophils. The intense intestinal inflammatory response in severe CDI may also result in fever, abdominal pain, thickening of the colon and paralytic ileus that can evolve into toxic megacolon. Profuse watery diarrhoea may also be associated with nausea, vomiting, dehydration or lethargy, in addition to severe hypoalbuminemia (serum albumin <35g/L) as a result of protein losing enteropathy (Sunenshine & McDonald, 2006).

2.1 Pseudomembraneous colitis

Pseudomembranes are characterised as discrete plaques of yellow-white exudate <10mm diameter separated by normal or mildly hyperaemic mucosa usually restricted to the colon, with occasional cases involving the small intestine (Figure 1A &B). These may progress to form a membraneous exudate covering a large degree of the colonic epithelial surface. Ulceration into the sub-mucosa can result in severe cases. The lesions are characterised histologically as discrete regions of necrotic surface epithelium with accumulation of fibrin, mucous and cell debris (Pothoulakis, 1996). Polymorphonuclear cells and neutrophils infiltrate into the lesion exudate and the underlying lamina propria from the systemic bloodstream (Kelly *et al.*, 1994a). Later stage lesions involve the superficial mucosa and crypts and further infiltration of polymorphonuclear cells and eosinophils. Lesions coalesce to create plaques covering larger areas of the mucosa. Rare complications involve deep necrosis and ulceration of the colon sub-mucosa which can lead to perforation, septicaemia and death.

A B

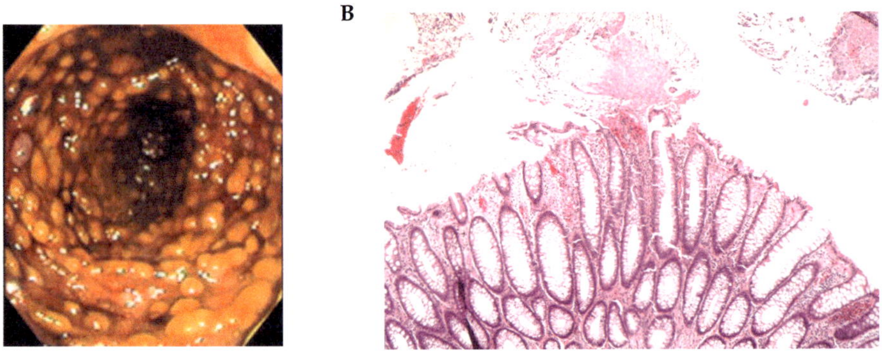

Fig. 1. (A) Pseudomembraneous colitis as confirmed by sigmoidoscopy. Discrete yellow plaques indicate the ulcerated lesions. (B) Histopathological features of pseudomembraneous colitis include loss of crypt structure, infiltration of polymorphonuclear cells and surface accumulation of fibrin, mucous and necrotic cell debris.

3. Risk factors

The major risk factors for CDI are increasing age, prolonged hospital stay and recent or current antimicrobial use. The most important risk factor is alteration of bowel microflora and subsequent loss of colonisation resistance associated with antimicrobial usage within the previous 2-3 months prior to infection (Bignardi, 1998; Dial *et al.*, 2008). There are particular classes of antimicrobials that are associated with the highest risk of *C. difficile* acquisition, including clindamycin, cephalosporins and β-lactam antimicrobials and more recently fluoroquinolones (Owens *et al.*, 2008). Recent outbreaks involving a particular epidemic strain of *C. difficile* have been predominantly associated with fluoroquinolone usage (Loo *et al.*, 2005; Pepin *et al.*, 2005). The risk of developing CDI increases with the use of multiple antibiotics and prolonged duration of therapy.

In addition to these traditional risk factors, other factors associated with CDI include; underlying comorbidities, including inflammatory bowel disease (IBD), gastrointestinal procedures and exposure to an environment contaminated with toxigenic *C. difficile*, usually via hospitalisation (Johnson & Gerding, 1998). Proton pump inhibitors have been associated with CDI risk but their use is often a marker of the severity of underlying disease, which is in itself a strong risk factor for CDI (Kyne *et al.*, 2000; Kyne *et al.*, 2001).

The host immune status is also important in determining the outcome of colonisation with *C. difficile*. Immuno-compromised patients are at increased risk for CDI (Yolken *et al.*, 1982) as are patients with a poor immune response to *C. difficile* toxins (Kyne *et al.*, 2000; Mulligan *et al.*, 1993). The role of protective host immunity in determining progression and severity of CDI, specifically the inability to mount an adequate colonic IgA and or serum IgG response to *C. difficile* toxins will be discussed further.

The incidence of CDI acquired in the community appears to be increasing. Cases have also been reported in which there has been no recorded exposure to antibiotics or recent hospitalisation. Similarly an increasing number of cases of CDI are occurring in lower age groups and children. This may be due to the emergence of a new strain that is more commonly associated with animal and non-hospital sources of infection, but this has yet to be fully substantiated (Goorhuis *et al.*, 2008).

4. Microbial virulence factors

4.1 Toxins A and B

The major virulence factors of toxigenic *Clostridium difficile* are two large protein toxins A (TcdA) and B (TcdB) that have both been shown to be responsible for the profound intestinal inflammatory response seen in CDI (Kuehne *et al.*, 2010; Thelestam & Chaves-Olarte, 2000). Toxins A and B are very similar in structure, with three functional domains: a receptor binding domain, a translocation domain and a catalytic domain involved in binding to the host cell, entry into the cytoplasm and inactivation of Rho GTPases respectively (von Eichel-Streiber *et al.*, 1996).

Most disease-causing *C. difficile* strains produce both toxins, encoded by the pathogenicity locus (PaLoc) (Braun *et al.*, 1996; Rupnik *et al.*, 2005). Genetic variations in the toxin genes leads to strains of different 'toxinotypes'(Rupnik, 2008). Most variation across toxinotypes is seen in the binding domain of toxin A, which can lead to so called TcdA-TcdB+ strains which have been found to demonstrate comparable cytotoxicity to normal toxin-producing strains and have been involved in clinical outbreaks (Drudy *et al.*, 2007). Up to 31 different toxinotypes have been identified so far (Rupnik, Feb 2011), highlighting the possibility of a wide variety of *C. difficile* toxin protein structures and cytotoxic activities. Infection with non-toxigenic strains that do not possess the pathogenicity locus can occur and is usually thought to result in asymptomatic colonisation.

The PaLoc also contains genes involved in regulation of transcription of the toxins (Braun *et al.*, 1996; Rupnik *et al.*, 2005). The epidemic strain BI/NAP-1/ribotype 027 has been shown to contain an 18bp deletion in one of these regulatory genes, *tcdC,* which results in increased toxin production (Dupuy *et al.*, 2008). This is thought to contribute to the virulence of this strain and its involvement in recent epidemics (Warny *et al.*, 2005).

Toxins A and B mediate their cytopathic effect by disrupting the cytoskeleton of intestinal epithelial cells and causing tight junctions to open, resulting in loss of integrity of the protective monolayer (Figure 2).

Once the intestinal epithelium is breached, the toxins are able to access the underlying lamina propria and come into contact with resident macrophages and circulating peripheral blood mononuclear cells (Pothoulakis, 2000; Thelestam & Chaves-Olarte, 2000).

C. difficile toxins are also capable of inducing the release of several classes of cytokines and neuroimmune pro-inflammatory mediators such as interleukin-8 (Il-8) and tumour necrosis factor-α (TNF- α) from intestinal epithelial cells, macrophages and mast cells. These recruit circulating inflammatory cells such as neutrophils into the site of infection and perpetuate the inflammation and fluid secretion associated with CDI (Pothoulakis, 2000).

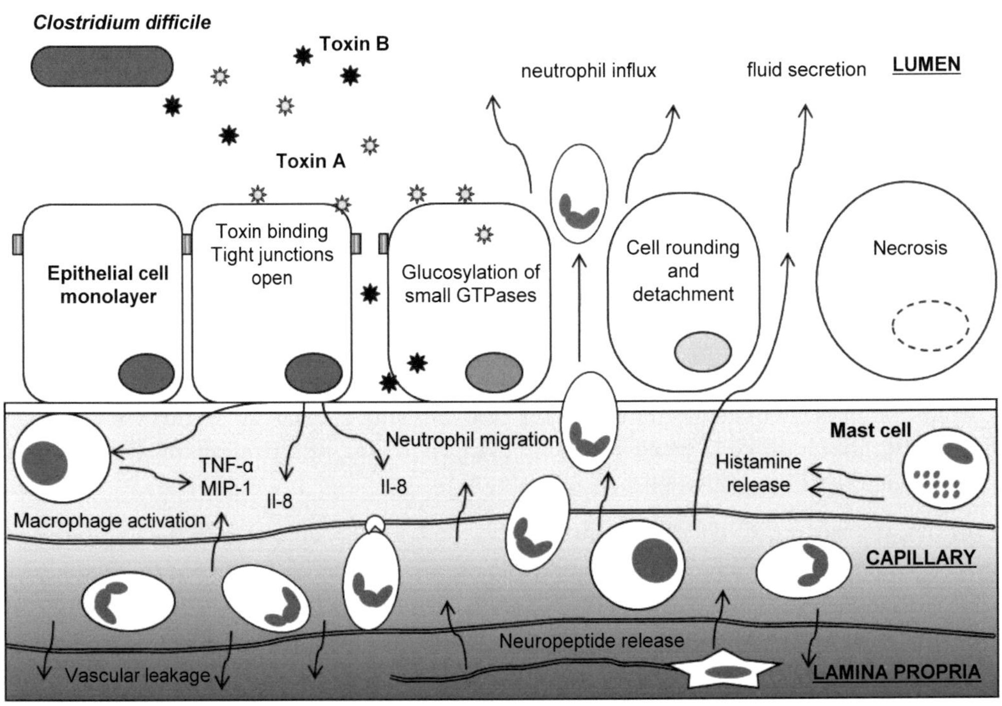

Fig. 2. The role of *C. difficile* toxins A and B in mediating the host inflammatory response

In addition to the indirect effect of the toxins on cells of the immune system, *C. difficile* toxin A has also been shown to directly bind to peripheral blood mononuclear cells, most notably monocytes and induce cell death by apoptosis (Modi *et al.*, 2011; Solomon *et al.*, 2005). This highlights the essential role that toxins play in initiating and prolonging bacterial infection by inactivating key elements of the host protective immune response.

4.2 Binary toxin

In addition to toxins A and B, a further toxigenic component, binary toxin, is expressed in a subset of toxigenic *C. difficile* strains, most notably the epidemic BI/NAP-1/ribotype 027 strain (Rupnik, 2008; Stubbs *et al.*, 2000). Although possessing an ADP-ribosylation function and cytotoxic activity against mammalian cell lines, the role of binary toxin in disease is unclear (Geric *et al.*, 2006).

4.3 Surface layer proteins

In addition to the major secreted toxins, the vegetative *C. difficile* bacterium produces other potential virulence factors. Surface layer proteins are considered to play a vital role in colonisation of the gut and bacterial adherence to the mucosa. They are also important immunogens and can induce the host inflammatory and antibody response (Ausiello *et al.*, 2006; Calabi *et al.*, 2002; Drudy *et al.*, 2004; Pechine *et al.*, 2005). As seen with the toxin proteins, surface layer proteins can be highly variable, particularly surface layer protein A (SlpA) resulting in varying degrees of bacterial adherence ability.

4.4 Flagella

Flagella are also major bacterial virulence factors that enable chemotaxis and penetration of the mucus layer and direct adherence of the bacterium to the epithelial cell surface for localised secretion of toxins. Pathogenic *C. difficile* strains display a range of flagella proteins and subsequent adhesion capabilities (Tasteyre *et al.*, 2001). The immunogenic potential of flagellin is widely appreciated and specific Toll-like receptors (TLRs) are present on the epithelial cell surface to detect flagellin as part of the host cell sensing of pathogens.

5. Host factors that influence outcome of infection

The host's ability to respond to *C. difficile* virulence factors plays a major role in determining the outcome of colonisation with this organism. Infection with the same toxigenic strain can result in a variety of outcomes, including asymptomatic carriage through to symptomatic or severe disease. Certain intrinsic host features, including toxin receptor density (Eglow *et al.*, 1992) and presence or absence of barrier flora (Borriello, 1990) are important in the initial stages of colonisation, however early host detection of infection and initiation of an appropriate immune response likely plays a role in preventing prolonged and severe disease and in providing protection from recurrence of infection.

5.1 Host protective microflora

The most important risk factor for the development of CDI is antimicrobial use, which leads to alteration of the commensal gut microflora and loss of colonisation resistance, enabling unrestricted growth of toxigenic *C. difficile.* It is proposed that the healthy gut microflora affords resistance by physical inhibition of pathogen adhesion to the mucosa, blocking production of microbial toxins, competition for nutrients and stimulation and development of the mucosal immune system (Mazmanian *et al.*, 2005; Weinstein & Cebra, 1991).

Recent metagenomic studies have provided a detailed insight into the various bacterial species groups involved in host protection against *C. difficile* and have identified an important role for members of the *Bifidobacterium* and *Bacteroides* species (Hopkins & Macfarlane, 2002; Hopkins *et al.*, 2002) Bacterial species diversity was markedly lower in CDI patients and consisted of a higher number of facultative anaerobes than in healthy controls (Hopkins & Macfarlane, 2002).

Healthy resident faecal microflora have been shown to directly suppress the growth of *C. difficile* introduced *in vivo*, possibly through production of volatile fatty acids and bacterial metabolic by-products (Rolfe, 1984). This may explain how approximately 5% of asymptomatic healthy adults carry low concentrations of *C. difficile* in their colon. They have been shown *in vitro* to be held in check by normal gut flora (Fekety & Shah, 1993). Non-toxigenic strains of *C. difficile* may colonise the gut and prevent infection with toxigenic strains (Borriello & Barclay, 1985; Sambol *et al.*, 2002) and even asymptomatic colonisation with toxigenic strains has been associated with a decreased risk of CDI (Shim *et al.*, 1998).

The precise mechanisms by which asymptomatic colonisation is able to protect against CDI have yet to be defined, however continuous immunological challenge with *C. difficile* bacterial peptides and/or low levels of toxins may prime the immune system to act efficiently in response to a subsequent infection (Viscidi *et al.*, 1983). The commensal microflora has also been shown to profoundly influence the development of the humoral components of the gut immune system, influencing IgA production by B cells (Weinstein & Cebra, 1991).

5.2 The innate immune response

0 - 12 hours post-infection

C. difficile toxins act quickly to breach the protective mucosal barrier in order to release nutrients for bacterial growth in to the lumen. The host needs to respond rapidly to circumvent further cellular damage and possible dissemination of toxins into the sub-mucosa and bloodstream. The early host pro-inflammatory response or inducible innate immune response is stimulated initially by the epithelial cells, the first and major cell type encountered by microorganisms in the mucosa.

The intestinal epithelium has developed a wide array of protective mechanisms to prevent bacterial adherence and maintain the integrity of the monolayer, including mucous secretion and tight junctions. Epithelial cells are also able to sense pathogen-associated molecules such as LPS, peptidoglycan and flagellin via specific cell surface TLR receptors. Epithelial cells intoxicated by *C. difficile* release pro-inflammatory mediators including Interleukin-8 (Il-8) and macrophage inflammatory protein-2 (MIP-2) into the underlying lamina propria (Flegel *et al.*, 1991; Mahida *et al.*, 1998).

The sub-mucosal macrophages, monocytes and dendritic cells then disseminate the inflammatory cascade, via the further release of pro-inflammatory cytokines and neuropeptides that recruit peripheral blood cells to the site of infection (Pothoulakis, 1996).

The combined action of cytokines and histamine increases permeability of the vascular endothelium causing fluid leakage and the symptomatic profuse watery diarrhoea associated with *C. difficile* infection. The expression of specific monocyte and leucocyte-adhesion molecules, including CD18 integrins and selectins are upregulated and enable migration of leukocytes and monocytes towards the site of cytokine release (Kelly *et al.*, 1994a). Phagocytosis and digestion of the bacteria with lysozyme, collagenase and peroxidise promotes clearance of the infection, but contributes to the extensive cellular necrosis characterised by the pseudomembraneous plaques.

5.3 The adaptive immune response

1 - 12 days post infection

The importance of the adaptive immune response in influencing the outcome of *C. difficile* colonisation has been appreciated for many years (Aronsson *et al.*, 1985; Johnson *et al.*, 1992; Warny *et al.*, 1994), however the contributions that individual immunoglobulin classes play in protection and prevention have taken longer to elucidate.

An initial challenge with *C. difficile* (irrespective whether this is associated with symptoms or not) will stimulate the maturation and multiplication of naive B-cells, generating antibody-producing plasma cells and specific memory B-cells. The process of immunoglobulin class switching is then induced by specific cytokines, to ensure that the full range of immunoglobulin classes are generated in response to specific *C. difficile* antigens. It is likely that the initial immune challenge occurs in infancy, as approximately 60% of healthy non-colonised or asymptomatic adults have detectable serum IgG and IgA antibodies to *C. diffiicle* toxins (Kelly *et al.*, 1992; Sanchez-Hurtado *et al.*, 2008; Viscidi *et al.*, 1983).

Certain immunoglobulin classes are more important than others in mediating immunity to *C. difficile*. IgA is mainly associated with the gut mucosa and prevention of pathogen colonisation, whereas IgM is released first in infection, followed by IgG, which provides the major protection against pathogens (Underdown & Schiff, 1986). A selective reduction in mucosal IgA has been shown to be associated with severe CDI and reduction in colonic IgA producing cells may predispose to recurrence of infection (Johal *et al.*, 2004).

Serum anti-toxin antibody levels have been found to play an important role in determining the outcome of colonisation and protection against CDI recurrence. Patients who are asymptomatically colonised with *C. difficile* have higher serum anti-toxin A IgG levels than colonised patients who develop diarrhoea (Kyne *et al.*, 2000). This suggests that high anti-toxin A IgG levels at the time of colonistion protect against CDI.

Once colonisation has progressed to CDI, serum IgM and IgG antibody responses to *C. difficile* toxins A, B and non-toxin antigens have been shown to be higher in patients who experience a single episode of CDI compared to patients with recurrent CDI (Kyne *et al.*, 2001). The importance of varying antibody levels during the course of infection was also highlighted, as early IgM responses and later IgG responses (day 3 and day 12 post onset of diarrhoea respectively) were significantly higher in those patients who did not experience recurrence of CDI (Kyne *et al.*, 2001). Deficiency in certain subclasses of IgG (IgG2 and IgG3) has also been found to be related to recurrence of disease (Katchar *et al.*, 2007). A high natural anti-toxin antibody response does not always however protect from symptomatic CDI. Patients who are critically ill are less likely to be protected than those who are less severely ill, despite similar antibody levels (Kyne *et al.*, 2000). This suggests that other host factors are also important in immune protection and should be considered when predicting outcome of colonisation on host immune status alone.

Immunity to *C. difficile* surface layer proteins (SLP's) would be expected to provide important protection during bacterial colonisation and prevention of symptomatic CDI. IgM, IgA and IgG antibody levels to SLP's were shown to be similar in control patients, asymptomatic carriers and CDI patients, however a lower anti-SLP IgM response was observed in patients with recurrent CDI compared to patients with a single episode of CDI (Drudy *et al.*, 2004). A separate study showed that anti-SLP IgG levels in patients with CDI and asymptomatic carriers were higher compared to levels in control patients without CDI (Sanchez-Hurtado *et al.*, 2008).

C. difficile bacterial flagellar proteins FliC and FliD, and the other surface-associated proteins expressed during the course of infection, have also been shown to be immunogenic. Antibodies against these proteins may be detected after CDI diagnosis and for at least 2 weeks following diagnosis (Pechine *et al.*, 2005).

5.4 Genetic predisposition to infection: Il-8 promoter mutations

Mucosal Il-8 and neutrophil recruitment have been shown to be essential for the pathogenesis of CDI and subsequent amplification of the acute inflammatory response. In particular, the neutrophil response to *C difficile* toxins is likely to play a role in determining the severity of CDI.

C. difficile toxins induce monocytes and epithelial cells to produce Il-8, by increasing binding of nuclear factors to the Il-8 promoter and up-regulating transcription of the Il-8 gene (Linevsky *et al.*, 1997). Some patients may have a genetic pre-disposition to severe CDI due to a single nucleotide polymorphism (SNP) in the Il-8 gene promoter. The presence of an AA (rather than AT or TT) genotype at position −251 has been shown to be associated with increased susceptibility to *C. difficile* toxins and increased fecal Il-8 levels (Jiang *et al.*, 2006; Jiang *et al.*, 2007). The Il-8 promoter AA genotype SNP is also associated with the lack of a protective adaptive antitoxin A antibody response in hospital patients with CDI (Jiang *et al.*, 2006; Jiang *et al.*, 2007).

6. Treatment strategies for CDI

6.1 Antimicrobial therapy

Non-severe CDI can be treated initially with metronidazole for 10-14 days (ASHP, 1998). For severe disease, vancomycin treatment for 10 -14 days is suggested. Reliance on antimicrobial agents for treatment of *C. difficile* infection would be expected to further damage the host microflora, increasing the risk of recurrence. Recurrence can occur in up to 25% of cases (Kelly *et al.*, 1994b) and may be due to persistence of initial infection after treatment or re-infection. Treatment for recurrences may follow vancomycin administration in a pulsed regimen (Mc Farland *et al.*, 2002) that allows the germination of spores in between antimicrobial administration to improve efficacy. Other antibiotics, nitazoxanide, teicoplanin and most recently fidaxomicin have been shown to be as effective as vancomycin treatment and have been indicated as possible alternative therapies (de Lalla *et al.*, 1992 ; Louie *et al.*; Musher *et al.*, 2009).

Non-antimicrobial approaches to management of CDI and in preventing colonisation, such as immune-mediated therapy would limit the effect on the gut microflora, lessening the risk of replapse.

Currently available antimicrobial and non-antimicrobial therapies in use for management of CDI and those under development are outlined in Table 1.

	Currently used	Under development
Antimicrobial agents	Metronidazole Vancomycin Nitazoxanide Teicoplanin Fidaxomicin	Ramplanin
Non-antimicrobial agents		
Toxin neutralising agents	Cholestyramine	Bovine whey protein 'Mucomilk' Tolevamer
Biotherapeutic agents	*Saccharomyces boulardii* Fecal transplants	Non-toxigenic *C. difficile*
Immune-mediated agents	Intravenous immunoglobulin (IVIG)	Human monoclonal antibodies (HuMabs) Toxoid vaccines (Toxins A & B) Active vaccines (SLP, flagella antigens)

Table 1. Treatment strategies for the management of CDI

7. Immune-mediated therapy

An effective antibody response to *C. difficile* toxins and non-toxin antigens is important in influencing the outcome of colonisation and symptomatic CDI and provides the basis for the development of antibody-mediated therapeutics and vaccines. An overview of immunisation strategies in CDI treatment and prevention has been examined in various studies and is reviewed below and illustrated in Figure 3.

7.1 Passive immunisation therapy

Passive immunotherapy, involving the direct transfer of antibodies has been studied in both humans and animals and has mainly focused on antibodies against *C. difficile* toxins A and B

7.1.1 Animal studies

Oral and parenteral administration of bovine anti-toxoid immunoglobulin concentrate (BIC) has been shown to prevent diarrhoea and death in both the hamster and mouse models of CDI (Kelly *et al.*, 1996; Lyerly *et al.*, 1991). Similarly, hen IgY antibodies to recombinant peptides of both toxins A an B have also been shown to prevent diarrhoea or death when administered orally to hamsters (Kink & Williams, 1998).

Parenteral immunisation with monoclonal antibodies against the binding region of toxin A was able to protect gnotobiotic mice from diarrhoea and death following toxigenic *C. difficile* challenge (Corthier *et al.*, 1991). The best protection against CDI and recurrence is however afforded by combination therapy with neutralising antibodies against both toxins A and B. Human monoclonal antibodies (HuMabs) have been developed after immunisation of human immunoglobulin gene transgenic mice with inactivated toxins A and B (Babcock *et al.*, 2006). Intraperitoneal administration of anti toxin A and B HuMabs protected hamsters from mortality and recurrence of CDI.

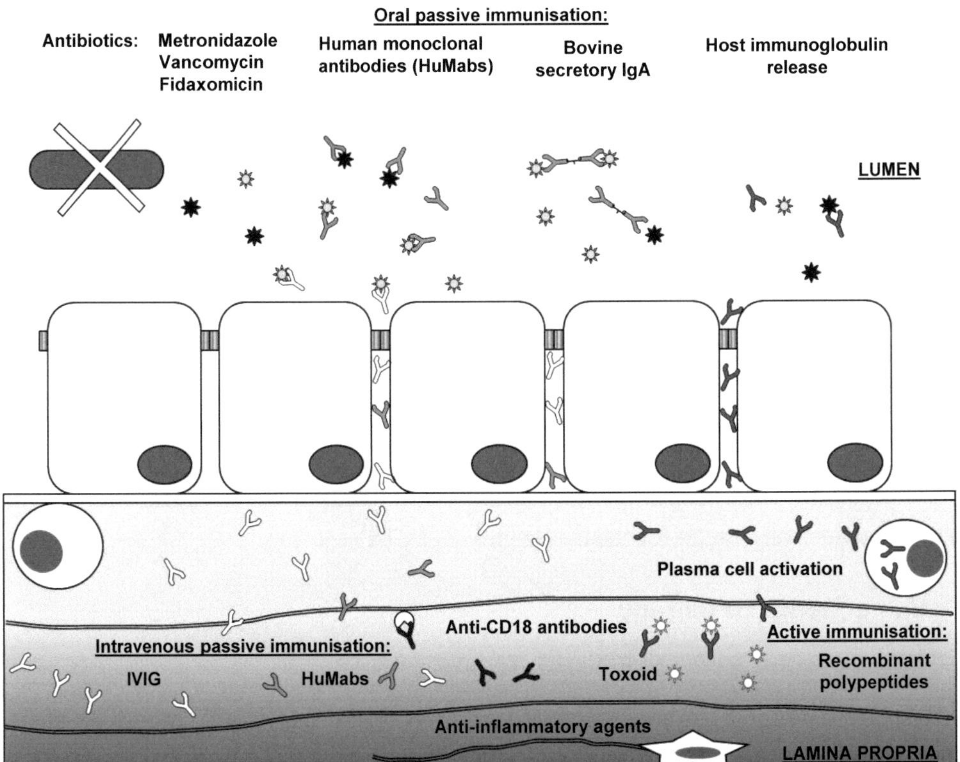

Fig. 3. An overview of immunisation, both active and passive and vaccination against *C. difficile.*

7.1.2 Human studies

Initial studies examining the efficacy of oral administration of bovine immunoglobulin (BIC) in preventing or treating human CDI were promising, but have not progressed further (Kelly *et al.*, 1996; Warny *et al.*, 1999). Bovine anti-*C. difficile* IgA purified from the milk of immunised cows (Mucomilk) was also found to be highly effective at reducing recurrent human CDI, but studies were also not continued further (Mattila *et al.*, 2008; van Dissel *et al.*, 2005).

Intravenous immunisation with pooled anti-toxin A and B IgG immunoglobulin (IVIG) has been the most widely studied mode of passive immunotherapy in humans (Abougergi *et al.*, 2010; O'Horo & Safdar, 2009; Wilcox, 2004). Administration of IVIG to children with low antitoxin antibody levels and relapsing CDI resulted in an increase in antibody levels and subsequent resolution of CDI (Leung *et al.*, 1991). IVIG has also been used for the treatment of severe or refractory CDI with varying success. There is a lack of consensus regarding the optimal dose (150 - 400mg/kg) and dosing regimen (1-3 doses) of IVIG. The lack of randomised controlled clinical trials for IVIG and an association with increased mortality when administered to critically ill patients with CDI in observational studies has served to limit its attractiveness as a possible therapy (Abougergi *et al.*, 2010).

Passive intravenous immunotherapy with HuMabs against toxins A and B has been shown to be well tolerated and effective in protecting patients from recurrence of CDI (Babcock *et al.*, 2006; Leav *et al.*, 2010; Lowy *et al.*, 2010). When used in symptomatic CDI patients in conjunction with standard antimicrobial therapy, recurrence rates were reduced by 72%, although severity of symptoms was not reduced (Lowy *et al.*, 2010). The circulating HuMabs provided protection from subsequent challenge or recurrence due to a half-life of up to 26 days. A role for HuMabs in reducing symptomatic CDI is less well defined however they may be useful as prophylaxis for patients at high risk of infection or in enabling clearance of persistent infection.

7.2 Active immunisation/vaccination

As soon as the importance of *C. difficile* toxins in initiating symptomatic infection was appreciated, studies into active immunisation with inactivated toxin protein toxoids as a means of protecting from CDI were carried out (Kim *et al.*, 1987; Libby *et al.*, 1982).

7.2.1 Animal studies

Hamsters vaccinated with formalin-inactivated *C. difficile* culture filtrate by combined parenteral and mucosal immunisation were found to be protected from CDI (Torres *et al.*, 1995). Similarly, parenteral administration of a toxoid vaccine to hamsters induced high serum levels of anti-toxin A and B antibodies that mediated immune protection against diarrhoea and death (Giannasca *et al.*, 1999). Anti-toxin antibodies were therefore confirmed as the major mediators of the protective response.

Vaccination of mice via transcutaneous administration of a toxin A toxoid derivative and cholera toxin as an immunoadjuvant also showed good induction of anti-toxin A IgG antibodies (Ghose *et al.*, 2007).

Subsequent studies have focused on the use of recombinant polypeptides from toxin A, thought at the time to be the main toxin mediator of intestinal injury in CDI. Immunisation with recombinant toxin A binding domain polypeptides was shown to partially protect hamsters against CDI, and induced a systemic neutralizing immune response in mice, when administered with an *E. coli* toxin adjuvant (Lyerly *et al.*, 1990; Ward *et al.*, 1999). Oral immunisation with an attenuated *Vibrio cholerae* live vector modified to express a fusion protein of the binding domain of toxin A was also shown to induce effective immunity against toxin A in rabbits (Ryan *et al.*, 1997). A DNA vaccine against the binding domain of toxin A has also been developed for human use. It was shown in a trial to be successfully expressed in host mice cells and induced the production of neutralising antibodies and protected from death (Gardiner *et al.*, 2009).

7.2.2 Human studies

Only one candidate *C. difficile* vaccine has progressed to human trials. A formalin-inactivated toxin A and B toxoid vaccine was safely tolerated in healthy individuals after intramuscular administration and was shown to induce high serum anti-toxin antibody levels (Aboudola *et al.*, 2003; Kotloff *et al.*, 2001). When used to treat patients with recurrent CDI, the vaccine was also successful (Sougioultzis *et al.*, 2005). Phase II clinical trials of a *C. difficile* toxoid vaccine are currently in progress. It is thought that this vaccine would be most cost effective when targeted at those at high-risk of developing CDI and in preventing recurrence thereby reducing the economic burden of *C. difficile* disease (Lee *et al.*, 2010).

7.3 Innate immunity-mediated therapy

The inflammatory response to CDI is mediated in the early stages by the innate immune response, most notably the release of Il-8 from intoxicated epithelial cells and the infiltration of neutrophils from the bloodstream. Pre-treatment of rabbits with monoclonal anti-CD18 antibodies was found to protect from severe inflammation and tissue necrosis, by preventing neutrophils from migrating across the vascular endothelium (Kelly *et al.*, 1994a). *C. difficile* toxins would still be able to cause intestinal epithelial damage in anti-CD18-treated patients via triggering infiltration of other inflammatory cells including monocytes and mast cells via Il-8 release from intoxicated intestinal epithelial cells. Amplification of the inflammatory response by neutrophils however would be greatly reduced. The symptoms of CDI in anti-CD18-treated patients would therefore be expected to be less severe and disease may resolve independently of treatment.

Inflammatory mediators have also been shown to reduce intestinal injury in CDI by blocking signals that perpetuate the inflammatory cascade (Kim *et al.*, 2007; Kokkotou *et al.*, 2009). Their use in conjunction with antibiotics or other therapies may be more effective in the most severe CDI cases.

8. Future strategies for prevention and treatment of CDI

Vaccination strategies currently under trial focus on inducing an immune response to *C. difficile* toxins A and B, however colonisation is the first step in pathogenesis. Other *C. difficile* targets, such as surface layer proteins and flagella antigens that have been developed as vaccine antigens to inhibit colonisation have proven to reduce *C. difficile* colonisation in mice and hamsters, but did not prevent it completely (Brun *et al.*, 2008; Ni Eidhin *et al.*, 2008; Pechine *et al.*, 2007). Widespread vaccination against *C. difficile* would be expected to reduce bacterial carriage and therefore spread of the organism, but may serve to inadvertently reduce other protective members of the *Clostridium* spp. in the gut microflora leading to unanticipated side-effects.

Development of toxoid vaccines against both toxin A and B should also take into account the variety in toxin protein structures exhibited by the 31 toxinotypes currently identified.

All vaccines currently under trial are based on inactivated toxoids from a reference strain of *C. difficile* (Aboudola *et al.*, 2003; Sougioultzis *et al.*, 2005), therefore would in theory only protect immunised patients from a proportion of the possible toxin proteins that would be encountered in infection with multiple strain types. This limited cross-reactivity could be further reduced in vaccines where recombinant polypeptides from the cell-binding domain have been used. This would be most important in recurrent cases, where a small proportion of patients can be infected with a different strain type to their initial infection, rather than re-infection or lack of clearance of their existing colonising strain.

The impact of aging on the efficient functioning of the immune system is also under-investigated with respect to CDI. Older patients are most at risk of developing CDI and therefore are the population most likely to be targeted for vaccination. Due to immune senescence many older patients may not mount an adequate antibody response to vaccination (Burns, 2004).

9. Conclusions

The outcome of *C. difficile* infection, whether it is asymptomatic colonisation or fulminant colitis, is mediated at every stage by the host immune system. The innate immune response plays the foremost role in CDI-induced inflammation and tissue injury, whilst the adaptive immune response mainly mediates protection, either from initial infection or subsequent recurrence. The most effective therapies against *C. difficile* would therefore augment a specific immunoglobulin response whilst suppressing the innate response that triggers neutrophil migration into the mucosa. Vaccine targets developed to protect the at-risk population have shown initial efficacy, however further trials are needed to determine whether they have the widespread cross-reactivity needed to protect patients from all possible strains of *C. difficile*. It also remains to be seen whether the majority of older patients will be able to mount an immune response of a sufficient magnitude to the vaccine, to provide adequate protection.

Until these conditions are met, antimicrobials (metronidazole, vancomycin and the newly FDA-approved Fidaxomicin) remain the mainstay of CDI treatment despite their limitations.

10. References

Aboudola, S., Kotloff, K. L., Kyne, L., Warny, M., Kelly, E. C., Sougioultzis, S., Giannasca, P. J., Monath, T. P. & Kelly, C. P. (2003). *Clostridium difficile* vaccine and serum immunoglobulin G antibody response to toxin A. *Infect Immun* 71, 1608-1610.

Abougergi, M. S., Broor, A., Cui, W. & Jaar, B. G. (2010). Intravenous immunoglobulin for the treatment of severe *Clostridium difficile* colitis: an observational study and review of the literature. *J Hosp Med* 5, E1-9.

Aronsson, B., Granstrom, M., Mollby, R. & Nord, C. E. (1985). Serum antibody response to *Clostridium difficile* toxins in patients with *Clostridium difficile* diarrhoea. *Infection* 13, 97-101.

ASHP (1998). ASHP therapeutic position statement on the preferential use of metronidazole for the treatment of *Clostridium difficile*-associated disease. *Am J Health Syst Pharm* 55, 1407-1411.

Ausiello, C. M., Cerquetti, M., Fedele, G., Spensieri, F., Palazzo, R., Nasso, M., Frezza, S. & Mastrantonio, P. (2006). Surface layer proteins from *Clostridium difficile* induce inflammatory and regulatory cytokines in human monocytes and dendritic cells. *Microbes Infect* 8, 2640-2646.

Babcock, G. J., Broering, T. J., Hernandez, H. J., Mandell, R. B., Donahue, K., Boatright, N., Stack, A. M., Lowy, I., Graziano, R., Molrine, D., Ambrosino, D. M. & Thomas, W. D., Jr. (2006). Human monoclonal antibodies directed against toxins A and B prevent *Clostridium difficile*-induced mortality in hamsters. *Infect Immun* 74, 6339-6347.

Bartlett, J. G. (1994). *Clostridium difficile*: history of its role as an enteric pathogen and the current state of knowledge about the organism. *Clin Infect Dis* 18 Suppl 4, S265-272.

Bignardi, G. E. (1998). Risk factors for *Clostridium difficile* infection. *J Hosp Infect* 40, 1-15.

Borriello, S. P. (1990). The influence of the normal flora on *Clostridium difficile* colonisation of the gut. *Ann Med* 22, 61-67.

Borriello, S. P. & Barclay, F. E. (1985). Protection of hamsters against *Clostridium difficile* ileocaecitis by prior colonisation with non-pathogenic strains. *J Med Microbiol* 19, 339-350.

Braun, V., Hundsberger, T., Leukel, P., Sauerborn, M. & von Eichel-Streiber, C. (1996). Definition of the single integration site of the pathogenicity locus in *Clostridium difficile*. *Gene* 181, 29-38.

Brun, P., Scarpa, M., Grillo, A., Palu, G., Mengoli, C., Zecconi, A., Spigaglia, P., Mastrantonio, P. & Castagliuolo, I. (2008). *Clostridium difficile* TxAC314 and SLP-36kDa enhance the immune response toward a co-administered antigen. *J Med Microbiol* 57, 725-731.

Burns, E. A. (2004). Effects of aging on immune function. *J Nutr Health Aging* 8, 9-18.

Calabi, E., Calabi, F., Phillips, A. D. & Fairweather, N. F. (2002). Binding of *Clostridium difficile* surface layer proteins to gastrointestinal tissues. *Infect Immun* 70, 5770-5778.

Cloud, J., Noddin, L., Pressman, A., Hu, M. & Kelly, C. (2009). *Clostridium difficile* strain NAP-1 is not associated with severe disease in a nonepidemic setting. *Clin Gastroenterol Hepatol* 7, 868-873 e862.

Corthier, G., Muller, M. C., Wilkins, T. D., Lyerly, D. & L'Haridon, R. (1991). Protection against experimental pseudomembranous colitis in gnotobiotic mice by use of monoclonal antibodies against *Clostridium difficile* toxin A. *Infect Immun* 59, 1192-1195.

de Lalla, F., Nicolin, R., Rinaldi, E., Scarpellini, P., Rigoli, R., Manfrin, V. & Tramarin, A. (1992). Prospective study of oral teicoplanin versus oral vancomycin for therapy of pseudomembranous colitis and *Clostridium difficile*-associated diarrhea. *Antimicrob Agents Chemother* 36, 2192-2196.

Dial, S., Kezouh, A., Dascal, A., Barkun, A. & Suissa, S. (2008). Patterns of antibiotic use and risk of hospital admission because of *Clostridium difficile* infection. *CMAJ* 179, 767-772.

Drudy, D., Calabi, E., Kyne, L., Sougioultzis, S., Kelly, E., Fairweather, N. & Kelly, C. P. (2004). Human antibody response to surface layer proteins in *Clostridium difficile* infection. *FEMS Immunol Med Microbiol* 41, 237-242.

Drudy, D., Fanning, S. & Kyne, L. (2007). Toxin A-negative, toxin B-positive *Clostridium difficile*. *Int J Infect Dis* 11, 5-10.

Dupuy, B., Govind, R., Antunes, A. & Matamouros, S. (2008). *Clostridium difficile* toxin synthesis is negatively regulated by TcdC. *J Med Microbiol* 57, 685-689.

Eglow, R., Pothoulakis, C., Itzkowitz, S. & al, e. (1992). Diminished *Clostridium difficile* toxin A sensitivity in newborn rabbit ileum is associated with decreased toxin A receptor. *J Clin Invest* 90, 822-829.

Fekety, R. & Shah, A. B. (1993). Diagnosis and treatment of *Clostridium difficile* colitis. *JAMA* 269, 71-75.

Flegel, W. A., Muller, F., Daubener, W., Fischer, H. G., Hadding, U. & Northoff, H. (1991). Cytokine response by human monocytes to *Clostridium difficile* toxin A and toxin B. *Infect Immun* 59, 3659-3666.

Gardiner, D. F., Rosenberg, T., Zaharatos, J., Franco, D. & Ho, D. D. (2009). A DNA vaccine targeting the receptor-binding domain of *Clostridium difficile* toxin A. *Vaccine* 27, 3598-3604.

Geric, B., Carman, R. J., Rupnik, M., Genheimer, C. W., Sambol, S. P., Lyerly, D. M., Gerding, D. N. & Johnson, S. (2006). Binary toxin-producing, large clostridial toxin-negative *Clostridium difficile* strains are enterotoxic but do not cause disease in hamsters. *J Infect Dis* 193, 1143-1150.

Ghose, C., Kalsy, A., Sheikh, A., Rollenhagen, J., John, M., Young, J., Rollins, S. M., Qadri, F., Calderwood, S. B., Kelly, C. P. & Ryan, E. T. (2007). Transcutaneous immunization with *Clostridium difficile* toxoid A induces systemic and mucosal immune responses and toxin A-neutralizing antibodies in mice. *Infect Immun* 75, 2826-2832.

Giannasca, P. J., Zhang, Z. X., Lei, W. D., Boden, J. A., Giel, M. A., Monath, T. P. & Thomas, W. D., Jr. (1999). Serum antitoxin antibodies mediate systemic and mucosal protection from *Clostridium difficile* disease in hamsters. *Infect Immun* 67, 527-538.

Goorhuis, A., Debast, S. B., van Leengoed, L. A., Harmanus, C., Notermans, D. W., Bergwerff, A. A. & Kuijper, E. J. (2008). *Clostridium difficile* PCR ribotype 078: an emerging strain in humans and in pigs? *J Clin Microbiol* 46, 1157; author reply 1158.

Hopkins, M. J. & Macfarlane, G. T. (2002). Changes in predominant bacterial populations in human faeces with age and with *Clostridium difficile* infection. *J Med Microbiol* 51, 448-454.

Hopkins, M. J., Sharp, R. & Macfarlane, G. T. (2002). Variation in human intestinal microbiota with age. *Dig Liver Dis* 34 Suppl 2, S12-18.

Jiang, Z. D., DuPont, H. L., Garey, K., Price, M., Graham, G., Okhuysen, P., Dao-Tran, T. & LaRocco, M. (2006). A common polymorphism in the interleukin 8 gene promoter is associated with Clostridium difficile diarrhea. *Am J Gastroenterol* 101, 1112-1116.

Jiang, Z. D., Garey, K. W., Price, M., Graham, G., Okhuysen, P., Dao-Tran, T., LaRocco, M. & DuPont, H. L. (2007). Association of interleukin-8 polymorphism and immunoglobulin G anti-toxin A in patients with *Clostridium difficile*-associated diarrhea. *Clin Gastroenterol Hepatol* 5, 964-968.

Johal, S. S., Lambert, C. P., Hammond, J., James, P. D., Borriello, S. P. & Mahida, Y. R. (2004). Colonic IgA producing cells and macrophages are reduced in recurrent and non-recurrent *Clostridium difficile* associated diarrhoea. *J Clin Pathol* 57, 973-979.

Johnson, S. & Gerding, D. N. (1998). *Clostridium difficile*--associated diarrhea. *Clin Infect Dis* 26, 1027-1034; quiz 1035-1026.

Johnson, S., Gerding, D. N. & Janoff, E. N. (1992). Systemic and mucosal antibody responses to toxin A in patients infected with *Clostridium difficile*. *J Infect Dis* 166, 1287-1294.

Katchar, K., Taylor, C. P., Tummala, S., Chen, X., Sheikh, J. & Kelly, C. P. (2007). Association between IgG2 and IgG3 subclass responses to toxin A and recurrent *Clostridium difficile*-associated disease. *Clin Gastroenterol Hepatol* 5, 707-713.

Kelly, C. P., Becker, S., Linevsky, J. K., Joshi, M. A., O'Keane, J. C., Dickey, B. F., LaMont, J. T. & Pothoulakis, C. (1994a). Neutrophil recruitment in *Clostridium difficile* toxin A enteritis in the rabbit. *J Clin Invest* 93, 1257-1265.

Kelly, C. P., Pothoulakis, C. & LaMont, J. T. (1994b). *Clostridium difficile* colitis. *N Engl Jour Med* 330, 257-262.

Kelly, C. P., Pothoulakis, C., Orellana, J. & LaMont, J. T. (1992). Human colonic aspirates containing immunoglobulin A antibody to *Clostridium difficile* toxin A inhibit toxin A-receptor binding. *Gastroenterology* 102, 35-40.

Kelly, C. P., Pothoulakis, C., Vavva, F., Castagliuolo, I., Bostwick, E. F., O'Keane, J. C., Keates, S. & LaMont, J. T. (1996). Anti-*Clostridium difficile* bovine immunoglobulin concentrate inhibits cytotoxicity and enterotoxicity of C. difficile toxins. *Antimicrob Agents Chemother* 40, 373-379.

Kim, H., Rhee, S. H., Pothoulakis, C. & Lamont, J. T. (2007). Inflammation and apoptosis in *Clostridium difficile* enteritis is mediated by PGE2 up-regulation of Fas ligand. *Gastroenterology* 133, 875-886.

Kim, P. H., Iaconis, J. P. & Rolfe, R. D. (1987). Immunization of adult hamsters against *Clostridium difficile*-associated ileocecitis and transfer of protection to infant hamsters. *Infect Immun* 55, 2984-2992.

Kink, J. A. & Williams, J. A. (1998). Antibodies to recombinant *Clostridium difficile* toxins A and B are an effective treatment and prevent relapse of *C. difficile*-associated disease in a hamster model of infection. *Infect Immun* 66, 2018-2025.

Kokkotou, E., Espinoza, D. O., Torres, D., Karagiannides, I., Kosteletos, S., Savidge, T., O'Brien, M. & Pothoulakis, C. (2009). Melanin-concentrating hormone (MCH) modulates *C difficile* toxin A-mediated enteritis in mice. *Gut* 58, 34-40.

Kotloff, K. L., Wasserman, S. S., Losonsky, G. A., Thomas, W., Jr., Nichols, R., Edelman, R., Bridwell, M. & Monath, T. P. (2001). Safety and immunogenicity of increasing doses of a *Clostridium difficile* toxoid vaccine administered to healthy adults. *Infect Immun* 69, 988-995.

Kuehne, S. A., Cartman, S. T., Heap, J. T., Kelly, M. L., Cockayne, A. & Minton, N. P. (2010). The role of toxin A and toxin B in *Clostridium difficile* infection. *Nature* 467, 711-713.

Kyne, L., Warny, M., Qamar, A. & Kelly, C. P. (2000). Asymptomatic carriage of *Clostridium difficile* and serum levels of IgG antibody against toxin A. *N Engl J Med* 342, 390-397.

Kyne, L., Warny, M., Qamar, A. & Kelly, C. P. (2001). Association between antibody response to toxin A and protection against recurrent *Clostridium difficile* diarrhoea. *Lancet* 357, 189-193.

Larson, H. E., Price, A. B., Honour, P. & Borriello, S. P. (1978). *Clostridium difficile* and the aetiology of pseudomembranous colitis. *Lancet* 1, 1063-1066.

Leav, B. A., Blair, B., Leney, M., Knauber, M., Reilly, C., Lowy, I., Gerding, D. N., Kelly, C. P., Katchar, K., Baxter, R., Ambrosino, D. & Molrine, D. (2010). Serum anti-toxin B antibody correlates with protection from recurrent *Clostridium difficile* infection (CDI). *Vaccine* 28, 965-969.

Lee, B. Y., Popovich, M. J., Tian, Y., Bailey, R. R., Ufberg, P. J., Wiringa, A. E. & Muder, R. R. (2010). The potential value of *Clostridium difficile* vaccine: an economic computer simulation model. *Vaccine* 28, 5245-5253.

Leung, D. Y., Kelly, C. P., Boguniewicz, M., Pothoulakis, C., LaMont, J. T. & Flores, A. (1991). Treatment with intravenously administered gamma globulin of chronic relapsing colitis induced by *Clostridium difficile* toxin. *J Pediatr* 118, 633-637.

Libby, J. M., Jortner, B. S. & Wilkins, T. D. (1982). Effects of the two toxins of *Clostridium difficile* in antibiotic-associated cecitis in hamsters. *Infect Immun* 36, 822-829.

Linevsky, J. K., Pothoulakis, C., Keates, S., Warny, M., Keates, A. C., Lamont, J. T. & Kelly, C. P. (1997). IL-8 release and neutrophil activation by *Clostridium difficile* toxin-exposed human monocytes. *Am J Physiol* 273, G1333-1340.

Loo, V. G., Poirier, L., Miller, M. A., Oughton, M., Libman, M. D., Michaud, S., Bourgault, A. M., Nguyen, T., Frenette, C., Kelly, M., Vibien, A., Brassard, P., Fenn, S., Dewar, K., Hudson, T. J., Horn, R., Rene, P., Monczak, Y. & Dascal, A. (2005). A predominantly clonal multi-institutional outbreak of *Clostridium difficile*-associated diarrhea with high morbidity and mortality. *N Engl J Med* 353, 2442-2449.

Louie, T. J., Miller, M. A., Mullane, K. M., Weiss, K., Lentnek, A., Golan, Y., Gorbach, S., Sears, P. & Shue, Y.-K. Fidaxomicin versus Vancomycin for *Clostridium difficile* Infection. *New England Journal of Medicine* 364, 422-431.

Lowy, I., Molrine, D. C., Leav, B. A., Blair, B. M., Baxter, R., Gerding, D. N., Nichol, G., Thomas, W. D., Jr., Leney, M., Sloan, S., Hay, C. A. & Ambrosino, D. M. (2010). Treatment with monoclonal antibodies against *Clostridium difficile* toxins. *N Engl J Med* 362, 197-205.

Lyerly, D. M., Bostwick, E. F., Binion, S. B. & Wilkins, T. D. (1991). Passive immunization of hamsters against disease caused by *Clostridium difficile* by use of bovine immunoglobulin G concentrate. *Infect Immun* 59, 2215-2218.

Lyerly, D. M., Johnson, J. L., Frey, S. M. & Wilkins, T. D. (1990). Vaccination against lethal *Clostridium difficile* enterocolitis with a nontoxic recombinant peptide of toxin A. *Current Microbiology* 21, 29-32.

Mahida, Y. R., Galvin, A., Makh, S., Hyde, S., Sanfilippo, L., Borriello, S. P. & Sewell, H. F. (1998). Effect of *Clostridium difficile* toxin A on human colonic lamina propria cells: Early loss of macrophages followed by T-cell apoptosis. *Infect Immun* 66, 5462-5469.

Mattila, E., Anttila, V. J., Broas, M., Marttila, H., Poukka, P., Kuusisto, K., Pusa, L., Sammalkorpi, K., Dabek, J., Koivurova, O. P., Vahatalo, M., Moilanen, V. & Widenius, T. (2008). A randomized, double-blind study comparing *Clostridium difficile* immune whey and metronidazole for recurrent *Clostridium difficile*-associated diarrhoea: efficacy and safety data of a prematurely interrupted trial. *Scand J Infect Dis* 40, 702-708.

Mazmanian, S. K., Liu, C. H., Tzianabos, A. O. & Kasper, D. L. (2005). An immunomodulatory molecule of symbiotic bacteria directs maturation of the host immune system. *Cell* 122, 107-118.

Mc Farland, L. V., Elmer, G. W. & Surawicz, C. M. (2002). Breaking the cycle: treatment strategies for 163 cases of recurrent *Clostridium difficile* disease. . *Am J Gastroenterol* 97, 1769.

Modi, N., Gulati, N., Solomon, K., Monaghan, T., Robins, A., Sewell, H. F. & Mahida, Y. R. (2011). Differential binding and internalisation of *Clostridium difficile* toxin A by human peripheral blood monocytes, neutrophils and lymphocytes. *Scand J Immunol.*

Mulligan, M. E., Miller, S. D., McFarland, L. V., Fung, H. C. & Kwok, R. Y. (1993). Elevated levels of serum immunoglobulins in asymptomatic carriers of *Clostridium difficile. Clin Infect Dis* 16 Suppl 4, S239-244.

Musher, D. M., Logan, N., Bressler, A. M., Johnson, D. P. & Rossignol, J.-F. o. (2009). Nitazoxanide versus Vancomycin in *Clostridium difficile* Infection: A Randomized, Double-Blind Study. *Clinical Infectious Diseases* 48, e41-e46.

Ni Eidhin, D. B., O'Brien, J. B., McCabe, M. S., Athie-Morales, V. & Kelleher, D. P. (2008). Active immunization of hamsters against *Clostridium difficile* infection using surface-layer protein. *FEMS Immunol Med Microbiol* 52, 207-218.

O'Horo, J. & Safdar, N. (2009). The role of immunoglobulin for the treatment of *Clostridium difficile* infection: a systematic review. *Int J Infect Dis* 13, 663-667.

Owens, R. C., Jr., Donskey, C. J., Gaynes, R. P., Loo, V. G. & Muto, C. A. (2008). Antimicrobial-associated risk factors for *Clostridium difficile* infection. *Clin Infect Dis* 46 Suppl 1, S19-31.

Pechine, S., Janoir, C., Boureau, H., Gleizes, A., Tsapis, N., Hoys, S., Fattal, E. & Collignon, A. (2007). Diminished intestinal colonization by *Clostridium difficile* and immune response in mice after mucosal immunization with surface proteins of *Clostridium difficile. Vaccine* 25, 3946-3954.

Pechine, S., Janoir, C. & Collignon, A. (2005). Variability of *Clostridium difficile* surface proteins and specific serum antibody response in patients with *Clostridium difficile*-associated disease. *J Clin Microbiol* 43, 5018-5025.

Pepin, J., Saheb, N., Coulombe, M. A., Alary, M. E., Corriveau, M. P., Authier, S., Leblanc, M., Rivard, G., Bettez, M., Primeau, V., Nguyen, M., Jacob, C. E. & Lanthier, L. (2005). Emergence of fluoroquinolones as the predominant risk factor for *Clostridium difficile*-associated diarrhea: a cohort study during an epidemic in Quebec. *Clin Infect Dis* 41, 1254-1260.

Pepin, J., Vo, T. T., Boutros, M., Marcotte, E., Dial, S., Dube, S., Vasilevsky, C. A., McFadden, N., Patino, C. & Labbe, A. C. (2009). Risk factors for mortality following emergency colectomy for fulminant *Clostridium difficile* infection. *Dis Colon Rectum* 52, 400-405.

Pothoulakis, C. (1996). Pathogenesis of *Clostridium difficile*-associated diarrhoea. *Eur J Gastroenterol Hepatol* 8, 1041-1047.

Pothoulakis, C. (2000). Effects of *Clostridium difficile* toxins on epithelial cell barrier. *Ann N Y Acad Sci* 915, 347-356.

Rolfe, R. D. (1984). Role of volatile fatty acids in colonization resistance to *Clostridium difficile. Infect Immun* 45, 185-191.

Rupnik, M. (2008). Heterogeneity of large clostridial toxins: importance of *Clostridium difficile* toxinotypes. *FEMS Microbiol Rev* 32, 541-555.

Rupnik, M. (Feb 2011). *Clostridium difficile* Toxinotypes, Date of access: 28 June 2011, Available from: http://www.mf.uni-mb.si/mikro/tox/. .

Rupnik, M., Dupuy, B., Fairweather, N. F., Gerding, D. N., Johnson, S., Just, I., Lyerly, D. M., Popoff, M. R., Rood, J. I., Sonenshein, A. L., Thelestam, M., Wren, B. W., Wilkins, T. D. & von Eichel-Streiber, C. (2005). Revised nomenclature of *Clostridium difficile* toxins and associated genes. *J Med Microbiol* 54, 113-117.

Ryan, E. T., Butterton, J. R., Smith, R. N., Carroll, P. A., Crean, T. I. & Calderwood, S. B. (1997). Protective immunity against *Clostridium difficile* toxin A induced by oral immunization with a live, attenuated Vibrio cholerae vector strain. *Infect Immun* 65, 2941-2949.

Sambol, S. P., Merrigan, M. M., Tang, J. K., Johnson, S. & Gerding, D. N. (2002). Colonization for the prevention of *Clostridium difficile* disease in hamsters. *J Infect Dis* 186, 1781-1789.

Sanchez-Hurtado, K., Corretge, M., Mutlu, E., McIlhagger, R., Starr, J. M. & Poxton, I. R. (2008). Systemic antibody response to Clostridium difficile in colonized patients with and without symptoms and matched controls. *J Med Microbiol* 57, 717-724.

Savidge, T. C., Pan, W. H., Newman, P., O'Brien, M., Anton, P. M. & Pothoulakis, C. (2003). *Clostridium difficile* toxin B is an inflammatory enterotoxin in human intestine. *Gastroenterology* 125, 413-420.

Shim, J. K., Johnson, S., Samore, M. H., Bliss, D. Z. & Gerding, D. N. (1998). Primary symptomless colonisation by *Clostridium difficile* and decreased risk of subsequent diarrhoea. *Lancet* 351, 633-636.

Solomon, K., Webb, J., Ali, N., Robins, R. A. & Mahida, Y. R. (2005). Monocytes are highly sensitive to *Clostridium difficile* toxin A-induced apoptotic and nonapoptotic cell death. *Infect Immun* 73, 1625-1634.

Sougioultzis, S., Kyne, L., Drudy, D., Keates, S., Maroo, S., Pothoulakis, C., Giannasca, P. J., Lee, C. K., Warny, M., Monath, T. P. & Kelly, C. P. (2005). *Clostridium difficile* toxoid vaccine in recurrent *C. difficile*-associated diarrhea. *Gastroenterology* 128, 764-770.

Stubbs, S., Rupnik, M., Gibert, M., Brazier, J., Duerden, B. & Popoff, M. (2000). Production of actin-specific ADP-ribosyltransferase (binary toxin) by strains of *Clostridium difficile*. *FEMS Microbiol Lett* 186, 307-312.

Sunenshine, R. H. & McDonald, L. C. (2006). *Clostridium difficile*-associated disease: new challenges from an established pathogen. *Cleve Clin J Med* 73, 187-197.

Tasteyre, A., Barc, M. C., Collignon, A., Boureau, H. & Karjalainen, T. (2001). Role of FliC and FliD flagellar proteins of *Clostridium difficile* in adherence and gut colonization. *Infect Immun* 69, 7937-7940.

Thelestam, M. & Chaves-Olarte, E. (2000). Cytotoxic effects of the *Clostridium difficile* toxins. *Curr Top Microbiol Immunol* 250, 85-96.

Torres, J. F., Lyerly, D. M., Hill, J. E. & Monath, T. P. (1995). Evaluation of formalin-inactivated *Clostridium difficile* vaccines administered by parenteral and mucosal routes of immunization in hamsters. *Infect Immun* 63, 4619-4627.

Underdown, B. J. & Schiff, J. M. (1986). Immunoglobulin-A - Strategic defense initiative at the mucosal surface. *Annu Rev Immunol* 4, 389-417.

van Dissel, J. T., de Groot, N., Hensgens, C. M., Numan, S., Kuijper, E. J., Veldkamp, P. & van 't Wout, J. (2005). Bovine antibody-enriched whey to aid in the prevention of a relapse of *Clostridium difficile*-associated diarrhoea: preclinical and preliminary clinical data. *J Med Microbiol* 54, 197-205.

Viscidi, R., Laughon, B. E., Yolken, R., Bo-Linn, P., Moench, T., Ryder, R. W. & Bartlett, J. G. (1983). Serum antibody response to toxins A and B of *Clostridium difficile*. *J Infect Dis* 148, 93-100.

von Eichel-Streiber, C., Boquet, P., Sauerborn, M. & Thelestam, M. (1996). Large clostridial cytotoxins--a family of glycosyltransferases modifying small GTP-binding proteins. *Trends Microbiol* 4, 375-382.

Ward, S. J., Douce, G., Dougan, G. & Wren, B. W. (1999). Local and systemic neutralizing antibody responses induced by intranasal immunization with the nontoxic binding domain of toxin A from *Clostridium difficile*. *Infect Immun* 67, 5124-5132.

Warny, M., Fatimi, A., Bostwick, E. F., Laine, D. C., Lebel, F., LaMont, J. T., Pothoulakis, C. & Kelly, C. P. (1999). Bovine immunoglobulin concentrate-*Clostridium difficile* retains *C. difficile* toxin neutralising activity after passage through the human stomach and small intestine. *Gut* 44, 212-217.

Warny, M., Pepin, J., Fang, A., Killgore, G., Thompson, A., Brazier, J., Frost, E. & McDonald, L. C. (2005). Toxin production by an emerging strain of *Clostridium difficile* associated with outbreaks of severe disease in North America and Europe. *Lancet* 366, 1079-1084.

Warny, M., Vaerman, J. P., Avesani, V. & Delmee, M. (1994). Human antibody response to *Clostridium difficile* toxin A in relation to clinical course of infection. *Infect Immun* 62, 384-389.

Weinstein, P. D. & Cebra, J. J. (1991). The preference for switching to IgA expression by Peyer's patch germinal center B cells is likely due to the intrinsic influence of their microenvironment. *J Immunol* 147, 4126-4135.

Wilcox, M. H. (2004). Descriptive study of intravenous immunoglobulin for the treatment of recurrent *Clostridium difficile* diarrhoea. *J Antimicrob Chemother* 53, 882-884.

Yolken, R. H., Bishop, C. A., Townsend, T. R., Bolyard, E. A., Bartlett, J., Santos, G. W. & Saral, R. (1982). Infectious gastroenteritis in bone-marrow-transplant recipients. *N Engl J Med* 306, 1010-1012.

5

Fulminant Amoebic Colitis: Role of the Innate and Adaptive Immune Responses

Ventura-Juárez Javier[1], Campos-Esparza María del Rosario[1], Muñoz-Ortega Martin-H[1] and Campos-Rodríguez Rafael[2]
[1]*Departamento de Morfología, Universidad Autónoma de Aguascalientes,*
[2]*Departamento de Bioquímica, Escuela Superior de Medicina, Instituto Politécnico Nacional, Ciudad de México, México*

1. Introduction

About 10% of the world population is affected by an invasion of the colon by *Entamoeba histolytica* (*E. histolytica*) that results in intestinal amebiasis. This pathogenesis is an important cause of death worldwide, ranking fourth among parasite related fatalities, behind malaria, Chagas disease and Leshmaniasis. Clinically speaking, *E. histolytica* causes amoebic dysentery, ameboma, amoebic appendicitis and fulminant amoebic colitis (FAC) (Espinosa-Cantellano & Martínez-Palomo, 2000; Pérez-Tamayo, 1986; Prathap & Gilman, 1970).

Amoebic dysentery, or ulcerative colitis, affects 90% of the population that is invaded by *E. histolytica.* By means of adhesins, amebapores and proteases, amebas induce the formation of two kinds of ulcers: nodular and irregular. Nodular ulcers are round, measuring 0.1 to 0.5 cm in diameter, and are slightly elevated compared to surrounding tissue. The necrotic center can appear sunken and hemorrhagic, but more frequently is covered with yellowish mucous material (Fig. 1, arrows) the ulcer is surrounded by edematous mucosa. Chronic and abundant nodular ulcers become irregular ulcers (Fig. 1, asterisk) that affect a greater area of the colon and can reach up to 5 cm in diameter. Irregular ulcers, surrounded by edematous mucosa, acellular proteinaceous material, erythrocytes and strand of fibrins, can even invade the submucosa cap, causing abundant infiltrate of neutrophils and macrophages, and a scarce quantity of eosinophils (Fig. 1, asterisk) (Espinosa-Cantellano & Martínez-Palomo, 2000). An appropriate treatment of metronidazole or its derivatives normally cures this type of amebiasis satisfactorily.

During intestinal amebiasis, it is unusual to find colonic ameboma, which is characterized by a great mass of well-defined tissue on the wall of the intestinal lumen. The ulcerated mucosa is a thin layer and the other layers of the colon are thicker than normal, edematous and hemorrhagic. The peritoneum is affected and there are adherences between one or more loops of the small intestine.

Another clinical manifestation of intestinal amebiasis is amebic appendicitis, in which there are nodular ulcers in the mucosa of the organ accompanied by acute inflammation. However, the histopathology is similar to other appendicitis and the parasite can only be detected through microscopic intestinal cuts (Pérez-Tamayo, 1986).

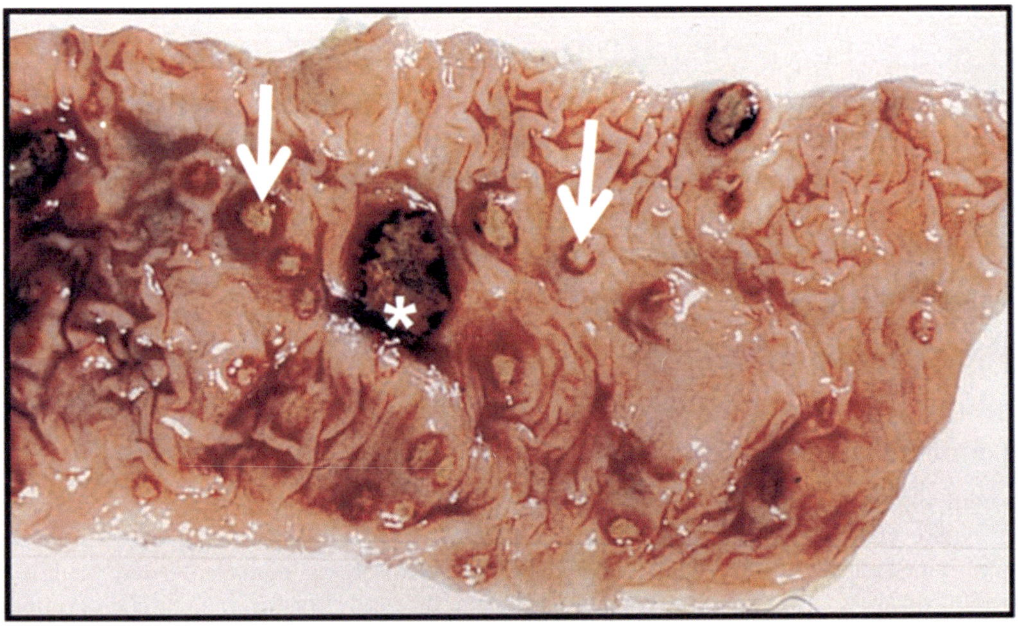

Fig. 1. **Amebic nodular necrotic ulcers (arrows) and amebic irregular ulcers (asterisk) in human colon** (Espinosa-Cantellano & Martínez Palomo, 2000).

FAC is the rarest intestinal amebiasis, with a morbidity rate of 0.01% and a mortality rate of 40 to 100%. It is characterized by the following clinical manifestations: stomach pain, diarrhea, rectal bleeding, peritonitis, fever and abdominal pain (Chun et al., 1994; Takahashi et al., 1997). In the colon of patients, FAC is characterized by inflammation and ulcerous necrotic lesions that extend to great areas, on occasions covering the entire organ (Chun et al., 1994; Natarajan et al., 2000). Various researchers have queried about the role played by the immune response in this pathology (Ventura-Juárez et al., 2002, 2007). For instance, perhaps the inflammatory response has the objective of eliminating the amebas, only to end up participating in the pathogenesis (Kammanadiminti et al., 2007; Seydel et al., 1998).

Different hypothesis have been proposed regarding the role of the immune response during the FAC:

a. The immune response of the host is inappropriate (Seydel et al., 1997, 1998, 2000).
b. The trophozoites of *E. histolytica* are capable of inhibiting the action of complement proteins (Petri et al., 2002; Que et al., 2003; Que & Reed, 2000).
c. Inflammation is induced by cytokines of colonic epithelial cells (Eckmann et al., 1995; Kammanadiminti et al., 2007; Seydel et al., 1997; Yu & Chadee, 1997).
d. A type 2 (Th2) immune response predominates during amebic colitis.

It is important to note that there are scant reports on the interaction between *E. histolytica* and elements of the immune response during FAC. Consequently, the physiopathology of this disorder deserves to be deeply analyzed. Like intestinal or hepatic amebiasis, a hallmark of FAC is that trophozoites of E. *histolytica* are capable of migrating through the intestine and of provoking perforations in intestinal tissue that cannot be repaired. An important question is why these lesions can be formed and later cannot be repaired, in spite of or perhaps to some extent because of the immune response.

On the other hand, there are other ways in which the immune response during the pathogenesis of FAC differs from that which occurs as a result of other types of amebiasis. With FAC there is never any contact between neutrophils and *E. histolytica* trophozoites, decreased levels exist of macrophages, eosinophils, mast cell, CD8 cells and IgM producing plasma cells, and INFγ is apparently not produced. Several researchers have suggested that it is precisely these special conditions of the immune response to FAC that are responsible for ability of E. *histolytica* trophozoites to induce mortal damage to the patient (Prathap & Gilman, 1970; Shetty et al., 1990; Ximénez et al., 1990; Haque et al., 2001; Valenzuela et al., 2001; Sánchez-Guillén et al., 2002; Ventura-Juárez et al., 2003). However, there are other elements of the immune response to FAC, as well as to other forms of amebiasis, that have yet to be studied, among which are IL-8, IL-4, IL-10, TGFβ and NK cells, nevertheless, the cellular immunological factors that underlie the pathogenesis of FAC, especially in the context of host-parasite interactions, are currently unknown. Therefore, the aim of this chapter is to approach the study of FAC firstly from a morphological point of view and secondly by considering the implications of the inflammatory and immune response in the host-parasite relation.

2. Materials and methods

2.1 Immunohistochemical techniques

Specimens were placed in 10% formaldehyde and processed by conventional histological technic for paraffin sectioning. Six-micron thick slices of healthy or FAC intestine specimens were deparaffinized and rehydrated with phosphate-buffered saline (PBS). The activity of endogenous peroxidase was inhibited for 30 min with a 1% H_2O_2 solution in 100% methanol. The specimens were then rehydrated in a graded alcohol series and placed in PBS for 5 min. An antigen-unmasking solution (Vector Laboratories, Inc., Burlingame, CA, USA) was applied at vapor pressure for 1 min. Next, the samples were washed in PBS for 5 min, incubated in 20% fetal bovine serum (Hyclone Laboratories, Logan, UT, USA) in PBS for 30 min and washed three times PBS-0.25% Tween for 10 min. The slides of infected and uninfected tissue were then incubated with the primary antibody for 12 h using the primary antibodies described in table 1.

After incubation all slides were washed with PBS-0.25% Tween for 10 min, then incubated for 1 h at 37 °C, at room temperature using the secondary antibodies: Anti-Polyvalent HRP Ultra Vision Plus Large Volume Detection System (Thermo Scientific TP-060-HLX). Once this incubation was finished, the slides were washed with PBS-0.25%-Tween for 10 min, and peroxidase activity was developed with diaminobenzidine for 5 min. Finally, the slides were counterstained for 7 min with 1:10 Harris' haematoxylin diluted in distilled water, washed with water, dehydrated in a graded alcohol series, passed twice through xylene and covered with synthetic resin. Control slides were prepared following the same protocol for each antibody, with the exception that the primary antibody was substituted with a nonspecific IgG antibody. Finally, immune-stained cells were counted from five slides for each sample. Five 40x fields were analyzed for each slide (viewing each corner and the center) with the aid of Image Pro-Plus imaging software (Image Pro Plus, Media Cybernetics, Silver Spring, MD, USA).

Primary antibody	Host	Antigen recognized	dilution	Trademark
Human CD15 (Neutrophils)	Ms	Lacto-N-fucose pentaosyl	1:50	Chemicon CBL-144
Human CD68 (Macrophages)	Ms	Glycoprotein	1:100	Vector VP-C364
Human CD4	Ms	Glycoprotein CD4	1:20	Novocastra MS392-5
Human CD8	Ms	Glycoprotein CD8	1:100	Novocastra RM9116-5
Human CD57 (NK Cells)	Ms	Glycoprotein	1:150	Chemicon CBL-519
E. histolytica	Rb		1:500	Obtained in our laboratory
Human IgG	Gt	Heavy chains of human	1:100	Chemicon AP112
Human IgA	Gt	Heavy chains of human	1:100	Sigma A-0295
Human IgM	Gt	Heavy chains of human	1:100	Sigma A-0420
Human TGF-β	Ms	TGF-β	1:100	Chemicon MAB1032
Human IFN-γ	Ms	IFN-γ	1:100	Pierce M701
Human IL-8	Ms	IL-8	1:100	US Biological 18430-15
Human IL-10	Rb	IL-10	1:100	Chemicon AB1416
Biotin- mouse IL-4 (biotylinated)	Rt	IL-4	1:100	US Biological 18426-004
Human CD59	Ms	Glycoprotein 17 a 25kDa	1:100	Chemicon MAB-1759

Table 1. Antibodies used for the localization of antigens. Mouse (Ms), rabbit (Rb), rat (Rt) and goat (Gt).

2.2 Histochemical technique

2.2.1 Eosinophil staining

In order to detect eosinophils in colonic tissue sections, paraffin embedded specimens were used. They were deparaffinized and rehydrated in a graded alcohol series to distilled water, then stained with Harris' haematoxylin for 1 min and washed in distilled water. Afterward, the slides were stained with 1.5% erythrosin B in 0.1 % of glycine buffer, pH 10, for 30 min, and, to remove the excess stain in the specimen, they were placed in a quick bath of 70% ethanol in Coplin jars. Finally, the specimens were dehydrated and covered with synthetic resin.

2.2.2 Mast cell staining

Six-micron-thick slices of specimens of normal or infected large intestine were deparaffinized and rehydrated with PBS. They were stained with Harris' haematoxylin for 5 min, washed in distilled water, and incubated for 1 hour with 0.7% toluidine blue in 0.2% acetic acid/sodium acetate. The slides were quickly dehydrated in 70% alcohol, passed to 100% alcohol for 5 min, passed twice through xylene and covered with synthetic resin.

3. Background of fulminant amoebic colitis

Although the histopathological characteristics of FAC are currently very well defined, the role played by inflammatory cells and other cells of the immune response during this usually mortal pathological process is unknown. Masliah & Perez-Tamayo (1984) made an analysis based on 10 patients with FAC characterized by an acute and fatal course of illness. They did staining with Haematoxilin and Eosin (H & E), and reaction with periodic acid Schiff (PAS), finding extensive necrosis with scarce inflammation on the colon walls, in the midst of abundant amebas in process of disintegration. The amoebic ulcers healed without scar tissue. The authors described the histopathological damage in four forms: **a)** ulcers with *E. histolytica* in the mucosa-submucosa showing inflammation and/or necrosis, but without *E. histolytica* in the external muscular layer; **b)** *E. histolytica* in mucosa-submucosa and in the *muscularis mucosae*, without alterations in the external muscular layer; **c)** *E. histolytica* in the mucosa-submucosa and the external muscular layer; **d)** necrosis in the mucosa-submucosa and external muscular layer, but without *E. histolytica*. In each case the *E. histolytica* trophozoites were found to be more abundant in the mucosa-submucosa than the external muscular layer.

A decade later, Chun et al. (1994) analyzed four patients who underwent surgery for acute abdominal pain, practicing a surgical resection of colon. Immediately after surgery there was 50% mortality. Macroscopically they discovered a pseudomembranous colitis characterized by an extremely friable intestinal wall, and the mucosa with innumerable ulcers covered by yellowish-green pseudomembranes. Although intact, the mucosa among the ulcers was hyperemic and the serous membrane presented fibrinopurulent exudate and discoloration of the tissue. By using H & E and immunohistochemical techniques, the lesion was described as acute transmural necrotizing colitis, where alterations were not found in the Lieberkhün crypts, but were indeed found in the lamina propria adjacent to the edges of the ulcers, with abundant lymphocytes and plasma cells. The pseudomembranes that covered the ulcers contained granular remains of eosinophils and/or basophils. The purulent exudate that covered the walls and base of the ulcers contained abundant trophozoites de *E. histolytica*, located principally at the edges of the ulcers and rarely in the blood vessels. In 50% of the cases *E. histolytica* trophozoites were observed in the pericolic fatty tissue, but not in the adjacent ischemic mucosa.

A few years later a report was published about 55 patients with FAC (Takahashi et al., 1997) treated in the Hospital de la Nutrición Salvador Zubirán in Mexico City (1943 to 1994). The operative mortality was 76% and the total mortality 89%, both associated mainly with a reduced level of leukocytes. Furthermore, 54% were found to have an association with amebic liver abscess (AHA), and the most common systemic illness was *Diabetes Mellitus*. Macroscopically the colon was observed to have multiple sites of perforation, with amebic appendicitis found in 5 cases and ameboma in 4 others. Microscopic analysis showed necrosis and the presence of *E. histolytica* in the upper and lower layers of the colon, with acute and/or chronic inflammation in the external muscular layer. Cases of FAC are uncommon, but the majority result in death of the patient. To the naked eye, the colon presents a great quantity of ulcers with robust necrosis and mucosa exudate, but surrounded by apparently normal tissue. The ulcers contain round or oblong *E. histolytica* (with erythrocytes and phagocytes) the size similarly to macrophages.

Recently associations have been reported between FAC and other pathologies such as tuberculosis (Park et al., 2000), co-infection with *Actinomyces* (Nishena et al., 2009) and *Histoplasmosis* (Koh et al., 2010). One case was published of FAC associated with a chemotherapy treatment for advanced gastric cancer (Hanaoka et al., 2009). What stands out from these reports is the association of FAC with a deficit in the immune system and malnutrition, which further emphasizes the need to analyze the role of the distinct cells of the immune response against the *E. histolytica*, and especially whether there is an active inflammatory response.

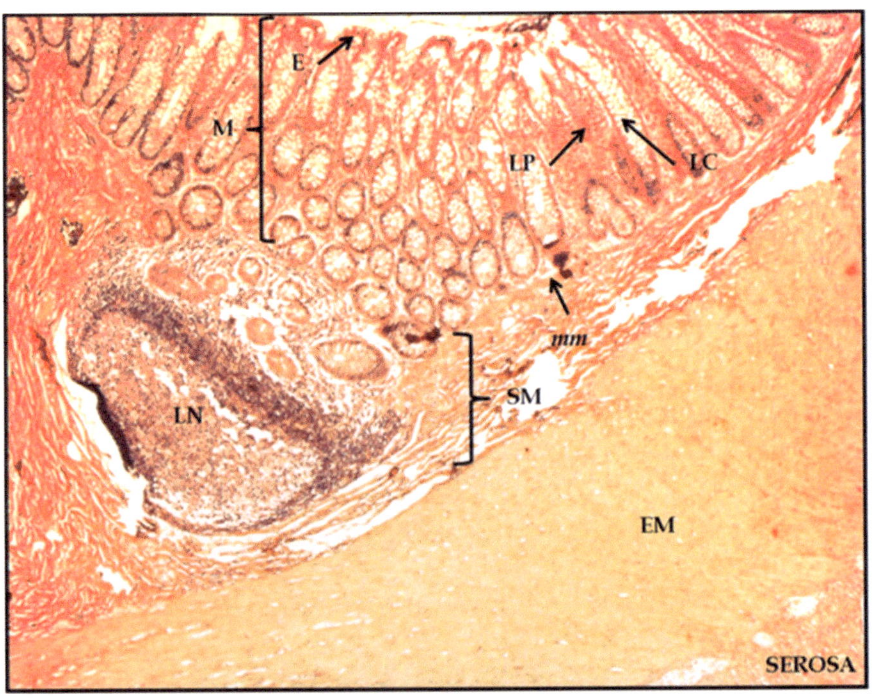

Fig. 2. **Histology of a healthy human colon.** The mucosa (M), epithelial tissue (E) and Lieberkhün crypts (LC), surrounded by the lamina propria (LP) and delimited by the *muscularis mucosae* (*mm*) from the submucosa (SM), which contains lymphatic nodes (LN). The external muscular tissue (EM) and serous tissue (H & E; X25).

3.1 The host-parasite interaction during FAC

Before describing the structure of the colon with amebiasis, the histological structure of a healthy colon must first be laid out.

The Ventura-Juárez group described (2007), in mucosa (M) and submucosa (SM) of healthy colon, the location of cells of the innate and adaptive immune response, by using histochemical and immunohistochemical techniques, finding macrophages, NK cells, eosinophils, mast cells, CD4 and CD8 lymphocytes, but without neutrophils (Fig 3 a-f). Additionally, abundant IgA, IgG and IgM producing cells were found (Fig 3 g-i), which had been previously described by Douglas & Rodger (1997).

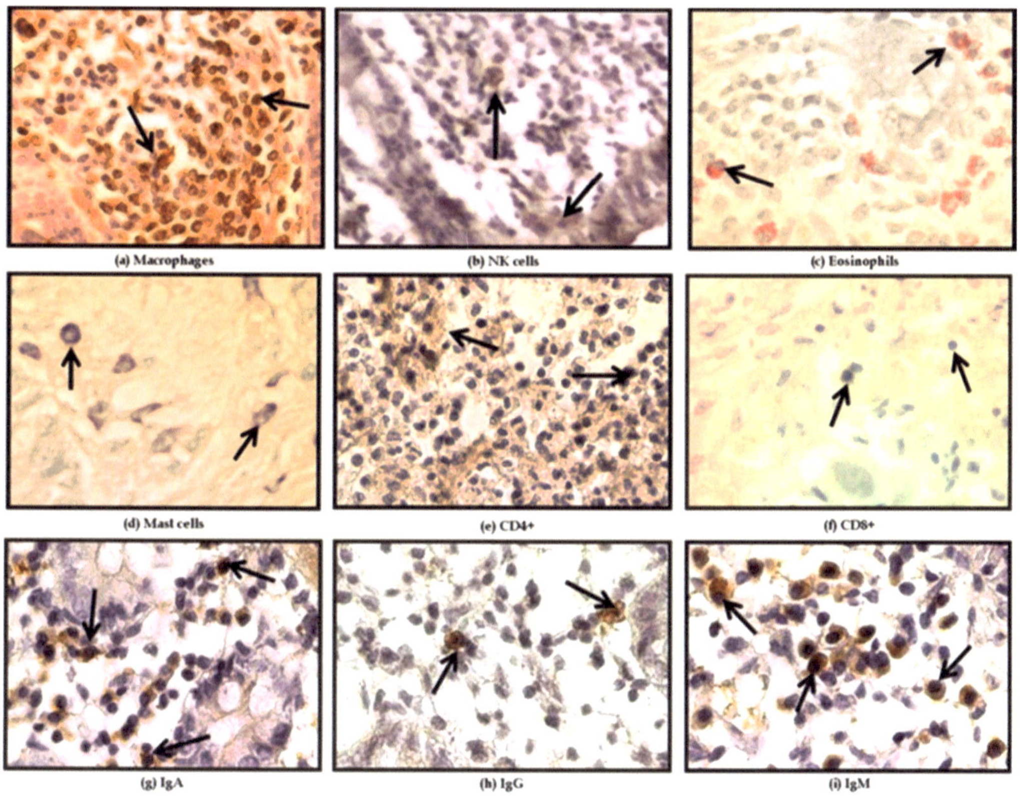

Fig. 3. **Cells from the innate and adaptive immune response in healthy human colon.** Cells from the innate (a-d) and adaptive (e-i) immune response located in the lamina propria and submucosa of healthy human colon tissue. (Histochemistry and Immunohistochemistry X400). (Ventura-Juárez et al., 2007).

3.2 Histopathology of amebic ulcers in fulminant amebic colitis

In order to describe the role of the immune response and inflammation during FAC, eleven tissue samples were analyzed (from 5 women and 6 men), originating from patients who underwent surgery of the ileum and colon during the period of 1999 to 2004 in three hospitals in Mexico (Ventura-Juárez et al., 2007). Macroscopic analysis of intestines with FAC showed, externally, intestinal perforations (arrows) with hemorrhagic necrosis (asterisk) (Fig. 4a), and internally, ample zones of necrosis with bloody-mucosa deposits (asterisk) and thickening of the mucosa with perforations (arrows) (Fig. 4b).

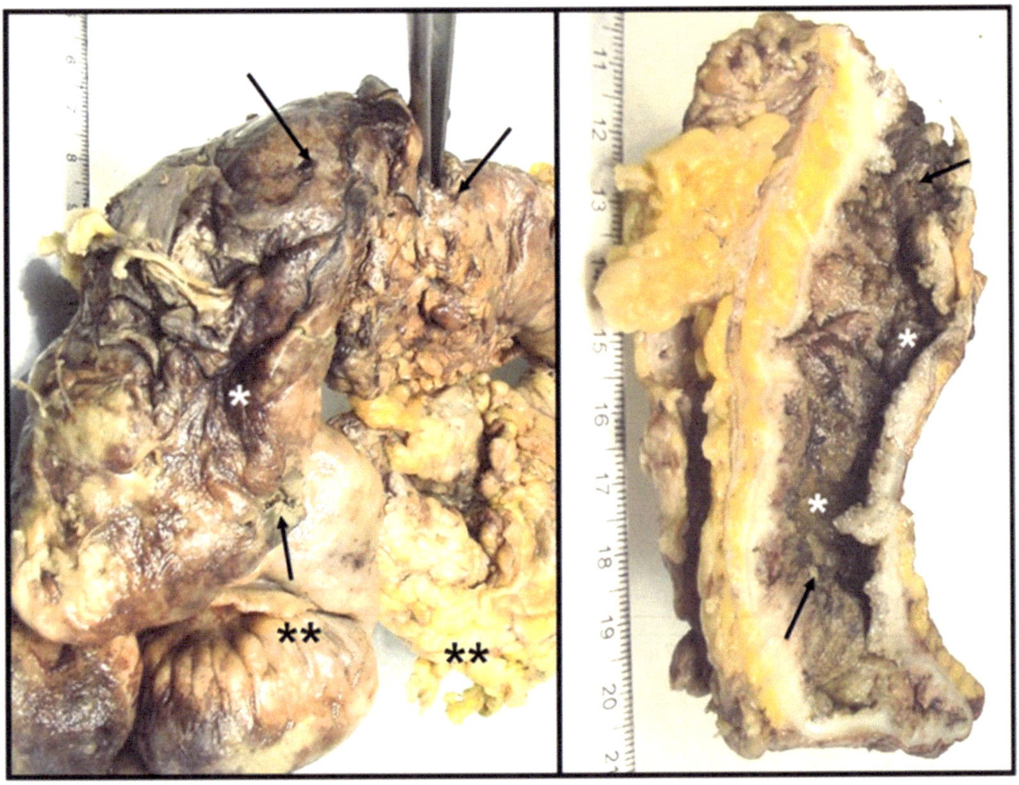

(a) (b)

Fig. 4. **Macroscopic characteristics of fulminant amebic colitis**: **(a)** External view of the colon, where large areas of hemorrhagic necrosis (*) and perforations can be appreciated (arrows); small normal-looking areas of the colon and the mesentery (**). **(b)** Internal view of the colon, where hemorrhagic necrosis and fibrinoid deposits are observed (*), along with amebic ulcers (arrows).

The amebic ulcer (Fig. 5) is characterized by the classic form of the "flask ulcer" delimited (blue line) laterally by Mucosa (M), Submucosa (SM), external muscular tissue (EM) and the peritoneum (P). The ulcer, viewed from the intestinal lumen (IL) toward the deep ulcer (DU), shows: 1) a thickened surface zone composed of lytic material mixed with mucous, (**) 2) a thickened intermediate zone with abundant proteinaceous material (PM), and 3) a deeper zone with the mucosa and submucosa damaged by the amebic invasion and an area where the mucosa and submucosa are fused together, which is termed the necrotic zone. At the center of this zone there is an area of discontinuity of the external muscular tissue and peritoneum, where the intestinal perforation is formed (arrow).

Histological cuts show *E. histolytica* located abundantly in the mucosa outside (Fig. 6a) and inside the amebic ulcer, mixed with cells of the inflammatory infiltrate. In the external muscular layer (EM) of the ulcer, abundant *E. histolytica* trophozoites were found, although

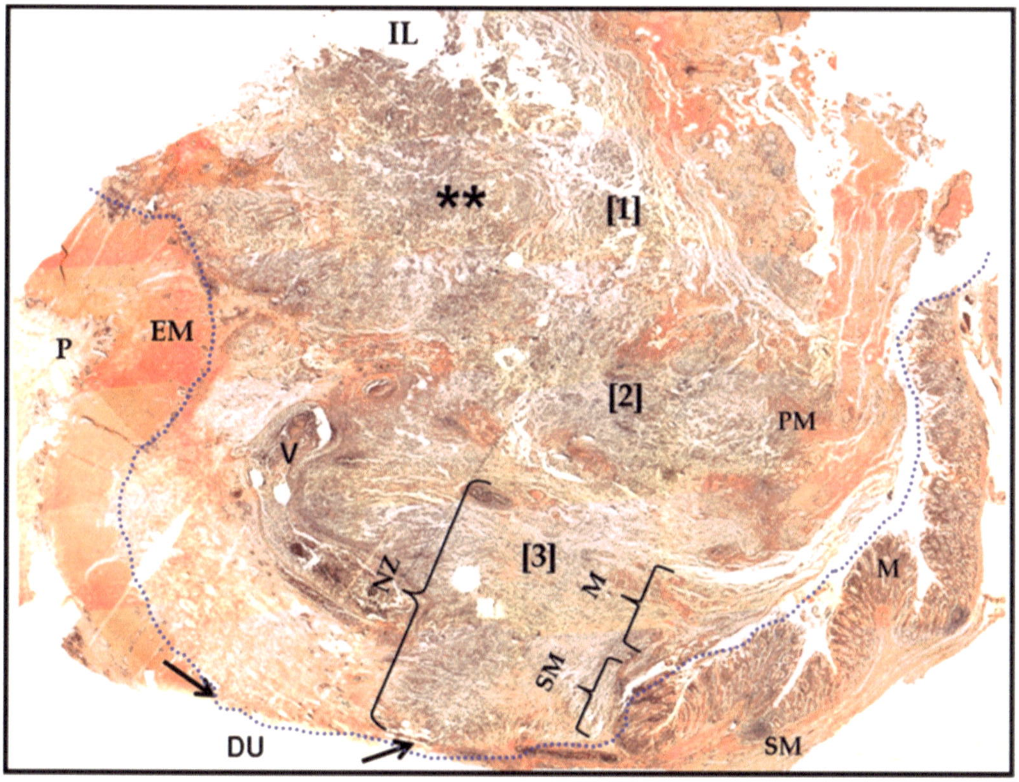

Fig. 5. **Amebic ulcer characteristic of FAC**. The amebic ulcer (dotted line) is delimited by the mucosa (M), submucosa (SM), external muscular tissue (EM) and the peritoneum (P). The ulcer consists of: (1) a surface zone formed by mucous (**), 2) an intermediate zone with proteinaceous material (PM), and 3) a deep zone that contains damaged mucosa (M) and submucosa (SM) and a necrotic zone (NZ). At the bottom of the ulcer is found a zone of discontinuity of the external muscular (EM) and the peritoneum (P), where the intestinal perforations are formed (arrow). View from the intestinal lumen (IL) and the deep ulcer (DU).

without inflammatory infiltrate, that caused the intestinal perforation (Fig. 6b). Curiously, *E. histolytica* trophozoites were observed on the edge of the ulcers or within them, even when these areas extended to the entire mucosa-submucosa with necrotic material, cellular debris and strands of fibrins. Nevertheless, inside some dilated blood vessels (bv) *E. histolytica* can indeed be observed (Fig. 6c).

4. Role of the cellular immune response

The mechanisms of damage caused by the *E. histolytica* in the mucosa of the colon of FAC patients are similar to those described in liver with invasive amebiasis (Aikat, 1979; Ventura-Juárez, 1997). It has been seen that when *E. histolytica* are present, tissue damage can be caused by *E. histolytica* adhesion, lysis of host cells, and effects of the proteolytic enzymes derived from the parasite (Huston, 2004; Stanley & Reed, 2001). However, when *E. histolytica* are not present in the tissue, damage probably arises from an ischemia or the immune response of the host (Campos-Rodríguez et al., 2009; Stanley & Reed, 2001).

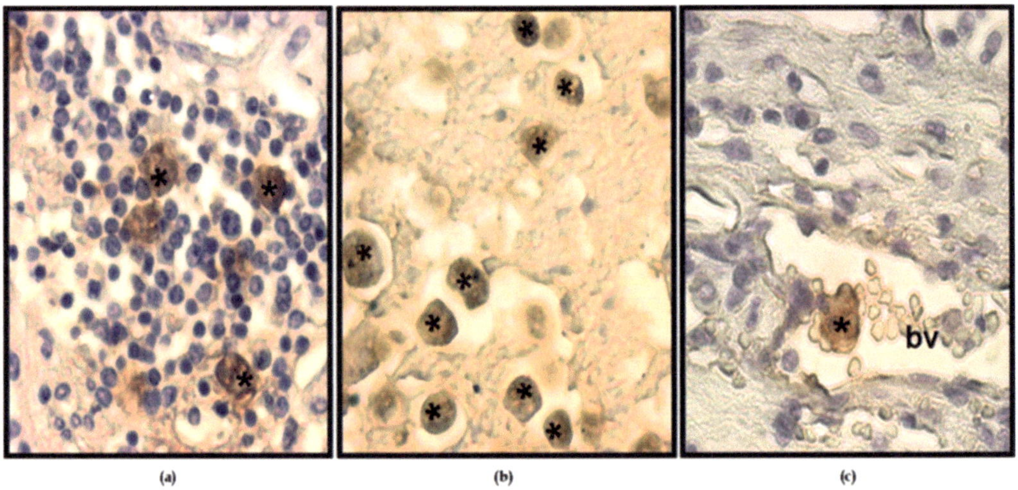

Fig. 6. ***E. histolytica* trophozoites in intestines with FAC.** *E. histolytica* (*) located in **(a)** The mucosa outside of the ulcer, mixed with abundant inflammatory infiltrate cells. **(b)** The external muscular of the ulcer without any associated inflammatory reaction. **(c)** The blood vessels (bv) of the muscular layer adjoining the ulcer (Immunoperoxidase, X400).

4.1 In FAC, the cellular immune response does not participate in the death of *E. histolytica* trophozoites

Neutrophils and macrophages are important effector cells in the defense of the host against *E. histolytica* (Cantellano & Martínez-Palomo, 2000; Ghadirian & Denis, 1992; Seydel et al., 1997; Tsutsumi et al., 1984; Velázquez et al., 1998).Ventura-Juárez et al (2007) demonstrated that during an amebic invasion, the inflammatory response is restricted to the areas without cellular damage. That is, the fact that neutrophils are abundant in the mucosa adjoining the ulcer (20.7272 ± 7.2950), absent in the zones distant from the ulcer, and are scarce and rarely in contact with the trophozoites in lytic zones of the ulcer that contain *E. histolytica* (7.2950 ± 4.6363) (Fig. 7 a, b, e), indicates that the amebic invasion does not prompt a generalized inflammatory response.

Macrophages, on the other hand, are scant in the amebic ulcer compared with a healthy intestine (56.8 ± 14.6697), and are principally in the lamina propria. They were found to be greatly diminished in the mucosa inside of the ulcer (1.7272 ± 1.4893) compared to mucosa outside (9.1818 ± 1.3280) (Fig. 7 c-e). This scarcity of macrophages in the amebic ulcer could be caused by their reduced migration as a consequence of the secretion of the locomotion inhibitory factor of monocytes (MLIF) (Kretschmer et al., 1985).

The fact that neutrophils and macrophages were not found in direct contact with *E. histolytica* (Fig. 7b, d) leads to the conclusion that these cells probably do not participate in the death of *E. histolytica* trophozoites, as this process is apparently dependent on direct contact (Burchard et al., 1993; Martínez-Palomo, 1987; Petri et al., 2002). Nevertheless, neutrophils and macrophages could be participating in the destruction of colonic tissue, as has been suggested by various researchers (Pittman, 1976; Tsutsumi et al., 1990; Tsutsumi et al., 2006) and confirmed by experiments conducted in animal models (Rivero-Nava 2002; Stanley & Reed 2001), in which it has been demonstrated that mucosa of healthy colon (without inflammation) do not present neutrophils (Lee et al., 1988).

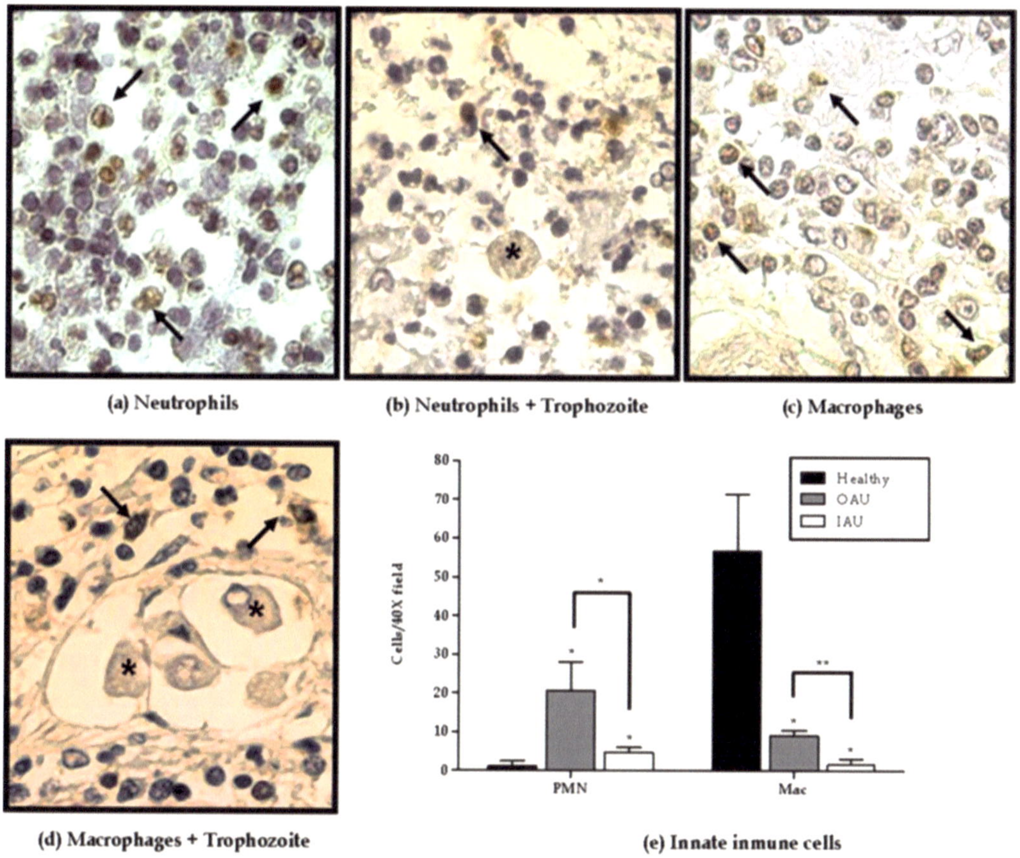

Fig. 7. **Distribution of neutrophils and macrophages in the intestine of patients with FAC.** **(a)** Abundant neutrophils (CD15+; arrows) in mucosa adjoining the amebic ulcer. **(b)** Trophozoites (*) surrounded by cells without any contact with neutrophils (CD15+; arrows) in a necrotic zone of the ulcer. **(c)** Macrophages (CD68+; arrows) in lamina propria outside of the ulcer. **(d)** Macrophages (arrows; CD68+) without contact with trophozoites (*). All photos were taken with a magnification of X400. **(e)** Graphic representation of the number of neutrophils (PMN) and macrophages (Mac) in healthy intestine, as well as areas outside (OAU) and inside (IAU) the ulcer of intestine with FAC. The bars represent the mean ± SD ($p < 0.05$; Students *t* Test).

Similarly, in the tissue of patients with FAC, a greater quantity of NK cells (CD57) were found than in healthy tissue (2.8 ± 0.8366). These cells in lamina propria outside the ulcer (5.6363 ± 1.8586) were abundant and were mixed with cellular debris. Inside the ulcer NK cells were less abundant (1.5454 ±1.0357) and had no contact with *E. histolytica* trophozoites, suggesting that they are not responsible for the elimination of the parasite (Fig. 8a y d). In an animal model of AHA in mice, it has also been observed that NK cells are not found in the inflammatory infiltrate or in cells that delimit the lesion (Jarillo-Luna, 2002). However, another study reported that NK cells activated by lipopeptidophosphoglicane from *E. histolytica* reduce the size of AHA (Lotter et al., 2009).

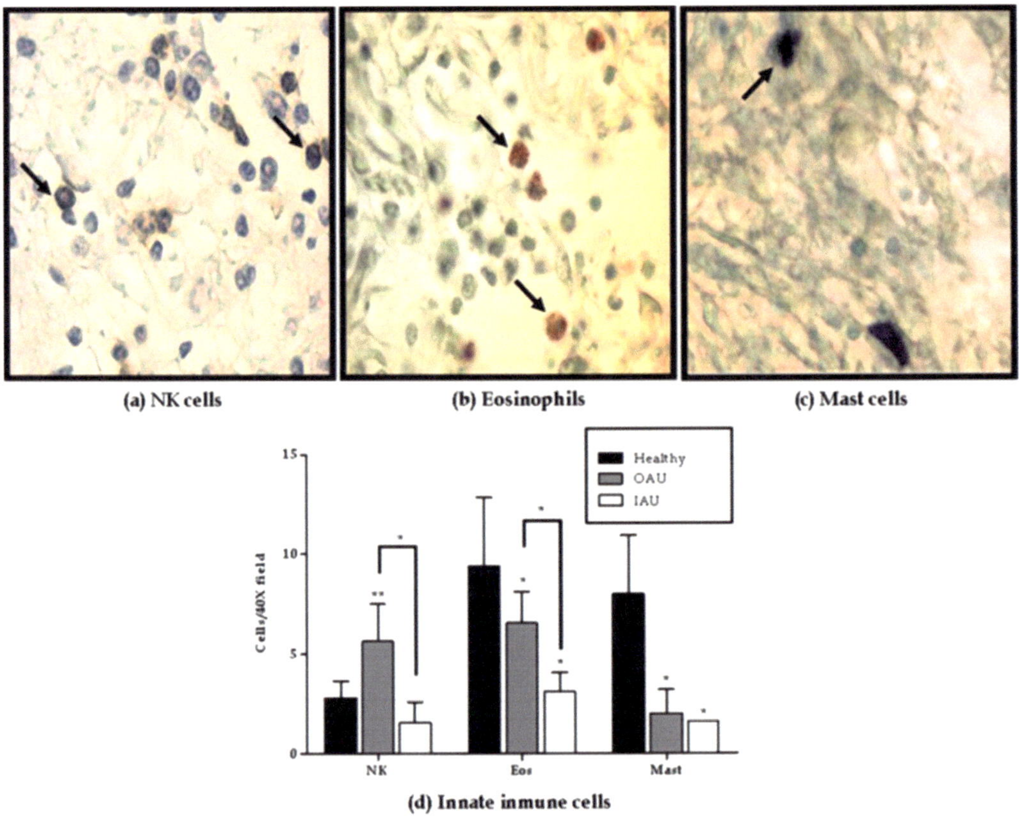

Fig. 8. **NK cells, eosinophils and mast cells are scarce in ulcers in the intestine of patients with FAC**. **(a)** NK cells (arrows) are distant from the trophozoites in the lamina propria (Immunoperoxidase, X400). **(b)** Eosinophils (arrows) are observed in the lamina propria outside of the ulcer remote from trophozoites (Histochemistry, X400). **(c)** Mast cells (arrows) in the lamina propria outside the ulcer, distant from trophozoites (Histochemistry, X400). **(d)** Graphic representation of the number of NK cells (NK), eosinophils (Eos) and mast cells (Mast) in healthy intestine, as well as in areas outside (OAU) and inside (IAU) the ulcer in the intestine of patients with FAC. Bars represent the mean ± SD ($p< 0.05$; Students *t* Test).

Moreover, eosinophils and mast cells are also implicated in the cellular response and have been found to be involved in the reduction of amebic damage in various *in vivo* models (Houpt, 2002; Jarillo-Luna, 2002; López-Osuna et al., 1997, 2002). By using histochemical techniques in human intestinal tissue with FAC, eosinophils were stained with eritrosine B 1.5% (Benítez et al., 1987) and mast cells with toluidine blue 0.7% (Enerback, 1986; Ventura-Juárez et al., 1990). Then, by using light microscopy, it was observed that both types of cells diminished significantly in the lamina propria and inside the ulcer with respect to healthy intestine (9.4 ±3.435; 8.0 ± 2.9154), suggesting that *E. histolytica* could participate in the destruction of these cells (Fig. 8d).

Eosinophils are located mostly in the lamina propria outside of the ulcer (6.5454 ± 1.5724) and only scantly (3.0909 ± 0.94387) in the lamina propria of the amebic ulcer (Fig. 8b y d). It has been shown by *in vitro* studies that the MLIF produced by *E. histolytica* do not affect the locomotion and respiratory burst of human eosinophils (Rico & Kretschmer, 1997). However, *E. histolytica* is capable of destroying normal eosinophils (not activated) (López-Osuna & Kretschmer, 1989).

Mast cells did not show significant changes between the lamina propria inside (2.0000 ± 1.1832) and outside (1.6124 ± 0.00009) the amebic ulcer (Fig. 8c y d). Some studies reveal that there is an association between the activity of mast cells and the deterioration of immunity. In mice infected by nematodes, mast cells and their proteases, specifically protease-1, increased the elimination of the parasite (Knight et al., 2000), possibly through increasing vascular permeability and epithelial permeability. Taking this into account, and considering that *E. histolytica* trophozoites favor zones of epithelial rupture, *E. histolytica* could be benefited by the permeability of the epithelial cells. Moreover, mast cells also could be a direct cause of proteases or proinflammatory cytokines, or perhaps through neutrophils dependent on IgE and the recruitment of monocytes (Wershil et al., 1996). In a model of amebic colitis in mice, it has been determined that mast cells do not protect against amebiasis (Houpt et al., 2002).

Cell type	**Function in intestinal immunity**	**Healthy intestine**		**Intestine in patients with FAC**					
				Outside the amebic ulcer			**Inside the amebic ulcer**		
		E	*LP*	*E*	*LP*	*SM*	*E*	*LP*	*SM*
				Cellular Immune Response					
PMN	First phagocytic cells attracted to the damaged site and inhibited by *E. histolytica.*		3.1510		20.727*			7.2950* #	
Mac	Phagocytic cell that presents antigens destroyed by *E. histolytica.*		56.800		9.1818*			1.7272*#	
NK	Cells responsible for activating macrophages and liberating IFN gamma, attracted to the damaged site and destroyed by *E. histolytica.*		2.8000		5.6363**			1.5454#	
Eos	Cells with anti-helminthic activity that are nevertheless inhibited by *E. histolytica.*		9.4000		6.5454*			3.0909*#	
Mast	Cells responsible for the repair of tissue that are inhibited by *E. histolytica*		7.4000		1.6124 *			2.0000*	
CD4	Cells that do not participate during FAC.		4.3441		3.6531			4.8112	
CD8	Cytotoxic cells inhibited by *E. histolytica* in necrotic zones of the ulcer.		6.7001			6.6			2.1411 *#

Table 2. Role of the Cellular Immune Response during fulminant amebic colitis. Neutrophils (PMN), Macrophages (Mac), NK cells (NK), Eosinophils (Eos), Mast cell (Mast). *Epithelium (E), Lamina propria (LP), Sub-mucosa (SM).** Significant values with respect to healthy intestinal tissue. # Significant values with respect to areas outside the ulcer of the intestine of patients with FAC.

In general, there were a lesser number of immune cells in areas inside the amebic ulcer than areas outside (see table 2). Various explanations could be given for this fact: (a) the immune cells are eliminated by products of *E. histolytica;* (b) migration of cells is inhibited by the locomotion inhibitory factor of monocytes, (c) the dysfunction of endothelial cells is induced by *E. histolytica*, which causes thrombosis and local ischemia, and consequently a reduced cellular migration (Campos-Rodríguez et al., 2009).

4.2 In FAC, *Entamoeba histolytica* inhibits the cytotoxic response of CD8 lymphocytes

By observing intestinal tissue of patients with FAC, descriptions have been made not only of the cells and molecules of the innate immune response, but also the cells of the acquired cellular immune response (T CD4+ lymphocytes, T CD8+ lymphocytes). These latter cells require at least two weeks to be able to differentiate and recognize antigens. No significant changes were found between the number of CD4+ lymphocytes of the lamina propria of healthy mucosa (4.3441 ± 1.1639), and the number of these cells in patients with FAC inside (4.8112± 0.8556) and outside (3.6531 ± 0.9011) the lamina propria of the intestine (Figs. 9a and 9c).

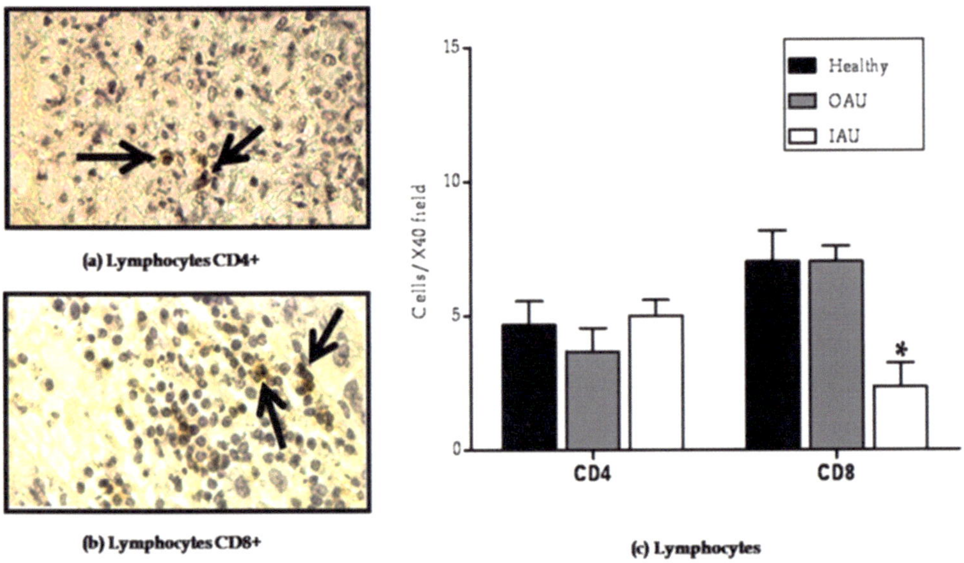

Fig. 9. **Decrease of T CD8+ cells in la amebic ulcers. (a)** T CD4+ cells located in the lamina propria of the amebic ulcer. **(b)** Scarce T CD8+ lymphocytes in the lamina propria the amebic ulcer (Immunoperoxidase, X400). **(c)** Graphic representation of CD4+ and CD8+ lymphocytes in healthy intestine, as well as areas outside (OAU) and inside (IAU) the ulcer in the intestine of patients with FAC. Bars represent the mean ± SEM ($p \leq 0.05$; Tukey Test).

These results suggest that the amebic invasion does not alter the activation of these T CD4+ cells. Moreover, there were no significant changes in the number of CD8+ cells of the lamina propria between healthy intestine (6.7001 ± 1.3101) and areas outside of the ulcer (6.6 ± 1.1), although a diminished recruitment of these cells was observed in the lamina propria of amebic ulcers (2.1411 ± 0.9111)(Figs. 9b and 9c).

The role of T CD4+ and CD8+ cells in intestinal amebiasis is unknown, although it has been proposed that T CD8+ cells are involved in the lysis by direct contact of *E. histolytica* (Martínez-Palomo, 1987). If so, the low number of T CD8+ lymphocytes given by the Th2 response could contribute to the persistence of amebas in the colonic mucosa (see table 2) (Ventura-Juárez et al., 2007).

5. Role of the humoral immune response

In the colon, immunoglobins (Igs) are in part responsible for maintaining equilibrium between the host and parasite. In the intestine the first immunoglobin to express itself, IgA, prevents microorganisms from penetrating the mucosa due to its anti-adherence properties. If the invasion succeeds in spite of this defense, IgG is produced and IgM begins to form binding complexes with the complement.

Ventura-Juárez (2007) studied intestine in patients with FAC and healthy human intestine by immunohistochemical techniques in order to localize the immunoglobins IgA, IgG and IgM, finding plasma cells IgA, IgG and IgM (Fig. 10) in the lamina propria outside and inside the amebic ulcer.

The number of cells positive for IgA and IgG in lamina propria outside the ulcer was significantly greater (38.5454 ± 4.8859, 40.0000 ± 7.2938) with respect to lamina propria inside the ulcer (4.8181 ± 1.6011; 1.7272 ± 1.42062) and in healthy intestine (22.0000 ± 4.3588; 4.8000 ± 0.8366) (Fig. 10a-d, g). However, both types of plasma cells significantly diminished in the lamina propria of the amebic ulcer with respect to healthy intestine.

In contrast, IgM plasma cells significantly diminished in the lamina propria of the amebic ulcer with respect to healthy intestine (29.6666 ± 2.5166). That is, in the lamina propria outside the ulcer (6.0909 ± 1.9211) there is a significantly greater number of IgM cells with respect to the ulcer (2.9090 ± 1.0444) (Fig. 10e-g). Additionally, no inflammatory cells were found in contact with trophozoites, meaning that they probably do not participate in resolving the amebic invasion. Indeed, these cells could contribute to tissue damage.

Plasma cells can be involved in the synthesis of antibodies against amebic antigens. About 64% of patients with amebic colitis have an increase in the titers of antibodies for *E. histolytica*, which are used in the diagnosis of the amebic invasion.

However, these antibodies do not protect against the pathogen. IgA is a central component of the immune defense, modulating the host-parasite interaction. It is the dominant immunoglobulin of the intestinal surface (see table 3). It has been seen that the cysteine proteases of *E. histolytica* break down IgA and IgG. Broken down IgG, in turn, reduces the affinity of antibodies for antigens. If the Fc portion is removed, the trophozoites could evade the immune response by encasing themselves in immunogenic surface molecules found in Fab fragments. This could prevent the activation of the complement by the classic pathway and attack the immune cells with the anchor corresponding to the Fc receptor. Thus, the parasite could move around the internal medium, ignoring the immune system of the host (Mortimer & Chadee, 2010).

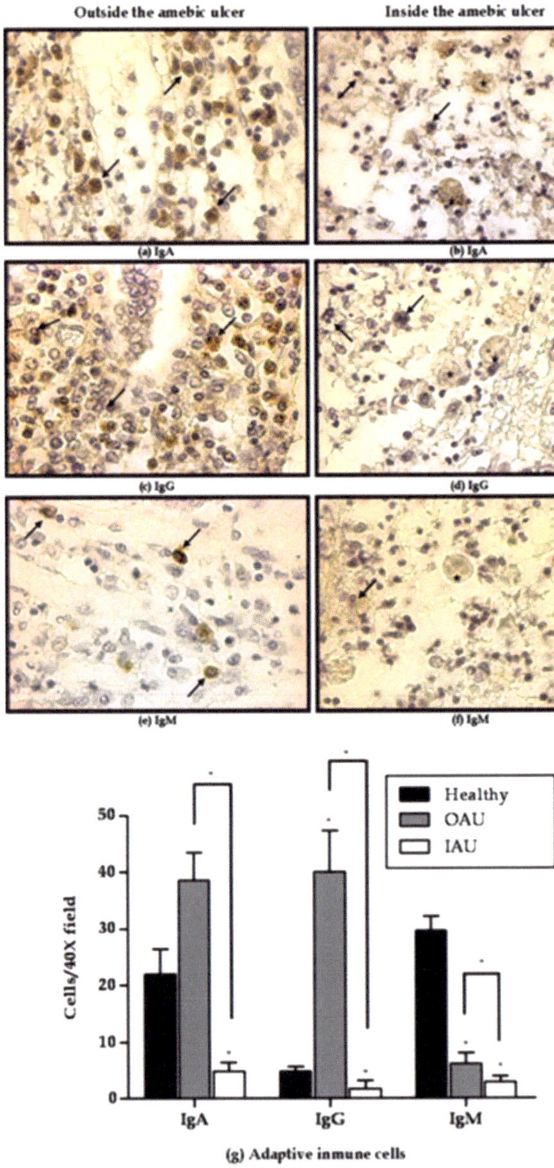

Fig. 10. **Distribution of plasma cells in intestines with FAC. (a)** Abundant IgA+ cells (arrows) are found in the lamina propria outside the ulcer. **(b)** Scarce IgA+ cells (arrows) in the lamina propria near the trophozoites (*) of the amebic ulcer. **(c)** Numerous IgG+ cells (arrows) are found en la lamina propria nearly the ulcer, close to the necrotic zone. **(d)** Scant IgG+ cells (arrows) in the lamina propria around the trophozoites (*). **(e)** Scarce IgM cells (arrows) in the lamina propria outside the amebic ulcer. **(f)** IgM+ cells in the lamina propria of the ulcer near trophozoites (*). (Immunoperoxidase, X400). **(g)** Graphic representation of the number of IgA+, IgG+ and IgM+ in healthy intestine, as well as areas outside (OAU) and inside (IAU) the ulcer of the intestine of patients with FAC. Bars represents the mean ± SD ($p < 0.05$; Student *t* Test).

Cell type	Function in intestinal immunity	Healthy intestine		Intestine in patients with FAC					
				Outside the amebic ulcer			Inside the amebic ulcer		
		E	*LP*	*E*	*LP*	*SM*	*E*	*LP*	*SM*
		Humoral Immune Response							
IgA	Principal Immunoglobulin of defense in the mucosa. Abundant during the processes of FAC, and destroyed by *E. histolytica*.		22.0000		38.5454*			4.8181*#	
IgG	Immunoglobulin responsible for activating the complement. Abundant during the processes of FAC.		4.8000		40.0000*			1.7272*#	
IgM	Immunoglobulin of defense in the mucosa. Its production is inhibited by *E. histolytica*.		29.6666		6.0909*			2.9090*#	

Table 3. Role of the Humoral Immune Response during fulminant amebic colitis. *Epithelium (E), Lamina propria (LP), Sub-mucosa (SM).** Significant values with respect to healthy intestinal tissue. # Significant values with respect to areas outside the ulcer of the intestine of patients with FAC.

6. Role of anti-inflammatory and pro-inflammatory cytokines in FAC

The role of the acquired cellular immune response in protecting against fulminant colitis has not yet been well defined. It is still not clear if the type 1 (Th1) or type 2 response (Th2) dominates the immune response in amebic colitis. Information is lacking in data from the literature about cytokine expression in the colon of patients with amebic colitis. According to results obtained from human intestine with FAC by the Sierra-Puente et al (2009), both pro-inflammatory cytokines (IL-8 e INFγ) and anti-inflammatory cytokines (IL-4, IL-10, TGF-β) were found, promoters of the Th1 and Th2 type response, respectively (Guo et al, 2008; Sierra-Puente et al., 2009).

6.1 In FAC, epithelial cells of the intestine produce IL-8

In vitro studies have demonstrated that *E. histolytica* stimulates the production of IL-8, a pro-inflammatory chemotactic cytokine for neutrophils (Yu & Chadee, 1997). Also using antibodies against human IL-8, cells positive to this cytokine were identified in the epithelial cells outside the ulcer from patients with FAC (2.200 ± 0.4667), while no cells positive to this cytokine were found in healthy intestine (Fig. 11a) (Sierra-Puente et al., 2009). In the model of SCID mice with intestinal xenografts from humans infected with virulent *E. histolytica* trophozoites, IL-8 was detected in epithelial cells distal of the ulcer (Seydel et al., 1997), which corroborates the findings by our workgroup.

In a previous study, Ventura-Juárez (2007) demonstrated that in human intestine with FAC, the mucosa adjoining the amebic ulcer presented a great quantity of neutrophils, which are related with IL-8 produced by epithelial cells located in the same area of the intestine. Some researchers support the hypothesis that the high production of IL-1 and IL-8 by epithelial cells could be a key contributor to the pathogenesis of amebic infection. This probably takes place through the attraction of neutrophils, which in turn increases inflammation and damage (see table 4) (Garcia-Zepeda et al., 2007; Seydel et al., 1997).

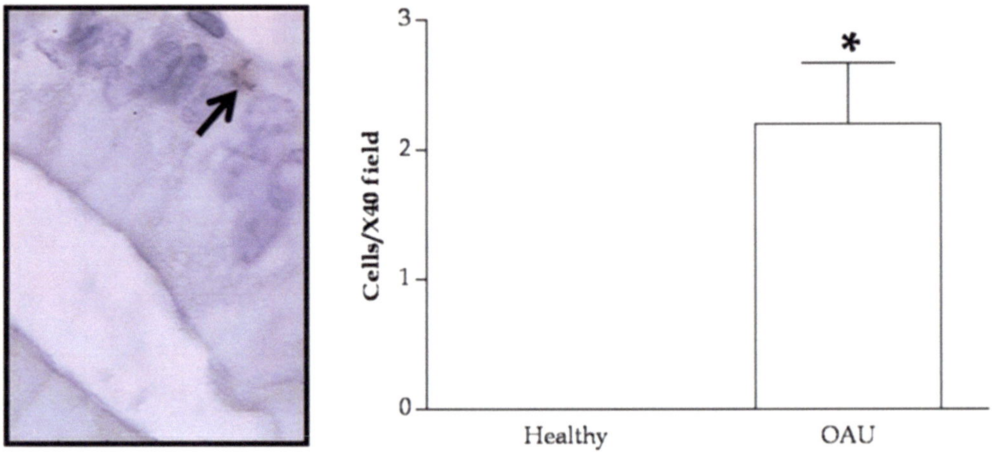

(a) IL-8 (b) IL-8

Fig. 11. ***E. histolytica*** **induces the overproduction of IL-8 by epithelial cells. (a)** IL-8+ epithelial cells outside the amebic ulcer (arrows) (Immunoperoxidase, X400). **(b)** Graphic representation of IL-8+ epithelial cells from healthy intestine and outside the ulcer in the intestine of patients with FAC. Bars represents the mean ± SEM ($p \leq 0.004$; Students *t* Test).

Cell type	Function in intestinal immunity	Healthy intestine		Intestine in patients with FAC					
				Outside the amebic ulcer			Inside the amebic ulcer		
		E	*LP*	*E*	*LP*	*SM*	*E*	*LP*	*SM*
Cytokines in FAC									
IL-8	Cytokine that attracts and activates neutrophils. Cytokine produced in processes of FAC.		0	2.200*					
IL-10	Stimulates the synthesis of IgA, antagonizes Th1 cells. Cytokine produced in processes of FAC.		2.3002	10.351*					
IL-4	Cytokine that promotes the development of B cells producing IgA and IgG. Cytokine produced in processes of FAC.		1.0001		12.3600*				
TGF-β	Cytokine that inhibits Th1 cells. TGF-beta-producing cells inhibited in the processes of FAC.	13.4100	5.0290	7.7880*	7.4740				
IFN-γ	Cytokine that activates the immune response. There is no production of IFN gamma in the process of FAC.							Few	Few

Table 4. Role of the cytokines during fulminant amebic colitis. *Epithelium (E), Lamina propria (LM), Sub-mucosa (SM).** Significant values with respect to healthy intestinal tissue. # Significant values with respect to areas outside the ulcer of the intestine of patients with FAC.

6.2 During FAC, the anti-inflammatory response is augmented, and thus the prevalence of a Th2 type response

IL-10, a cytokine of the Th2 response with pleiotropic functions, has immunosuppressive properties and acts in various immunological settings. The augmenting of this cytokine in amebiasis is probably responsible for enabling ample amebic invasion of intestine as well as liver (Bansal et al., 2005; Sierra-Puente et al., 2009). Sierra-Puente et al (2009) were the first to publish that IL-10 is produced by epithelial cells in the intestine of patients with FAC. By using antibodies from rabbit anti-human IL-10, it was observed in intestinal tissue of patients with FAC that this cytokine was intensely expressed by epithelial cells outside the ulcer (10.3512 ± 1.9220) (Fig. 12a) compared to healthy intestine (2.3002 ± 0.5814). On the other hand, in lymphoid cells of the lamina propria infected by *E. histolytica*, there was no positive reaction to this cytokine (Fig. 12b).

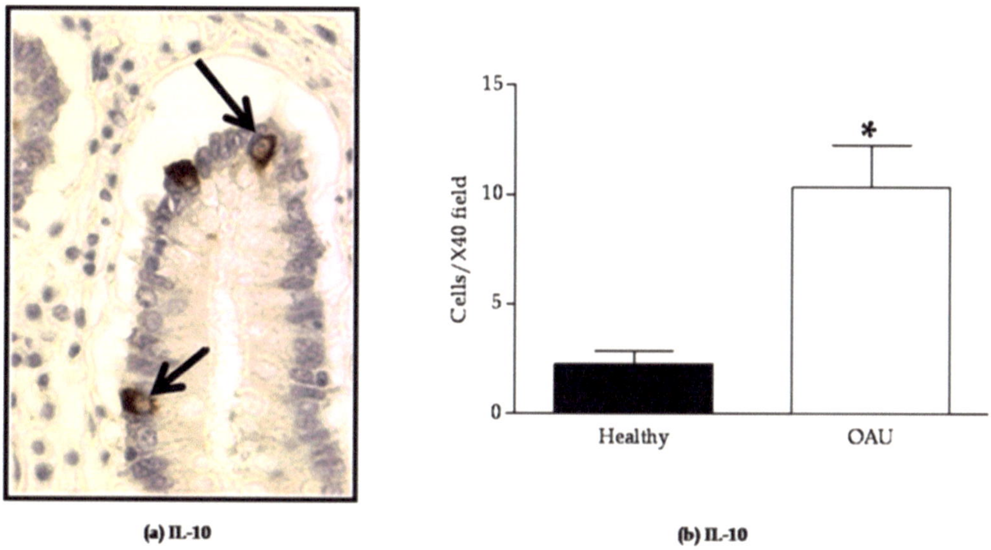

Fig. 12. **Increase of IL-10 in epithelial cells during FAC. (a)** Epithelial cells positive to IL-10 (arrows) outside the amebic ulcer (Immunoperoxidase, X400). **(b)** Graphic representation of IL-10+ cells in healthy intestines and outside the ulcer (OAU) in the intestine of patients with FAC. Bars represents the mean ± SEM ($p \leq 0.01$; Students *t* Test).

In different experimental models, an important role has been suggested for IL-10 in the stimulation of innate resistance to *E. histolytica* infection, although the possible mechanisms are still unknown (Hamano et al., 2006). One possible mechanism could be the participation of IL-10 in the stimulation of the production of mucous by goblet cells in the epithelium (Schwerbrock et al., 2004), which in turn maintains the protective mucous barrier. Another possible mechanism is based on the immunosuppressive effects of IL-10 from epithelial cells on leukocytes (García-Zepeda et al., 2007). Reports in the literature indicate that patients with invasive amebiasis (colitis and AHA) have a greater expression of IL-10 by mononuclear cells of peripheral blood (Bansal et al., 2005).

IL-4 is another cytokine classically generated by Th2 lymphocytes whose principal function is to induce a humoral response. In patients with amebiasis, this cytokine probably is responsible for suppressing the IFN-γ producing Th1 cells, and in this way contributing to the resistance to amebic invasion (Guo et al., 2008). Sierra Puente et al (2009) found, by employing specific antibodies, that IL-4 is expressed in numerous lymphocytes located in the lamina propria adjoining the amebic ulcer (12.3600 ± 1.6660) (Fig. 13a-b). No positive reaction to this cytokine was found in lymphocytes located in the ulcer near trophozoites (figure 13a), although there were traces found in lymphocytes from healthy intestines (1.0001 ± 0.4082) (Fig. 13b).

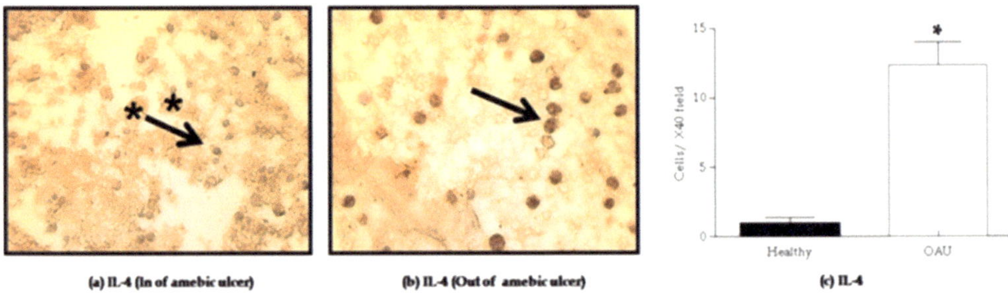

Fig. 13. **Presence of IL-4+ lymphocytes during FAC. (a)** Lymphocytes (arrows) in the lamina propria and near *E. histolytica* trophozoites (*) do not express IL-4+ in the amebic ulcer. **(b)** Lymphocytes located in the lamina propria outside the ulcer and far from the trophozoites show reactivity to IL-4 (arrows) (Immunoperoxide, X400). **(c)** Graphic representation of IL-4+ cells located in healthy intestine and outside the ulcer in the intestine of patients with FAC. Bars represents the mean ± SEM ($p \leq 0.01$; Students *t* Test).

In peripheral blood of individuals infected with *E. histolytica*, it has been demonstrated that mononuclear cells express IL-4 to a significantly greater degree than healthy individuals (Sánchez-Gillén et al., 2002). Furthermore, in a study on a cecal loop mice model of amebiasis, a rapid and sustained increase was shown in the cytokines type Th2 (IL-4 +, IL-5+ IL-13+) as well as an inhibition of the production of IFN-γ (Guo & Houpt, 2008).

It is well-known that the immunoregulation phenomenon in the intestine is mainly driven by TGF-β producing Th3 cells, which also have regulating functions for the inflammatory response (Houpt et al., 2002).

Sierra-Puente et al (2009) identified TGF-β producing cells with mouse anti-human TGF-β antibodies (Fig. 14a), noting a significant diminishment of positive epithelial cells in patients with FAC (7.7880 ± 1.1410) with respect to the epithelium of healthy intestinal tissue (13.4100 ± 1.1400). However, no significant difference was found in the lamina propria of intestines of patients with FAC (7.4740 ± 1.2740) compared to samples from healthy intestinal tissue (5.0290 ± 1.3030) (Fig. 14b). The decrease in TGF-β producing epithelial cells in intestines with FAC perhaps owes itself to the fact that the presence of *E. histolytica* causes the loss of immunological homeostasis in the intestinal lumen and mucosa. In patients with FAC, the presence of *E. histolytica* trophozoites induces a decrease in TGF-β production in the epithelium of the mucosa and an increase in the synthesis of IL-1 and IL-8, which are chemotactic and pro-inflammatory cytokines (Houpt et al., 2002; Sierra-Puente et al., 2009).

IFN-γ plays an important role in the pathogenesis of amebiasis in patients, rodent models and *in vitro* experiments. In general, in humans with amebiasis (Sierra-Puente et al., 2009) and in

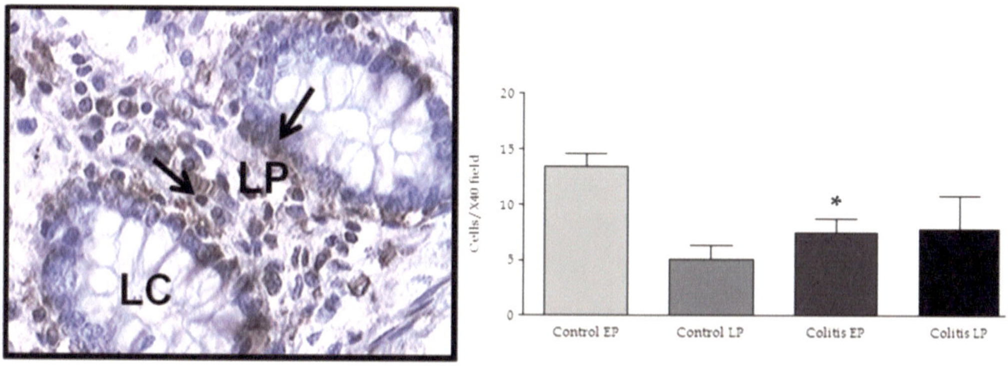

(a) TGF-β (b) TGF-β

Fig. 14. **TGF-β-producing cells of the mucosa in intestines of patients with FAC. (a)** Epithelial cells positive to TGF-β (arrows) were detected in the Lieberkhün crypts (LC) and the lamina propria (LP) (Immunoperoxidase, X400). **(b)** Graphic representation of TGF-β - cells located in epithelium of the Lieberkhün crypts (LC) and the lamina propria (LP) of healthy intestinal tissue and areas outside of the ulcer in the intestine of patients with FAC. Bars represents the mean ± SEM ($p \leq 0.01$; Students *t* Test).

experimental models (Seydel et al., 2000), the production of high levels of IFN-γ is associated with resistance to infection, and the production of low levels to greater susceptibility to intestinal and hepatic amebiasis (Guo et al., 2008). *In vitro* studies suggest that macrophages and neutrophils activated with IFN-γ increase their amoebicidal capacity (Campbell & Chadee, 1997; Ghadirian & Denis, 1992).

In studies conducted in the intestine of patients with FAC, Sierra-Puente (2009) did not find IFN-γ expression in inflammatory cells, coinciding with the finding of scarce macrophages in amebic ulcers reported by Ventura-Juárez (2007). Hence, the amoebicidal factor mediated by IFN-γ is inhibited in the intestine, a phenomenon probably related to the increase in the production of IL-4 and IL-10, which in turn principally inhibit IFN-γ producing Th1 cells (Sierra-Puente et al., 2009). It is worth noting that IFN-γ was not expressed in inflammatory infiltrate cells, whether near to or distant from amebas, but was indeed detected in the majority of *E. histolytica* trophozoites (Fig. 15) (see table 4). The positive reaction of trophozoites to IFN-γ could be due to the presence of T cells phagocyted by amebas.

7. CD59 could be linked to *E. histolytica* resistance to the innate immune response

It can be seen that during the processes of FAC, the activity of the cellular and humoral immune response (Ig) is inhibited in necrotic zones of ulcers. On the other hand, in areas outside the amebic ulcer and in absence of trophozoites, the cellular response and IgA and IgG producing plasma cells are active. This leads to the conclusion that *E. histolytica* possibly has some component on its membrane that allows it to protect itself from the immune response, and thus proceed to damage the intestine.

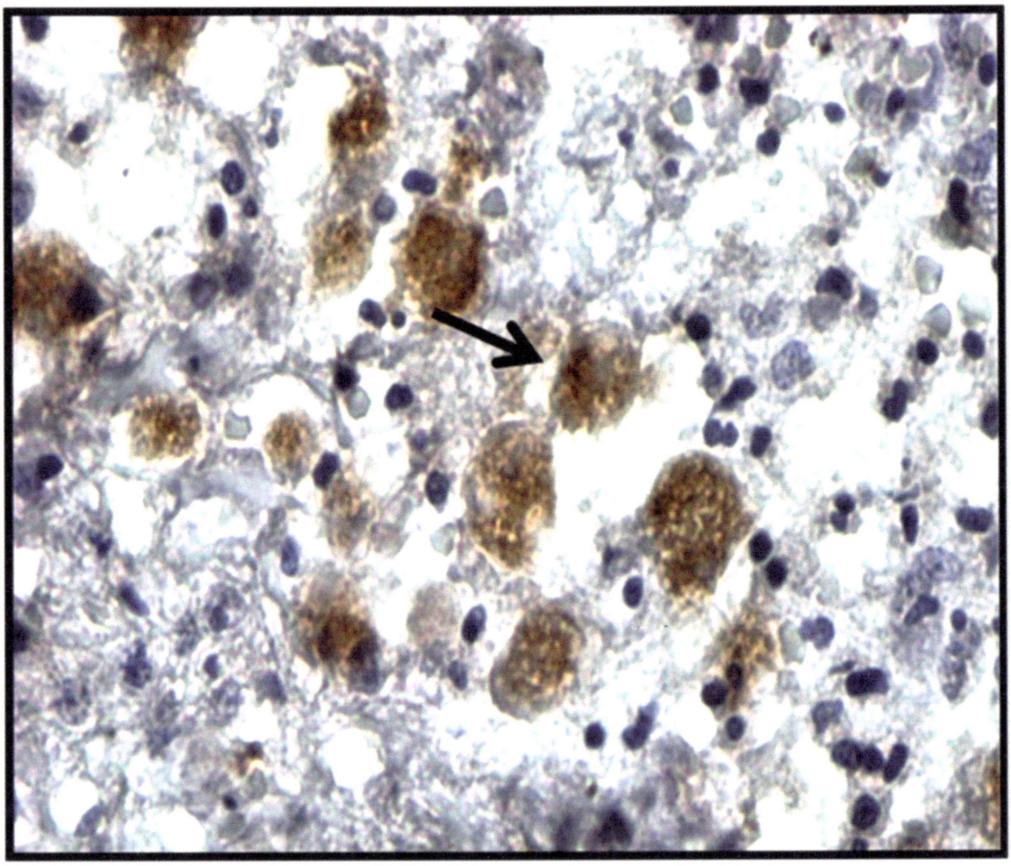

Fig. 15. ***E. histolytica*** **trophozoites positive to IFN-γ in the intestine of patients with FAC.** It can be seen that the trophozoites (arrow) with inflammatory infiltrate in the mucosa adjoining the ulcer (Immunoperoxidase, X400).

CD59 is a widely distributed membrane glycoprotein weighing 18-20 kDa. It covalently binds the membrane of the trophozoites to the surface of a host cell through an anchor called phosphatidil inositol. CD59 inhibits the cytolytic activity of the complement by binding to C8 and C9, and thus blocking the formation of the complex that could attack the membrane of the trophozoites (Lachmann, 1991).

Previous studies with pathogenic *E. histolytica* trophozoites have demonstrated the presence of proteins that share epitopes with human CD59, which probably protects amebas against lysis by the complement (Braga et al., 1992; Flores-Romo et al., 1994; Petri et al., 2002; Fritzinger et al., 2006). Nevertheless, the group of Ventura-Juárez (2009) found the antigen of CD59 by using immunohistochemical and immune-gold techniques. By light microscopy they observed that all trophozoites of *E. histolytica* immunostained with the CD59 antibody existed individually in necrotic zones of the amebic ulcer in the presence or absence of inflammatory infiltrate (Fig. 16a). By Electron Transmission Microscopy, trophozoites CD59 immunostained were identified, principally on their cellular membrane and to a lesser extent in the cytoplasm and vacuoles (Fig. 16b). However, *in vitro* it was observed that only some trophozoites express the CD59 protein (Fig. 16c), suggesting that only the trophozoites positive to CD59 manage to evade the immune response and thus induce cellular damage in the intestine.

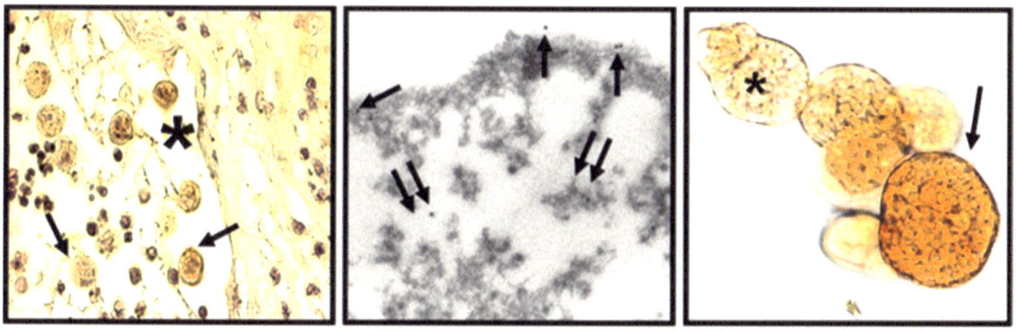

(a) CD59 in E. histolytica *in vivo* (b) CD59 in the cell membrane and citoplasm (c) CD59 in E. histolytica *in vitro*

Fig. 16. ***E. histolytica*** **trophozoites present CD59+ on their membrane during FAC. (a)** In human intestines with FAC, CD59 is found on the plasmatic membrane of whole trophozoites (arrow), surrounded by a halo without tissue or cellular debris (*) (Immunoperoxidase, X400). **(b)** Trophozoite marked with CD59+ presents abundant immunostaining on the cell membrane (arrow) and to a lesser extent on the cytoplasm (double arrows) located in the intestine of patients with FAC (Immune-gold, Electron Transmission Microscopy, X9450). **(c)** Some *E. histolytica* trophozoites *in vitro* present positive immunoreaction to CD59 on the plasmatic membrane (Immunoperoxidase, X1000).

On the other hand, on extract proteins of *E. histolytica* trophozoites, it was confirmed by Western Blot that the protein located on the surface of trophozoites corresponds to a molecular weight of approximately 21 kDa, similar to CD59 of mammalian cells (18–20 kDa) (Davies & Lachmann, 1993) as well as to the CD59 protein on *N. fowleri* (Fritzinger et al., 2006). In spite of this information, the source of these CD59 molecules in intestines with FAC is not clear. The presence of immunoreactive material in cytoplasm and vacuoles could indicate an endogenous synthesis. Another possibility is that CD59 recaptures intestinal fluid or phagocytes erythrocytes (Gutierrez-Kobeh et al., 1997). Therefore, the CD59 protein on the surface of *E. histolytica* trophozoites that invade human colon probably have an important mechanism of protection against the action of macrophages that enable their pathogenic mechanism to later do damage (Ventura-Juárez et al., 2009).

So far the precise mechanisms that allow *E. histolytica* to invade the intestine and cause peritonitis have not been clearly identified. However, it is known that there is no production of INFγ and IgM is decreased in intestinal tissue, which indicates the importance of determining these two immunological parameters in the serum of patients.

8. Conclusion

Although fulminant amebic colitis affects a tiny number of patients, it is a mortal manifestation of invasive intestinal amebiasis, and is generally associated with other pathologies. *E. histolytica* induces the activation of the innate immune response, which is not capable of eliminating the parasite, but is indeed capable of contributing to the pathogenesis by causing cellular damage on the walls of the colon. At the same time, *E. histolytica* partially induces an adaptive immune response that has immunosuppressive features. Much remains to be elucidated, as there is still no model that enables researchers to reproduce all of the aspects of the host-parasite interaction taking place in humans.

9. Acknowledgments

We are grateful to Bruce Allan Larsen for his support in translating the manuscript to English. We give our thanks to the Universidad Autónoma of Aguascalientes for the support given to the projects PIBB01-10N, PIBB05-2, PIBB06-2, PIBB07-6n and PIBB07-4. Also our thanks to CONACYT for support given to the projects 34611M (basic science awards, 2001), 49749 (2005) and 134487 (2009). Finally, we again thank CONACYT for support given to PhD María del Rosario Campos-Esparza in the second year of her postdoctoral fellowship (2010).

10. References

Aikat, B., Bhusnurmath, S., Pal, A., Chhuttani, P. & Datta, D.(1979). The pathology and pathogenesis of fatal hepatic amebiasis: a study based on 79 autopsy cases. *Trans R Soc Trop Med Hyg*, 73, 188–192.

Bansal, D., Sehgal, R., Chawla, Y., Malla, N. & Mahajan, RC. (2005). Cytokine mRNA expressions in symptomatic vs. Asymptomatic amoebiasis patients. *Parasite Immunol*, 27, 37–43.

Benítez B,L., Pérez, A. & Freyre, H. (1987) Tinción histoquímica para la proteína básica mayor mediante eritrosina B alcalina, en granulocitos eosinófilos y espermatozoides. *Arch Invest Med (Méx)*, 18, 213.

Braga, L., Ninomiya, H., McCoy, J., Eacker, S., Wiedmer, T., Pham, C., Wood, S., Sims, P. & Petri, WJr. (1992). Inhibition of the complement membrane attack complex by the galactose-specific adhesion of Entamoeba histolytica. *J Clin Invest,* 90, 1131–1137.

Burchard, G., Prange, G. & Mirelman, D. (1993). Interaction between trophozoites of *Entamoeba histolytica* and the human intestinal cell line HT-29 in the presence or absence of leukocytes. *Parasitol Res*, 79, 140–145.

Campbell, D. & Chadee, K. (1997) Interleukin (IL)-2, IL-4, and tumor necrosis factor-alpha responses during *Entamoeba histolytica* liver abscess development in gerbils. *J. Infect Dis*, 175, 1176-83.

Campos-Rodríguez, R., Jarillo-Luna, RA., Larsen, BA., Rivera-Aguilar, V. & Ventura-Juárez, J. (2009). Invasive amebiasis: A microcirculatory disorder?. *Medical Hypotheses*, 73, 687-697.

Chun, D., Chandrasoma, P. & Kiyabu, M. (1994). Fulminant amebic colitis. A morphologic study of four cases. *Dis Colon Rectum,* 37, 535-9.

Douglas, SL. & Rodger, CH. (1997). Colon, In: *Histology for Pathologists,* second edition, Stephen S Stenberg, 520-528, Lippincot-Raven, ISBN:0-397-51718-1, New York, USA.

Eckmann, L., Reed, S., Smith, J. & Kagnoff, M. (1995). Entamoeba histolytica trophozoites induce an inflammatory cytokine response by cultured human cells through the

paracrine action of cytolytically released interleukin-1 alpha. *J Clin Invest*, 96, 1269–1279.
Enerback, L., Miller, H. & Mayrhofer, G. (1986) Methods for the identification and characterization of mast cells by light microscopy, In *Mast Cells Differentiation and Heterogeneity*, Befus, A., Bienenstock, J., Denburg, J, 405–417, Raven Press, ISBN 0890048967, New York,
Espinosa-Cantellano, M. & Martínez-Palomo, A. (2000). Pathogenesis of intestinal amebiasis. From molecules to disease. *Clin. Microbiol. Rev*, 13, 318-331.
Flores-Romo, L., Tsutsumi, V., Estrada-García, T., Shibayama, M., Aubry, J., Bacon, K. & Martinez-Palomo, A. (1994). CD59 (protectin) molecule, resistance to complement, and virulence of *Entamoeba histolytica. Trans R Soc Trop Med Hyg*, 88, 116–117.
Fritzinger, A., Toney, D., MacLean, R. & Marciano-Cabral, F. (2006). Identification of a Naegleria fowleri membrane protein reactive with anti-human CD59 antibody. *Infect Immun* 74, 1189–1195.
García-Zepeda, EA., Rojas-López, A., Esquivel-Velázquez, M. & Ostoa-Saloma, P. (2007). Regulation of the inflammatory immune response by the cytokine/chemokine network in amoebiasis. *Parasite Immunol*, 29, 679-84.
Ghadirian, E. & Denis, M. (1992) In vivo activation of macrophages by IFN-gamma to kill Entamoeba histolytica trophozoites in vitro. *Parasite Immunol*, 14, 397–404.
Guo, X., Houpt, E., Petri, WA Jr. (2007). Crosstalk at the initial encounter: interplay between host defense and ameba survival strategies. *Curr Opin Immunol*, 19, 376–384.
Guo, X., Stroup, S. & Houpt, E. (2008). Persistence of Entamoeba histolytica infection in CBA mice owes to intestinal IL-4 production and inhibition of protective IFN-γ. *Mucosal Immuno*, 1, 139–146.
Gutierrez-Kobeh, L., Cabrera, N. & Perez-Montfort, R. (1997), A mechanism of acquired resistance to complement-mediated lysis by Entamoeba histolytica. *J Parasitol*, 83, 234–241.
Hamano, S., Asgharpour, A., Stroup, SE., Wynn, TA., Leiter, EH. & Houpt, E. (2006). Resistance of C57BL/6 mice to amoebiasis is mediated by nonhemopoietic cells but requires hemopoietic IL- 10 production. *J Immunol*, 177: 1208–1213.
Haque, RIM. Ali, RB., Sack, BM., Farr, GR. & Petri, WJr. (2001). Amebiasis and mucosal IgA antibody against the *Entamoeba histolytica* adherence lectin in Bangladeshi children. *J Infect Dis*, 183, 1787- 93.
Houpt, ER., Glembocki, DJ., Obrig, TG., Moskaluk, CA., Lockhart, LA., Wright, RL., Seaner, RM., Keepers, TR., Wilkins, TD. & Petri, WJr. (2002). The mouse model of amebic colitis reveals mouse strain susceptibility to infection and exacerbation of disease by CD4+ T cells. *J Immunol*, 169, 4496–4503.
Huston, CD. (2004). Parasite and host contributions to the pathogenesis of amoebic colitis. *Trends Parasitol*, 20, 23–26.
Jarillo-Luna, R., Campos-Rodríguez, R. & Tsutsumi, V. (2002). *Entamoeba histolytica*: immunohistochemical study of hepatic amoebiasis in mouse. Neutrophils and nitric oxide as possible factors of resistance. *Exp Parasitol*, 101, 40–56.
Kammanadiminti, S., Dey, I. & Chadee, K. (2007). Induction of monocyte chemotactic protein 1 in colonic epithelial cells by Entamoeba histolytica is mediated via the phosphatidylinositol 3-kinase/p65 pathway. *Infect Immun*, 75, 1765–1770.

Knight, PA., Wright, S., Lawrence E., Paterson, Y. & Miller, R. (2000). Delayed expulsion of the nematode *Trichinella spiralis* in mice lacking the mucosal mast cell-specific granule chymase, mouse mast cell protease-1. *J Exp Med,* 192: 1849.

Koh, PS., Roslani, AP., Vimal, KV., Shariman, M., Umasangar, R. & Lewellyn, R. (2010). Concurrent amoebic and histoplasma colitis. A rare cause of massive lowergastrointestinal bleeding. *World J. Gaestroenterol,* 16: 1296-1298.

Kretschmer, R., Collado, M., Pacheco, M., Salinas, M., López-Osuna, M., Lecuona, M., Castro, E. & Arellano, J. (1985). Inhibition of human monocyte locomotion by products of axenically grown E. histolytica. *Parasite Immunol,* 7, 5, 527-43.

Lachmann, P. (1991). The control of homologous lysis. *Immunol Today,* 12, 312–315.

Lee, E., Schiller, L. & Fordtran, J. (1988) Quantification of colonic lamina propria cells by means of a morphometric point-counting method. *Gastroenterology,* 94, 409–418.

López-Osuna, M. & Kretschmer, R. (1989). Destruction of normal human eosinophils by Entamoeba histolytica. *Parasite Immunol,* 1, 403-11.

Lopez-Osuna, M., Cardenas, G., Arellano, J., Fernandez-Diez, J. & Kretschmer, R. (2002). Eosinopenia induced by anti-IL-5 antibody, but not *Eimera nieschulzi* extract, increases susceptibility to experimental amoebic abscess of the liver (EAAL) in gerbils. *Arch Med Res;* 33, 316.

López-Osuna, M., Velázquez, J. & Kretschmer, R. (1997). Does the eosinophil have a protective role in amebiasis? *Mem Inst Oswaldo Cruz,* 92, 237-40.

Lotter, H., González-Roldán, N., Lindner, B., Winau, F., Isibasi, A., Moreno-Lafont, M., Ulmer, A., Holst, O., Tannich, E. & Jacobs, T. (2009). Natural killer T cells activated by a lipopeptidophosphoglycan from *Entamoeba histolytica* are critically important to control amebic liver abscess. *PLoS Pathog,* 5(5): e1000434.

Martínez-Palomo, A. (1987). The pathogenesis of amoebiasis. *Parasitol Today,* 3, 111–118.

Masliah, E. & Pérez-Tamayo, R. (1984). Nota sobre la histopatología de la amibiasis invasora del intestino grueso. *Patología (Mex.),* 22, 233-245.

Mortimer, L. & Chadee, K. (2010). The immunopathogenesis of Entamoeba histolytica. *Exp Parasitol,* 126, 366-80.

Natarajan, A., Souza, R., Lahoti, N. & Candrakala, S. (2000). Ruptured liver abscess with fulminant amoebic colitis: case report with review. *Trop Gastroenterol,* 21, 201–203.

Park, S., Jeon, H., Kim, J., Kim, W., Kim, K., Oh, S., Kim, E., Chang, S. & Lee E. (2000). Toxic amebic colitis coexisting with intestinal tuberculosis. *J. Korean Med Sci,* 15, 708-11.

Pérez-Tamayo, R. (1986). Patología de la Amibiasis. In *Amibiasis,* Martínez-Palomo A, 42-78. Editorial Médica Panamericana, ISBN: 968-7157-29-1, México.

Petri, W Jr., Haque, R. & Mann, B. (2002). The bittersweet interface of parasite and host: lectin-carbohydrate interactions during human invasion by the parasite *Entamoeba histolytica. Annu Rev Microbiol,* 56, 39–64.

Pittman, F., Pittman, J. & El-Hashimi, W. (1976). Human amebiasis: Light and electron microscopic findings in colonic mucosal biopsies from patients with acute amebic colitis. In *Proceedings of the International Conference on Amebiasis,* Sepúlveda B, Diamond LS, 398–417, México.

Prathap, K. & Gilman, R. (1970). The histopathology of acute intestinal amebiasis. A rectal biopsy study. *American Journal of Pathology,* 60, 229-245.

Que, X. & Reed, S. (2000). Cysteine proteinases and the pathogenesis of amebiasis. *Clin Microbiol Rev,* 13, 196–206.

Que, X., Kim, S., Sajid, M., Eckmann, L., Dinarello, C., McKerrow, J. & Reed, S. (2003). A surface amebic cysteine proteinases inactivates interleukin-18. *Infect Immun* 71, 1274–1280.

Rico, G. & Kretschmer, R. (1997). The monocyte locomotion inhibitory factor (MLIF) produced by axenically grown Entamoeba histolytica fails to affect the locomotion and the respiratory burst of human eosinophils in vitro. *Arch Med Res*, 28, 233-4.

Rivero-Nava, L., Aguirre-Garcia, J., Shibayama-Salas, M., Hernandez-Pando, R., Tsutsumi, V. & Calderón, J. (2002). *Entamoeba histolytica*: acute granulomatous intestinal lesions in normal and neutrophil depleted mice. *Exp Parasitol*, 101, 183–192.

Sánchez-Guillén, MC., Perez-Fuentes, R. & Salgado-Rosas, H. (2002). Differentiation of *Entamoeba histolytica / Entamoeba dispar* by PCR and their correlation with humoral and celular immunity in individuals with clinical variants of amoebiasis. *Am J Trop Med Hyg*, 66, 731–737.

Schwerbrock, NM., Makkink, MK. & Van der Sluis, M. (2004). Interleukin 10-deficient mice exhibit defective colonic Muc2 synthesis before and after induction of colitis by comensal bacteria. *Inflamm Bowel Dis*, 10: 811–823.

Seydel, K., Li, E., Swanson, P. & Stanley, SJr. (1997). Human intestinal epithelial cells produce proinflammatory cytokines in response to infection in a SCID mouse-human intestinal xenograft model of amebiasis. *Infect Immun*, 65, 1631–1639.

Seydel, K., Li, E., Zhang, Z. & Stanley, SJr. (1998). Epithelial cell-initiated inflammation plays a crucial role in early tissue damage in amebic infection of human intestine. *Gastroenterology*, 115, 1446–1453.

Seydel, KB, Smith, SJ. & Stanley, SJr. (2000). Innate immunity to amebic liver abscess is dependent on gamma interferon and nitric oxide in a murine model of disease. *Infect Immun*, 68, 400–402.

Shetty, N., Nagpal, S., Rao, S. & Schröder, H. (1990). Detection of IgG, IgA, IgM and IgE Antibodies in Invasive Amoebiasis in Endemic Areas. *Scandinavian Journal of Infection Diseases*, 22, 4, 485-491.

Sierra-Puente, R., Campos-Rodríguez, R., Jarillo-Luna, R., Muñoz-Fernández, L., Rodríguez, M., Muñoz-Ortega, M. & Ventura-Juárez, J. (2009). Expression of immune modulator cytokines in human fulminant amoebic colitis. *Parasite Immunol*, 31, 384-91.

Stanley, S. & Reed, S. (2001). Microbes and microbial toxins: Paradigms for microbial-mucosal infections. VI. *Entamoeba histolytica*: parasite–host interactions. *Am J Physiol Gastrointest Liver Physiol*, 280, G1049–G1054.

Takahashi, T., Gamboa-Domínguez, A., Gómez-Méndez, T., Remes, J., Rembis, V., Martínez-González, D., Gutiérrez-Saldívar, J., Morales J., Granados, J. & Sierra-Madero, J. (1997). Fulminant amebic colitis: analysis of 55 cases. *Dis Colon Rectum*, 40, 1362-7.

Tsutsumi, V. & Shibayama, M. (2006). Experimental amoebiasis: A selected review of some *in vitro* models. *Arch Med Res*, 37, 210–220.

Tsutsumi, V., Anaya-Velázquez, F. & Martínez-Palomo, A. (1990). Amibiasis intestinal experimental: invasión y extensión de la lesión amibiana. *Arch Invest Med*, 21, 47–52.

Tsutsumi, V., Mena-López, R., Anaya-Velázquez, F. & Martínez- Palomo, A. (1984). Cellular bases of experimental amoebic liver abscess formation. *Am J Pathol*, 117, 81–91.

Valenzuela, O., Ramos, F., Morán, P., González, E., Valadez, A., Gómez, A., Melendro, E., Ramiro, M., Muñoz, O. & Ximénez, C. (2001). Persistence of secretory antiamoebic antibodies in patients with past invasive intestinal or hepatic amoebiasis. *Parasitol Res*, 87, 10, 849-52.

Velázquez, C., Shibayama-Salas, M., Aguirre-García, J., Tsutsumi, V. & Calderón, J. (1998). Role of neutrophils in innate resistance to *Entamoeba histolytica* liver infection in mice. *Parasite Immunol*, 20, 255–262.

Ventura-Juárez, J., Barba-Gallardo, LF., Muñoz-Fernández L., Martínez-Medina, L., Márquez-Díaz, F., Sosa-Díaz, SJ., Gerardo-Rodríguez, M., González-Romo, R. & Campos-Rodríguez, R. (2007). Immunohistochemical characterization of human fulminant amoebic colitis. *Parasite Immunol*, 29, 201–209.

Ventura-Juárez, J., Campos-Rodríguez, R. & Tsutsumi, V. (2002). Early interactions of Entamoeba histolytica trophozoites with parenchymal and inflammatory cells in the hamster liver: animmunocytochemical study. *Can J Microbiol*, 48, 123–131.

Ventura-Juárez, J., Campos-Rodríguez, R., Jarillo-Luna, RA., Muñoz-Fernández, L., Escario-G-Trevijano, J., Pérez-Serrano, J., Quintanar, J., Salinas, E. & Villalobos-Gómez, F. (2009). Trophozoites of *Entamoeba histolytica* express a CD59-like molecule in human colon. *Parasitol Res*, 104, 821-6.

Ventura-Juárez, J., Campos-Rodríguez, R., Rodríguez-Martínez, H., Rodríguez-Reyes, A., Martínez-Palomo, A. & Tsutsumi, V. (1997). Human amoebic liver abscess: Expression of ICAM-1, ICAM- 2 and Von Willebrand factor endothelial cells. *Parasitol Res*, 83, 510–514.

Ventura-Juárez, J., González-Pérez, S., Jarillo-Luna, R. & Campos-Rodríguez, R. (1990). Mast cells in Peyer's patches in the Mouse. *Arch Invest Med (Mex)* 21, 2, 139-43.

Ventura-Juárez, J., Jarillo-Luna, R., Fuentes-Aguilar, E., Pineda-Vázquez, A., Muñoz-Fernández, L., Madrid-Reyes, J. & Campos-Rodríguez, R. (2003). Human amoebic hepatic abscess: *in situ* interactions between trophozoites, macrophages, neutrophils and T cells. *Parasite Immunol*, 25, 503–511.

Wershil, B., Furuta, T., Wang, S. & Galli, J. (1996). Mast celldependent neutrophil and mononuclear cell recruitment in immunoglobulin Einduced gastric reactions in mice. *Gastroenterology*, 110:1482.

Ximénez, C., Hernández, J., Melendro, E. & Ramiro, M. (1990). Fecal and serum anti-amebic antibodies in acute intestinal amebiasis. *Arch Invest Med (Mex)*, 21, 1, 239-44.

Yu, Y. & Chadee, K. (1997). *Entamoeba histolytica* stimulates interleukin 8 from human colonic epithelial cells without parasiteenterocyte contact. *Gastroenterology*, 112, 1536–154.

Part 3

Drug-Induced Colitis

6

Chemotherapy–Induced Colitis

Carlos H. Barcenas and Nuhad K. Ibrahim
University of Texas MD Anderson Cancer Center, Houston, USA

1. Introduction

Colitis is a very complex disease entity with several etiologic and pathogenesis charactistics. It may have acute or chronic forms that may be with significant morbidity and negative effect on the quality of life of the patient. While the most common and recognizable forms are those of infectious etiologies, however, other forms include ulcerative, Crohn's, immunologic, vascular, pseudo membranous, lymphocytic and collagenous types, to name some. Many different classes of pharmaceutical agents, including non-steroidal anti-inflammatory agents, cyclooxygenase-2 inhibitors, statins, triptans, anti-viral agents, hormone replacement therapies, antidepressants, and antibiotics, are known to induce colitis.[1-4] Colitis is also a well documented side effect of chemotherapy. Chemotherapy-induced colitis may manifest in different clinical settings and have serious sequelae that may impact patient care and outcomes.

Over the past few decades, several novel cytotoxic agents have been found to cause significant gastrointestinal toxicity. The presentation and pathological characteristics of the colitis induced by these novel agents do not necessarily adhere to the traditional description of neutropenic enterocolitis. These newer forms of colitis include taxane-induced colits[5-10] and anti-cytotoxic T-lymphocyte antigen-4 antibody immune-breakthrough enterocolitis.[11-14]

Description of colitis induced by other commonly used cytotoxic agents include reports of cases caused by vinorelbine,[15] capecitabine,[16] interferon,[17] bevacizumab,[18,19] rituximab,[20] dasatinib,[21] and topotecan.[22-24] Given the increasingly frequent use of chemotherapeutic agents capable of causing colitis, clinicians and oncologists should be knowledgeable of this complex condition and its various pathogeneses, risk factors, and prognoses to enhance patient care.

In this chapter we will review the clinical characteristics of the well-known and traditional neutropenic colitis; in addition, we will discuss the more recently described colitis induced by taxanes and by anti-CTLA-4 antibody.

2. Neutropenic enterocolitis

Netropenic colitis is a well recognized entity, however, encountered among cancer patients undergoing chemotherapy treatment. It was the first form of chemotherapy-induced colitis to be described in literature and is a well-known clinical syndrome. Mortality among patients with neutropenic enterocolitis, mainly due to sepsis and bowel perforation, has been reported at rates exceeding 50%.[25, 26] Early recognition of this condition may lead to lower mortality rates, but no prospective studies have explored this topic.

Neutropenic enterocolitis has been known by several names, including typhlitis (from the Greek *typhlon*),[27] neutropenic colitis, necrotizing enterocolitis, ileocecal syndrome, and cecitis.[25, 28] In 1962, neutropenic enterocolitis was described as "necrotizing enteropathy" in autopsy pathology findings of 65 leukemia patients and 7 lymphoma patients.[29, 30]

In 1970, Wagner et al[27] described the clinical characteristics and radiographic findings in a group of pediatric patients with advanced neutropenic enterocolitis identified using postmortem findings, and concluded that specific radiographic findings could suggest the diagnosis of typhlitis. Katz et al performed an updated postmortem review of 33 pediatric patients in 1990, and concluded that improved awareness of the signs and symptom of typhlitis, and the setting in which it occurs, may allow for early effective intervention.[31] Sloas et al[32] retrospectively identified 24 pediatric patients with neutropenic enterocolitis treated at a single institution over 30 years and found that the condition occurred more frequently in patients with acute leukemias, and also had the following conclusions: a) computed tomography (CT) scans and ultrasonography (US) were more sensitive for diagnosis than the plain radiography; b) the increase in the incidence of typhlitis may have been due to the wider availability of this imaging technology and to the increase in the intensity of the chemotherapeutic regimens; c) most patients responded to aggressive medical management, in contrast to prior case reports.

Neutropenic enterocolitis has also been reported in adult patients.[33, 34] The increase in number of reported adult cases was likely due to increased physician awareness and to increase in the use of more aggressive chemotherapy. Some authors suggested that surgical outcomes may be better in adults compared to pediatric patients.[33, 34] Otherwise the clinical presentation, radiographic findings and prognosis has been reported as similar in both adults and in pediatric cases.

Besides being primarily associated with acute leukemia, neutropenic enterocolitis has also been reported in patients with aplastic anemia, multiple myeloma, myelodysplastic syndromes, AIDS, cyclic neutropenia, and neutropenia induced by chemotherapy for solid tumors or stem cell transplants.[25, 31, 35-39]

A recent single-institution retrospective review of pediatric patients with neutropenic enterocolitis who had previously received intensive chemotherapy regimens revealed that cytarabine was associated with greater mortality compared to other chemotherapeutic agents.[40] Cytarabine is considered a prototype drug for the development of chemotherapy-induced neutropenic colitis as it is the most common agent associated with episodes of neutropenic enterocolitis reported in various studies.[26, 41]

2.1 Epidemiology

The true incidence of neutropenic enterocolitis is unknown. Based on autopsy reports, its incidence among children with leukemia has been reported as high as 46%.[26,31] After a systematic review of the literature that included 21 studies, Gorschluter et al[41] calculated the pooled incidence rate of neutropenic enterocolitis among adult patients hospitalized for hematological malignancies, high-dose chemotherapy for solid tumors, or aplastic anemia to be 5.3% (95% confidence interval, 4.7%–5.9%), which was similar to the pooled incidence rate of a subgroup of patients with acute leukemias who were treated with myelosuppressive chemotherapy (5.6%; 95% confidence interval, 4.6%–6.9%).

Initial publications of neutropenic enterocolitis cases reported associated mortality rates of 40–50%.[41] A more recent publication reported a mortality rate of 37.5%.[42] However, one publication reported a mortality rate of 11.7% among pediatric patients.[40] Earlier recognition of this condition and improvement in its management may have lowered the mortality rates associated with neutropenic enterocolitis over the years; however, large series on this subject are lacking.

2.2 Pathogenesis

The pathogenesis of neutropenic enterocolitis remains unclear but may involve several factors including mucosal injury by direct chemotherapy toxicity or leukemic infiltration; severe neutropenia; and/or a weakened host defense to intestinal microorganisms.[25,36] Leukemic infiltrates may rarely be implicated, however.[31] Neutropenia and infection are essential causative factors. Bacteria may invade the bowel wall—a process that neutropenia may facilitate—and bacterial endotoxins may infiltrate the bowel, resulting in bacteremia, sepsis, necrosis, and hemorrhage. Anatomically, neutropenic enterocolitis almost always affects the cecum, possibly because of the cecal dispensability and its low blood supply, but can extend to the ascending, transverse, descending, and/or sigmoid colon, as well as the terminal ileum.[31] Pathology specimens may show mucosal edema, mucosal loss, intramural edema, bowel wall thickening (BWT), ulcerations, focal hemorrhage, and/or transmural necrosis. Surgical specimens may contain multiple microorganisms, including gram-negative rods, gram-positive cocci, anaerobes, enterococci, *Candida*, and/or cytomegalovirus. [25, 31, 32] Polymicrobial infection is possible.

Several cytoxic therapies have been associated with neutropenic enterocolitis. In the earliest case reports of neutropenic enterocolitis, the condition was associated with cytotoxic agents used to treat leukemias and lymphomas, such as cytarabine, vincristine, doxorubicin, methotrexate, cyclophosphamide, etoposide, and prednisone.[25,26,31,32] Later studies implicated other agents used to treat solid tumors, such as vinorelbine, taxanes, carboplatin, cisplatin, gemcitabine and fluorouracil.[25,38,43-48] Avigan et al[49] reported neutropenic enterocolitis in 2 patients who underwent autologous stem cell transplant for solid tumors.

2.3 Clinical presentation

The onset of neutropenic enterocolitis symptoms usually occurs 10–14 days after the initiation of chemotherapy, when the neutropenia is at its nadir and the patient becomes febrile.[25] Neutropenic enterocolitis should be suspected in any patient with profound neutropenia (absolute neutrophil count <500 neutrophils/μl), fever, and right lower quadrant abdominal pain. Nausea, vomiting, abdominal distention, and watery or bloody diarrhea may also be present.[26,31,50,51] An acute surgical abdomen with peritoneal signs and septic shock may suggest bowel perforation.

2.4 Diagnosis

Currently, there is no consensus on standardized diagnostic criteria for neutropenic enterocolitis. A recently published diagnostic criteria for neutropenic enterocolitis was proposed by Gorschluter et al[41]:

- Presence of fever (axillary temperature >38.0°C or rectal temperature >38.5°C)
- Abdominal pain (self reported as grade 3 or more using a visual analogous pain score ranging from 1 to 10)
- US or CT demonstration of BWT of >4 mm (transverse scan) over >30 mm (longitudinal scan) in any segment

Pathologic examination of the cecum or affected area would be considered the gold standard but is not practical as colonoscopy and colonic biopsy are generally contraindicated because of the increased risk of bowel perforation, intraabdominal infection, and (especially in thrombocytopenic patients) bleeding.

Imaging studies are recommended to support the clinical diagnosis. Abdominal CT scan (without oral contrast) tends to be preferred over plain abdominal films because CT scan seems to have a lower false-negative rate of diagnosis and is better able to differentiate neutropenic enterocolitis from acute appendicitis or appendiceal abscess.[32] However, CT scan cannot be performed easily in severely ill patients. Therefore, ultrasonography may complement CT or replace it as the diagnostic modality of choice in select patients. In one prospective study, US revealed BWT of >4 mm in all 4 patients with neutropenic colitis and in 1 patient with mucositis, leading the authors to conclude that BWT of >4 mm is a good discriminator to make a clinical diagnosis of neutropenic enterocolitis.[52]

Radiological findings suggestive of neutropenic enterocolitis include BWT, a dilated and fluid-filled cecum, diffuse cecal wall thickening, an inflammatory mass in the right-lower quadrant, pericecal fluid, and inflammatory changes in the pericecal soft tissues.[25,32] Plain films may be normal or show nonspecific findings and occasionally reveal a fluid-filled, distended cecum with dilated adjacent small bowel loops, thumb printing, or localized pneumatosis intestinalis.[26] Barium enemas are usually contraindicated, as they could lead to bowel perforation.

Using an US-measured BWT of >5 mm as the cutoff point for diagnosis, Cartoni et al[53] demonstrated that patients with a positive US had a significantly longer mean duration of symptoms (7.9 days vs. 3.8 days) and a higher mortality rate (29% vs. 0%) than patients with a negative US. Furthermore, among patients with a positive US, the mortality rate among patients with a BWT of >10 mm (60%) was significantly higher than the mortality rate among patients with a BWT of ≤10 mm (4.2%).

However, BWT may not be specific for neutropenic enterocolitis alone. For example, a retrospective review of abdominal CT findings in 76 neutropenic patients revealed that BWT was most common in patients with *C. difficile* colitis, whereas the primary finding in patients with neutropenic enterocolitis and bowel ischemia was pneumatosis.[54] The specific use of BWT to diagnose neutropenic enterocolitis is thus a matter of debate, and a prospective validation study is needed.

2.5 Treatment

There is no standardized treatment guideline for neutropenic enterocolitis because of a lack of prospective randomized trials. Treatment decisions for patients with neutropenic enterocolitis are therefore based on descriptive or retrospective studies and clinical experts' opinions. A conservative treatment approach consisting of a combination of blood products support, broad-spectrum antibiotics, and bowel rest achieved by intravenous fluids and total parenteral nutrition has been recommended for patients who present without complications such as peritonitis, perforation, or massive bleeding.[55,56] Antibiotic coverage for *C. difficile* infection should be added if this infection has not been ruled out.[32] Antifungal treatment should also be considered, as per the guidelines for the management of neutropenic fever. Granulocyte colony-stimulating factor (G-CSF) may also be used to accelerate recovery from neutropenia.[25,26,47,57] Although case report series have reported the benefit of granulocyte transfusions,[58] such therapy is not recommended by consensus. Anticholinergic, anti- diarrheal, and opioid agents should be avoided because they may worsen ileus.

In 1979, Varki et al[59] reported a case of severe neutropenic enterocolitis in which early clinical recognition and surgical intervention resulted in survival advantage. Surgical intervention is recommended for patients with refractory gastrointestinal bleeding (after correcting cytopenias or coagulopathy), peritonitis, bowel perforation and patients who continue to deteriorate despite medical management.[25,26] The standard surgical approach is a 2-stage right hemicolectomy,[25] as neutropenia may impede primary bowel anastomoses.[60]

Because the likelihood of developing a second episode of neutropenic enterocolitis during a subsequent cycle of chemotherapy is notable, patients should be allowed to completely recover from an episode of neutropenic enterocolitis before subsequent chemotherapy is administered.[25]

3. Taxane-induced (ischemic) Colitis

Taxane-induced colitis is a recognized and a distinguished entity of the classically recognized neutropenic colitis or typhlitis. As its name suggest, patients with neutropenic colitis are neutropenic and commonly febrile, occurring at about 2 weeks of the administration of chemotherapy; on the otherhand, taxane- induced colitis occurs at a shorter interval, and is not necessarily associated with neutropenia or fever. Lower abdominal pain with or without diarrhea or blood per rectum should alert the physician to its occurrence.

In 2000, our group reported 6 patients with docetaxel-associated ischemic colitis.[5] Because of the early onset of symptoms, these patients did not fit the classic picture of neutropenic enterocolitis; besides, not all these patients were neutropenic or febrile, the cardinal features of neutropenic enterocolitis. Three patients had received docetaxel in combination with vinorelbine in a phase I trial. The other 3 patients were identified during a scheduled review of toxic effects in subjects enrolled in clinical trials receiving docetaxel: one of the patients received docetaxel as single agent, another patient received it in combination with pamindronate and the last one received it in combination with cyclophosphamide. Other studies have also noted as well the association of taxane-induced colitis with docetaxel with or without its combination with vinorelbine, another antitubulin agent.[6] There have been several case reports of patients who developed ischemic colitis and had a normal or high white blood cell counts after receiving paclitaxel[7, 8] or nab-paclitaxel (Dr. Nuhad Ibrahim, personal communication).

Of the 1,350 breast cancer patients who received taxane-based chemotherapy at MD Anderson Cancer Center between 1997 and 1999, 14 were diagnosed with colitis.[9] Of the 520 patients who received docetaxel, 10 patients (1.9%) developed colitis, and of the 830 patients who received paclitaxel, 4 patients (0.5%) developed colitis. The clinical data of these 14 patients were used to describe the characteristics of taxane-induced colitis. Colitis recurred in 2 patients who were re-challenged with the same taxane and at the same dose-schedule. CT scan findings typically showed diffuse or localized thickening of the colonic wall and revealed pneumoperitoneum in 1 patient. Colonoscopy confirmed ischemic colitis in 2 patients. Blood cultures were positive for coagulase-negative *Staphylococcus* in 3 (20%) of the colitis events, in addition to *Stenotrophomonas maltophilia* in 1 of these events. All patients had negative C. defficile titers. All patients who developed colitis received supportive care with intravenous fluids and broad-spectrum antibiotics. One patient died of septic shock. Two patients underwent hemicolectomy, the pathology of which revealed bowel perforation secondary to transmural necrosis.

3.1 Pathogenesis

The mechanism of taxane-induced colitis is unknown. Bowel necrosis or perforation may be a direct effect of the drug's rendering microtubule bundles nonfunctional, resulting in transient mitotic arrest. Paclitaxel is also known to have antiangiogenic activity and can induce apoptosis, which could account for the necrosis observed in biopsy samples of affected bowel; however, this has not been validated.[9, 10]

3.2 Clinical presentation and diagnosis

The diagnosis of taxane-induced colitis is based on the presence of acute, usually supra pubic abdominal pain with or without neutropenia, fever, diarrhea, or hematochezia. While blood cultures may or not be positive, *C. difficile* titers are always negative. Taxane-induced colitis tends to occur early in the course of the chemotherapy, with a reported median onset of 6 days after the start of a taxane administered every 3 weeks. Colitis onset occurs within 72 hours when the taxane is given weekly, however (Not published data, DR Nuhad Ibrahim).

The radiographic findings of taxane-induced colitis are not specific. CT scan of abdomen and pelvis may reveal involvement of any segment of the bowel or pan colitis as well as BWT, peritoneal stranding, and/or ascites.[10] The cecum may not be involved, as is almost always the case in patients with neutropenic enterocolitis. Histological analysis of a biopsied sample typically reveals ischemic features. Colonoscopy is not recommended because of the risk of bowel perforation.

3.3 Treatment

Aggressive supportive care with intravenous fluids, broad-spectrum antibiotics, and close surgical monitoring until the symptoms have resolved is recommended. Because taxane-induced colitis seems to be dose-related, the taxane dose should be reduced or discontinued to prevent a recurrence.

4. Anti-cytotoxic T-lymphocyte antigen-4 antibody–induced enterocolitis

One novel method of treating cancer is using monoclonal antibodies to target molecules that enhance antitumor immunity. One such molecule, cytotoxic T-lymphocyte antigen-4 (CTLA-4) is a T-cell receptor whose primary role is to down regulate T-cell activation, which results in immune-tolerance to self-antigens and prevents damage to normal host tissue.[61] Preclinical data have shown that CTLA-4 antibodies induce antitumor activity. Anti-CTLA-4 therapy indirectly targets tumor cells by activating the immune system against the tumor.[62] Two human monoclonal antibodies against CTLA-4 have been developed: ipilimumab, which was recently approved by the U.S. Food and Drug Administration for the treatment of metastatic melanoma, and tremelimumab.[63]

4.1 Pathogenesis

Clinical trials of anti-CTLA-4 therapy have revealed a relationship between tumor response and immune-related adverse events, suggesting that the anti-CTLA-4 antibody's mechanism of antitumor action may also affect the normal tissue and explain why this therapy is associated with a spectrum of side effects, including enterocolitis.[12,13] Several mechanisms by which the CTLA-4 blockade exerts its antitumor activity have been proposed: anti-CTLA-4 agents may block CD4+ and CD25+ regulatory T cells, which normally suppress the function and proliferation of tumor-specific $CD4^+$ and $CD8^+$ effector T cells and natural killer cells; or the CTLA-4 blockade may enable the proliferation and enhance the function of effector $CD4^+$ and $CD8^+$ cells, thereby inducing antibody responses; or anti-CTLA-4 antibodies may also cause direct cytotoxicity by directly binding to tumor cells that constitutively express CTLA-4.[14, 62]

The reported safety profiles of CTLA-4 blockade in melanoma patients and in patients with other cancers such as lung, prostate, and renal cancer are similar, which suggests the therapy has class-specific toxicity. The immune-related adverse events in patients receiving anti-CTLA-4 therapy are thought to be the result of nonspecific or cross-reactive tissue damage caused by activated T cells.[13]

Others have suggested that intestinal micro flora and bacterial antigens may be contributing factors to the enterocolitis seen in patients with graft-versus-host disease .[64] This type of enterocolitis may have a similar pathogenesis to the enterocolitis associated with anti-CTLA-4 antibodies. Future clinical research should evaluate the role of prophylactic antibiotics in this entity.

Studies have found an association between enterocolitis and objective tumor regression in melanoma patients and renal cell carcinoma patients, suggesting that enterocolitis could be a surrogate marker of drug efficacy.[11]

4.2 Clinical presentation

The most common grade 3 or 4 adverse events reported in clinical trials of anti-CTLA-4 therapy are enterocolitis, dermatitis, hepatitis, hypophysitis, and uveitis. The most frequent gastrointestinal adverse event in patients with anti-CTLA-4 antibody-induced immune-breakthrough enterocolitis is diarrhea.

Beck et al[11] found that of 198 patients with metastatic melanoma or renal cell carcinoma that were treated with ipilimumab, 41 patients (21%) had been diagnosed with enterocolitis. The hallmark symptom was diarrhea, which occurred in 40 patients (98%) and whose occurrence ranged from 3 soft stools per day to 20 watery stools daily. Other presenting symptoms included abdominal pain (20%), nausea/vomiting (15%), fever (12%), anal pain (10%), rectal bleeding (2%), and constipation (2%). The median time from the last dose of ipilimumab to the onset of symptoms was 11 days (range, 0–59 days), and there was no predictable pattern of symptomology.

Other studies have reported that diarrhea occurs in up to 44% of patients treated with ipilimumab, with grade 2 or worse diarrhea occurring in about 35% of patients and grade 3 or 4 diarrhea occurring in around 18% of patients.[14] One study reported a median time to diarrhea onset of 14 days (range, 5-36 days).[13] Generally, patients have watery or loose diarrhea that occurs 4–8 times a day without blood, fever, nausea, vomiting, or weight loss. Some patients may have abdominal pain.

4.3 Diagnosis

This clinical entity should be suspected in patients receiving a CTLA-4 antibody who develop diarrhea, and in whom other causes of diarrhea have been ruled out. Infectious diarrhea, such as that caused by parasites or *C. difficile*, should be excluded. Beck et al[11] considered patients to have enterocolitis if they had biopsy findings showing enterocolitis or had sudden-onset diarrhea with no alternative etiology, which lessened or resolved with steroids. Macroscopic findings include erythema, edema, friability, and erosions.[13] Histopathological analysis typically reveals neutrophilic inflammation (46% of patients), lymphocytic inflammation (15% of patients), or a combination of neutrophilic and lymphocytic inflammation (38% of patients).[11]

4.4 Treatment

The management of anti-CTLA-4 antibody–induced immune-breakthrough enterocolitis is based on the severity of the diarrhea. Guidelines and treatment algorithms have been published.[12,14] Patients who develop grade 1 diarrhea should receive symptomatic treatment and supportive care. In patients with grade 2 diarrhea, stool studies and colonoscopy can be used to determine whether enterocolitis is present; once the condition is confirmed, treatment is initiated with oral budesonide or prednisone tapering over a minimum of 4 weeks. Patients with grade 3 or 4 diarrhea should be given high-dose steroids such as intravenous methylprednisolone (2 mg/kg) once or twice a day with a minimum taper of 4 weeks. Patients whose enterocolitis is steroid-refractory should be given infliximab.[65] Patients on long-term immunosuppressive therapy should be given prophylactic antimicrobials. Patients receiving anti-CTLA-4 antibody should be educated about immune-related adverse events, which can occur at any time during therapy and require timely treatment.[13]

	Neutropenic Enterocolitis	Ischemic Colitis	Anti-CTLA4 Antibody Enterocolitis
Incidence, %	5.3 [a]	1.03[b]	21,[c] 44[d]
Chemotherapy	Various	Taxanes	Ipilimumab Tremelimumab
Symptoms	Neutropenia, fever, and RLQ abdominal pain	Lower (suprapubic) abdominal pain with or without diarrhea or hematochezia and the absence of *C. difficile*. Fever and neutropenia are not sufficient but not necessary features.	Diarrhea (watery or loose, without blood) occurring 4–8 times a day without fever, nausea, vomiting, or weight loss. Some patients have abdominal pain.
Median time to symptom onset, days (range)	12 (10-14)[e]	6 (3–8)	11 (0–59)
Diagnosis	Clinical presentation and radiologic finding.	Clinical presentation and radiologic findings. Ischemic colitis is the hallmark pathologic finding.	Clinical presentation. Histopathology evaluation may reveal neutrophilic and/or lymphocytic inflammation.
Radiologic findings	Cecal involvement is necessary and/or sufficient; additional colonic segments, pan-colonic, or distal ileum may be involved. US or CT may reveal bowel wall thickening > 4 mm (transverse scan) over more than 30 mm (longitudinal scan) in any.	Not specific. Any segment of the bowel may be involved; disease may be pan-colonic. Cecal involvement may be sufficient but not necessary. CT scan may reveal bowel wall thickening, peritoneal stranding, or ascites	Not specific

Treatment	Conservative management includes bowel rest, IV fluids, antibiotics, and G-CSF. Surgical intervention is reserved for patients with peritonitis, bowel perforation, or massive bleeding.	Supportive care with IV fluids, antibiotics, and close surgical monitoring.	Symptomatic treatment, steroids, or infliximab, depending on the severity of the symptom

CTLA 4, cytotoxic T-lymphocyte antigen 4; RLQ, right lower quadrant; CT, computed tomography; US, ultrasonography; IV, intravenous; G-CSF, granulocyte-colony stimulating factor.
[a] Gorschluter M, Mey U, Strehl J, et al, Eur J Haematol 2005
[b] Li Z, Ibrahim NK, Wathen JK, et al, Cancer 2004
[c] Beck KE, Blansfield JA, Tran KQ, et al, J Clin Oncol 2006
[d] Kaehler KC, Piel S, Livingstone E, et al, Semin Oncol 2010
[e] Davila ML, Curr Opin Gastroenterol 2006

Table 1. Comparison of characteristics of three types of chemotherapy-induced colitis

5. Conclusion

Chemotherapy-induced colitis is a significant complication of multiple chemotherapeutic agents. Its occurrence adds not only to the morbidity of the patient, but also may impact the treatment choices of the patient's cancer management. Early recognition may help the patient avoid grave consequences including death related to its severity. It is therefore essential that it is recognized in its different forms and the various drugs it may be associated with. It remains an uncommon event, however, but early appraisal of the presenting symptom complex in the context of chemotherapy administration is prudent.

6. References

[1] Cappell MS: Colonic toxicity of administered drugs and chemicals. Am J Gastroenterol 99:1175-90, 2004
[2] Schwartz DC, Smith DJ: Colonic ischemia associated with naratriptan use. J Clin Gastroenterol 38:790-2, 2004
[3] Westgeest HM, Akol H, Schreuder TC: Pure naratriptan-induced ischemic colitis: a case report. Turk J Gastroenterol 21:42-4, 2010
[4] Zervoudis S, Grammatopoulos T, Iatrakis G, et al: Ischemic colitis in postmenopausal women taking hormone replacement therapy. Gynecol Endocrinol 24:257-60, 2008
[5] Ibrahim NK, Sahin AA, Dubrow RA, et al: Colitis associated with docetaxel-based chemotherapy in patients with metastatic breast cancer. Lancet 355:281-3, 2000
[6] Kreis W, Petrylak D, Savarese D, et al: Colitis and docetaxel-based chemotherapy. Lancet 355:2164, 2000
[7] Daniele B, Rossi GB, Losito S, et al: Ischemic colitis associated with paclitaxel. J Clin Gastroenterol 33:159-60, 2001

[8] Tashiro M, Yoshikawa I, Kume K, et al: Ischemic colitis associated with paclitaxel and carboplatin chemotherapy. Am J Gastroenterol 98:231-2, 2003
[9] Li Z, Ibrahim NK, Wathen JK, et al: Colitis in patients with breast carcinoma treated with taxane-based chemotherapy. Cancer 101:1508-13, 2004
[10] Kaur H, Loyer EM, David CL, et al: Radiologic findings in taxane induced colitis. Eur J Radiol 66:75-8, 2008
[11] Beck KE, Blansfield JA, Tran KQ, et al: Enterocolitis in patients with cancer after antibody blockade of cytotoxic T-lymphocyte-associated antigen 4. J Clin Oncol 24:2283-9, 2006
[12] Weber J: Review: anti-CTLA-4 antibody ipilimumab: case studies of clinical response and immune-related adverse events. Oncologist 12:864-72, 2007
[13] Di Giacomo AM, Biagioli M, Maio M: The emerging toxicity profiles of anti-CTLA-4 antibodies across clinical indications. Semin Oncol 37:499-507, 2010
[14] Kaehler KC, Piel S, Livingstone E, et al: Update on immunologic therapy with anti-CTLA-4 antibodies in melanoma: identification of clinical and biological response patterns, immune-related adverse events, and their management. Semin Oncol 37:485-98, 2010
[15] Olithselvan A, Gorard DA: Vinorelbine and ischaemic colitis. Clin Oncol (R Coll Radiol) 15:166-7, 2003
[16] Alexandrescu DT, Dutcher JP, Wiernik PH: Capecitabine-induced pancolitis. Int J Colorectal Dis 22:455, 2007
[17] Wenner WJ, Jr., Piccoli DA: Colitis associated with alpha interferon? J Clin Gastroenterol 25:398-9, 1997
[18] Schellhaas E, Loddenkemper C, Schmittel A, et al: Bowel perforation in non-small cell lung cancer after bevacizumab therapy. Invest New Drugs 27:184-7, 2009
[19] Lecarpentier E, Ouaffi L, Mir O, et al: Bevacizumab-induced small bowel perforation in a patient with breast cancer without intraabdominal metastases. Invest New Drugs, 2010
[20] Ardelean DS, Gonska T, Wires S, et al: Severe ulcerative colitis after rituximab therapy. Pediatrics 126:e243-6, 2010
[21] Shimokaze T, Mitsui T, Takeda H, et al: Severe hemorrhagic colitis caused by dasatinib in Philadelphia chromosome-positive acute lymphoblastic leukemia. Pediatr Hematol Oncol 26:448-53, 2009
[22] Sears S, McNally P, Bachinski MS, et al: Irinotecan (CPT-11) induced colitis: report of a case and review of Food and Drug Administration MEDWATCH reporting. Gastrointest Endosc 50:841-4, 1999
[23] Sandmeier D, Chaubert P, Bouzourene H: Irinotecan-induced colitis. Int J Surg Pathol 13:215-8, 2005
[24] Takaoka E, Kawai K, Ando S, et al: Neutropenic colitis during standard dose combination chemotherapy with nedaplatin and irinotecan for testicular cancer. Jpn J Clin Oncol 36:60-3, 2006
[25] Davila ML: Neutropenic enterocolitis. Curr Opin Gastroenterol 22:44-7, 2006
[26] Wade DS, Nava HR, Douglass HO, Jr.: Neutropenic enterocolitis. Clinical diagnosis and treatment. Cancer 69:17-23, 1992

[27] Wagner ML, Rosenberg HS, Fernbach DJ, et al: Typhlitis: a complication of leukemia in childhood. Am J Roentgenol Radium Ther Nucl Med 109:341-50, 1970
[28] Williams N, Scott AD: Neutropenic colitis: a continuing surgical challenge. Br J Surg 84:1200-5, 1997
[29] Amromin GD, Solomon RD: Necrotizing enteropathy: a complication of treated leukemia or lymphoma patients. JAMA 182:23-9, 1962
[30] Gildenhorn HL, Springer EB, Amromin GD: Necrotizing enteropathy: roentgenographic features. Am J Roentgenol Radium Ther Nucl Med 88:942-52, 1962
[31] Katz JA, Wagner ML, Gresik MV, et al: Typhlitis. An 18-year experience and postmortem review. Cancer 65:1041-7, 1990
[32] Sloas MM, Flynn PM, Kaste SC, et al: Typhlitis in children with cancer: a 30-year experience. Clin Infect Dis 17:484-90, 1993
[33] Ikard RW: Neutropenic typhlitis in adults. Arch Surg 116:943-5, 1981
[34] Alt B, Glass NR, Sollinger H: Neutropenic enterocolitis in adults. Review of the literature and assessment of surgical intervention. Am J Surg 149:405-8, 1985
[35] Pokorney BH, Jones JM, Shaikh BS, et al: Typhlitis. A treatable cause of recurrent septicemia. JAMA 243:682-3, 1980
[36] Urbach DR, Rotstein OD: Typhlitis. Can J Surg 42:415-9, 1999
[37] Quigley MM, Bethel K, Nowacki M, et al: Neutropenic enterocolitis: a rare presenting complication of acute leukemia. Am J Hematol 66:213-9, 2001
[38] Cunningham SC, Fakhry K, Bass BL, et al: Neutropenic enterocolitis in adults: case series and review of the literature. Dig Dis Sci 50:215-20, 2005
[39] Bremer CT, Monahan BP: Necrotizing enterocolitis in neutropenia and chemotherapy: a clinical update and old lessons relearned. Curr Gastroenterol Rep 8:333-41, 2006
[40] Rizzatti M, Brandalise SR, de Azevedo AC, et al: Neutropenic enterocolitis in children and young adults with cancer: prognostic value of clinical and image findings. Pediatr Hematol Oncol 27:462-70, 2010
[41] Gorschluter M, Mey U, Strehl J, et al: Neutropenic enterocolitis in adults: systematic analysis of evidence quality. Eur J Haematol 75:1-13, 2005
[42] Dorantes-Diaz D, Garza-Sanchez J, Cancino-Lopez JA, et al: [Prevalence of neutropenic enterocolitis in adults with severe neutropenia and associated mortality.]. Rev Gastroenterol Mex 74:224-9, 2009
[43] Furonaka M, Miyazaki M, Nakajima M, et al: Neutropenic enterocolitis in lung cancer: a report of two cases and a review of the literature. Intern Med 44:467-70, 2005
[44] D'Amato G, Rocha Lima C, Mahany JJ, et al: Neutropenic enterocolitis (typhilitis) associated with docetaxel therapy in a patient with non-small-cell lung cancer: case report and review of literature. Lung Cancer 44:381-90, 2004
[45] Gadducci A, Gargini A, Palla E, et al: Neutropenic enterocolitis in an advanced epithelial ovarian cancer patient treated with paclitaxel/platinum-based chemotherapy: a case report and review of the literature. Anticancer Res 25:2509-13, 2005
[46] Ferrazzi E, Toso S, Zanotti M, et al: Typhlitis (neutropenic enterocolitis) after a single dose of vinorelbine. Cancer Chemother Pharmacol 47:277-9, 2001

[47] Kouroussis C, Samonis G, Androulakis N, et al: Successful conservative treatment of neutropenic enterocolitis complicating taxane-based chemotherapy: a report of five cases. Am J Clin Oncol 23:309-13, 2000
[48] Cardenal F, Montes A, Llort G, et al: Typhlitis associated with docetaxel treatment. J Natl Cancer Inst 88:1078-9, 1996
[49] Avigan D, Richardson P, Elias A, et al: Neutropenic enterocolitis as a complication of high dose chemotherapy with stem cell rescue in patients with solid tumors: a case series with a review of the literature. Cancer 83:409-14, 1998
[50] Cloutier RL: Neutropenic enterocolitis. Hematol Oncol Clin North Am 24:577-84, 2010
[51] Aksoy DY, Tanriover MD, Uzun O, et al: Diarrhea in neutropenic patients: a prospective cohort study with emphasis on neutropenic enterocolitis. Ann Oncol 18:183-9, 2007
[52] Gorschluter M, Marklein G, Hofling K, et al: Abdominal infections in patients with acute leukaemia: a prospective study applying ultrasonography and microbiology. Br J Haematol 117:351-8, 2002
[53] Cartoni C, Dragoni F, Micozzi A, et al: Neutropenic enterocolitis in patients with acute leukemia: prognostic significance of bowel wall thickening detected by ultrasonography. J Clin Oncol 19:756-61, 2001
[54] Kirkpatrick ID, Greenberg HM: Gastrointestinal complications in the neutropenic patient: characterization and differentiation with abdominal CT. Radiology 226:668-74, 2003
[55] Davila ML: Neutropenic enterocolitis. Curr Treat Options Gastroenterol 9:249-55, 2006
[56] Davila ML: Neutropenic enterocolitis: current issues in diagnosis and management. Curr Infect Dis Rep 9:116-20, 2007
[57] Pestalozzi BC, Sotos GA, Choyke PL, et al: Typhlitis resulting from treatment with taxol and doxorubicin in patients with metastatic breast cancer. Cancer 71:1797-800, 1993
[58] O'Brien S, Kantarjian HM, Anaissie E, et al: Successful medical management of neutropenic enterocolitis in adults with acute leukemia. South Med J 80:1233-5, 1987
[59] Varki AP, Armitage JO, Feagler JR: Typhlitis in acute leukemia: successful treatment by early surgical intervention. Cancer 43:695-7, 1979
[60] Glenn J, Funkhouser WK, Schneider PS: Acute illnesses necessitating urgent abdominal surgery in neutropenic cancer patients: description of 14 cases and review of the literature. Surgery 105:778-89, 1989
[61] Liu Z, Geboes K, Hellings P, et al: B7 interactions with CD28 and CTLA-4 control tolerance or induction of mucosal inflammation in chronic experimental colitis. J Immunol 167:1830-8, 2001
[62] Fong L, Small EJ: Anti-cytotoxic T-lymphocyte antigen-4 antibody: the first in an emerging class of immunomodulatory antibodies for cancer treatment. J Clin Oncol 26:5275-83, 2008
[63] Ribas A, Hanson DC, Noe DA, et al: Tremelimumab (CP-675,206), a cytotoxic T lymphocyte associated antigen 4 blocking monoclonal antibody in clinical development for patients with cancer. Oncologist 12:873-83, 2007

[64] Beelen DW, Elmaagacli A, Muller KD, et al: Influence of intestinal bacterial decontamination using metronidazole and ciprofloxacin or ciprofloxacin alone on the development of acute graft-versus-host disease after marrow transplantation in patients with hematologic malignancies: final results and long-term follow-up of an open-label prospective randomized trial. Blood 93:3267-75, 1999
[65] Minor DR, Chin K, Kashani-Sabet M: Infliximab in the treatment of anti-CTLA4 antibody (ipilimumab) induced immune-related colitis. Cancer Biother Radiopharm 24:321-5, 2009

Part 4

Therapeutic Strategy of Colitis

7

Drug and Cell Delivery Systems in the Treatment of Colitis

Kristina Mladenovska
University "Ss Cyril and Methodius", Faculty of Pharmacy, Republic of Macedonia

1. Introduction

The term colitis describes variety of inflammatory diseases of the colon which can be differentiated according to their etiology, clinical, endoscopic and histological characteristics. In general, they can be classified as inflammatory bowel diseases (IBD) and infectious colitis (Hemstreet & Diprio, 2008; Novaneethan & Giannella, 2011), and non-IBD and non-infectious colitis, including ischemic colitis, chemical colitis, microscopic colitis, segmental colitis, radiation colitis, diversion colitis, eosinophilic colitis and Behcet's colitis (Koutroubakis, 2008). The two forms of idiopathic IBD, ulcerative colitis (UC), a mucosal inflammatory condition restricted to the rectum and colon, and Crohn's disease (CD), a transmural inflammation of the GIT affecting any part from the mouth to anus, are the most prevalent, especially in the western countries and in areas of northern latitude. Other forms, such as diversion colitis, eosinophilic colitis and Behcet's colitis are rare, with unknown ethiopathogenesis and limited epidemiological data. Clinical presentation of all forms is very similar and includes mild, moderate or severe local complications, such as diarrhea, abdominal pain or cramping, rectal bleeding and weight loss, and systemic ones, including hepatobiliary, joint, ocular, renal, dermatologic and mucosal complications.

The goals of the treatment include resolving of the acute inflammation and associated complications, alleviation of the systemic manifestations and maintenance of remission. Besides non-pharmacologic therapy, which includes nutritional support and surgical intervention, pharmacologic therapy is an integral part of the overall treatment of colitis. All the drugs are aimed to control the disease allowing the patient to perform normal daily activities. The main pharmacologic groups of drugs used for colitis treatment include aminosalycilates, corticosteroids, immunosuppressive agents, antimicrobials and inhibitors of TNF-α.

In addition, for maintaining remission in various GI diseases, including colitis, live bacterial cell biotherapeutics i.e probiotics, alone or combined with prebiotics as synbiotics, are also administered. Probiotics are defined as "viable microorganisms which alter the microflora (by implantation or colonization) in a compartment of the host and by that exert beneficial effects in the host", while prebiotics as "non-digestible food ingredients that beneficially affect the host by selectively stimulating the growth and/or activity of one or a limited number of bacteria in the colon" are considered (Gibson & Roberfroid, 1995). For prevention and maintaining of remission in colitis, various probiotics were clinically examined during the last decade, among which non-pathogenic *E. coli*, strains of bifidobacteria, lactobacilli, *Streptococcus thermophilus*, enterococci, coliforms, *Bacteroides* and *Clostridium perfringens*. From the prebiotics, the commercially available fructooligosaccharides (FOS), inulin and galactooligosaccharides are frequently used and many other potential prebiotics are still under investigation, among which xylooligosaccharides, soy-oligosacharides, pesticooligosaccharides, glucooligosaccharides, isomaltooligosaccharides and gentiooligosaccharides (Table 1).

Probiotic strain	Therapeutic effect	References
B. bifidium, B. breve, B. infantis, B. lactis LA 303, B. longum infantis UCC35624, B. longum, L. acidophilus LA 201, L. acidophilus, L. casei Shirota, L. casei subsp. Rhamnosus, L. delbruecki subsp. Bulgaricus, L. fermentum BR11, L. plantarum 299V, L. plantarum LA 301, L. paracasei, L. reuteri, L. rhamnosus GG, L. salivarius LA 302, L. salivarius UCC118, Lactococcus lactis, non-pathogenic E. coli Nisle 1917, Sacharomyces boulardi, Str. boulardi, Str. salivarius subsp. Thermophilus	Maintain balance of beneficial *vs.* aggressive commensal enteric microflora: inhibit pathogenic enteric bacteria (decrease luminal pH, secrete bactericidal proteins, resist colonization, block epithelial binding-induction of MUC2, inhibit epithelial invasion–Rho (in)dependent pathways); improve function of epithelial and mucosal barrier (produce short chain fatty acids (SCFAs), enhance mucus production, increase barrier integrity); alter immune-regulation (induce IL-10 and transforming growth factor β expression and secretion, stimulate secretory IgA production, decrease tumor necrosis factor expression).	Geier et al., 2007; Peran et al., 2007; Prakash, 2008.
Prebiotic		
Inulin, lactulose, goat's milk oligosacaccharides, fructo-oligosaccharide, hemi-celluloses- and glutamine-rich extract, maltodextrin	Decrease level of the pro-inflammatory cytokine IL-1β, increase anti-inflammatory TGF-β, increase caecal lactobacillus and bifidobacterium levels, decrease *E. coli* colonization, decrease clostridium and enterobacterium levels, increase levels of SCFAs.	Geier et al., 2007; Gibson & Roberfroid, 1995.

Table 1. Health benefits of different probiotic strains and prebiotics in colitis

Considering the pharmacologic treatment, many patients experience significant undesired effects (Table 2) which require discontinuation of the therapy. Avoiding or minimizing these effects is one of the great challenges in the pharmaceutical industry in which great effort is put on design of an ideal drug delivery system that would deliver the drug at a rate dictated by the needs of the patient within the period of treatment and target it to the specific i.e. inflamed site of the colon. Considering probiotics, the greatest achievement with these advanced delivery systems is their potential to protect the probiotics not only in the pro- or syn-biotic food or pharmaceutical product, but also from the harsh environment of the GIT, and to maintain their functionality unaltered on arrival to the colon. All these prerequisites require modified drug and/or cell release technologies which can improve the therapeutic efficacy and safety by precise temporal and spatial placement in the colon, thereby reducing both the dose and the frequency of administration.

Drug	Adverse effects	References
Aminosalycilates		
Sulfasalazine Mesalamine (5-Aminosalicylic acid; 5-ASA)	Agranulocytosis, pancreatitis, interstitial nephritis, hepatitis, male infertility, arthralgia, pneumonitis. Mesalazaine derivatives manifest lower frequency of adverse effects in comparison with sulfasalazine.	Hemstreet & Diprio, 2008; Linares et al., 2011; Sonu al., 2010.
Corticosteroids		
Budesonide Prednisone Prednisolone Dexamethasone	Hyperglycemia, hypertension, electrolyte disturbances, cataracts, osteoporosis, myopathy, conditions associated with immune suppression, adrenal insufficiency (long-term administration).	Ford et al., 2011.
Imunosupressive agents		
Azathioprine	Pancreatitis, fever, rash, arthralgia, diarrhea, infectious complications, hepatitis, myelo-suppression, known carcinogen.	Gisbert et al., 2009; Hemstreet & Diprio, 2008; Wahed et al., 2009.
Methotrexate	Diarrhea, skin reactions, bone marrow suppression, lung lesions, kidney dysfunction, hepatotoxicity, folic acid deficiency.	
Cyclosporine	Paresthesias, hypertension, nephrotoxicity, seizures.	
Antimicrobial agents		
Metronidazole	Urticaria, glossitis; long-term use may develop paresthesia, reversible peripheral neuropathy.	Hemstreet & Diprio, 2008; Khan et al., 2011.
Vancomycin	Infusion related events, nephrotoxicity, pseudo-membranous colitis, ototoxicity, reversible neutropenia, infrequently anaphylaxis, eosinophilia, rashes including exfoliative dermatitis, linear IgA bullous dermatosis, Steven-Johnson syndrome, vasculitis.	
Ciprofloxacin	Diarrhea, vomiting and rash. Other side effects (e.g. headache, abdominal pain, pain in extremities, injection site reaction, cardiovascular, gastrointestinal, etc.) in less than 1% of the patients.	
Tobramycin	Ototoxicity, nephrotoxicity, neurotoxicity, anemia, granulocytopenia, thrombocytopenia, fever, rash, exfoliative dermatitis, itching, urticaria, diarrhea, headache, lethargy, pain at the injection site, mental confusion, disorientation.	
Inhibitors of TNF-α		
Infliximab Adalimubab Etanercept Certolizumab	Acute infusion reactions, serum sickness, increase in serious infections (e.g. sepsis, pneumonia, tuberculosis), worsening of existing heart failure and even death.	Tursi et al., 2010; Talley et al. 2011.

Table 2. Adverse effects of drugs most commonly used for the treatment of colitis

2. Colon as a target for drug and probiotic cell delivery in colitis; biological and (patho)physiological factors

The principal goals of colon-specific delivery after oral administration are to prevent biodegradation of drugs and maintain viability of the probiotic cells in the stomach and small intestine where acid- or enzyme-labile drugs and cells are degraded, to avoid absorption of drugs in the upper intestine and accordingly, to release the drugs or to provide colonization of the cells in the lower intestine. Motility of the GIT, high surface area of the small intestine, pH of the intestinal fluids, bacterial flora, they all can affect and to a certain instance be an obstacle for efficacious colon targeted and controlled drug/cell delivery after oral administration. The segmental contractions of the colon increase the contact with the mucosa, which in turns promotes the design of mucoadhesive drug delivery systems for colon targeted and prolonged drug/cell release. Colonic transit time of a single-unit delivery systems varies significantly within a day; app. 6 hours are needed for the form to reach the transverse colon in the morning at fasting state, while in the evening, the colonic transfer is slower and app. 11 hours are needed for the dosage form to reach the transverse colon. The transit time from the stomach to the large intestine is 2-4 h and from the small intestine to the anus 6-48 h. This transit time may be altered by many factors, such as age, sex, dietary and disease factors (Washington et al., 2001).

The pH in the GIT ranges from 1.3-1.7 in the resting human stomach to 6.4 in duodenum, and then drops to the range of 5.0-6.5. In the colon, pH ranges from 6.4±06 in the ascending part to 6.6±08 in the transverse colon and 7.0±0.7 in the descending part (Washington et al., 2001). The literature data related to the colonic pH values in the state of colitis are controversial, pointing to increase, decrease or no change of pH at all (Nugent et al., 2001). Unpredictable alteration of the pH profile may significantly affect the viability of the cells and local bioavailability of the drugs by changing their chemical stability and degree of ionization i.e. absorption. This effect is particularly emphasized when delivery systems composed of pH sensitive polymers as drug or cell carriers for colon targeted and controlled release are used.

The total metabolic activity of the colonic wall is much lower than the one in the upper gut, so, the enzymatic degradation of drugs and cells is insignificant. However, the low redox potential favors the growth of low number of fungi and around 10^{12} viable bacteria/g of large bowel content in human. App. 400-500 bacterial are present, dominantly obligate anaerobic species which produce enzymes for lot of metabolic reactions that affect the drug and cell release from their delivery systems. This effect is especially emphasized when biodegradable polymers/systems are used. The predominant anaerobic species in the colon are *Bacteroides, Bifidobacterium, Clostridium, Euboacterium, Fusobacterium, Peptococcus, Peptostreptococcus,* whilst facultative aerobes are represented by *E. coli, Klebsiella, Streptococcus, Staphylococcus, Bacillus and Lactobacillus*. The enzymes they produce are β-glucuronidase, β-galactosidase, nitroreductase, azoreductase, etc. Number of mucosal bacteria increases progressively in the state of inflammation, with concentrations relatively higher in patients with active disease (Prakash & Urbanska, 2008).

The goblet cells, which together with absorptive and endocrine cells make up the colonic epithelial layer, are responsible for the production of mucus. In the inflamed state, patients manifest reduced thickness of the colonic mucus layer due to the reduced number of the goblet cells. The mucus layer is nearly free of bacteria in the mid to distal murine colon, but this is not true for the mucosa-adjacent and luminal regions of the caecum and proximal colon. Microorganisms co-aggregate and form biofilms that adhere to the epithelial surface (Strugala et al., 2008). Fast mucus turnover in colitic patients followed by increased activity of the bacterial enzymes and high concentrations of positively charged amino acids in the peptide core of the mucins may affect the affinity of charged drugs and cells and/or drug and cell delivery systems towards mucosa. Electrostatic interactions that occur may intensify adhesion to the inflamed mucosa and prolong the residence time of the delivery system or drug or cell in the colon. This effect is especially emphasized when bioadhesive polymers as drugs and cell carriers are used. Providing intimate contact with the mucosa, systems composed of bioadhesive polymers become resistant to GI motility, whilst the drug or cell release rate is controlled by the polymers' hydration, erosion and biodegradation.

It is well known that adaptive immune system relays on the lymphocytes, which are organized in Peyer's patches and isolated follicles. M-cells, a constitutional part of the follicle-associated epithelium, are responsible for sampling of particulate materials, including microbial cells. In inflamed mucosa, M cells get damaged and increased, which can significantly affect the selective retention of the small particles in the colon. This is especially significant when multi-particulate dosage forms, with different size distribution, as drug or cell carriers are administered (Washington et al., 2001).

Considering above mentioned, a design and development of advanced drug and cell carrier systems that react exclusively to the conditions in the colon and deliver their content with a controlled rate is of paramount importance. These systems can be optimized by using pH-sensitive and biodegradable polymers that provide selective adhesivity to the colonic mucosa. Delivery to the proximal colon may be achieved only when these systems remain intact for app. first 5 hours after administration and release their content within 10-24 hours.

3. Drug and cell delivery systems in colitis; strategies for targeted and controlled delivery

Advanced systems for colon-targeted and controlled drug and cell delivery in colitis are designed to modify drug and cell release and induce desired local effect by releasing the drug/cells in high concentrations close to the disease area, thereby minimizing systemic side effects. With these modified release dosage forms, not only therapeutic, but also safety and convenience objectives are accomplished, which are not typical for the conventional dosage forms. In conventional (non-parenteral) delivery, when using so called immediate-release dosage forms, blood concentrations of the drug rise after drug administration, than peak and decline. In such dosage forms, only the dose and dosing interval can vary and, for each drug, there exists a therapeutic window of plasma concentration below which the therapeutic effect is insufficient and above which toxic side effects occur.

An ideal form of colon drug delivery is a sustained or controlled form of drug release, which provides extended release, keeps plasma concentrations constant within the therapeutic window, and in this way, reduces dosage frequency at least two fold in comparison with the immediate release dosage form. The goal of the controlled release dosage forms is usually accomplished by attempting to obtain zero-order drug release. Drug carriers generally do not achieve this type of release considering lot of difficulties in dosage form design and production, but providing drug release in a slow first-order fashion results also in prolonged therapeutic effect. Delayed release dosage forms (e.g., enteric coated forms) are designed to release the drug at a time different than immediately after administration. The delay may be controlled by the influence of the environmental factors (e.g., GI pH, bacteria, temperature, pressure, etc) and time-controlled, such as in pulsatile release systems. The pressure controlled colon delivery utilizes the increase in pressure of the luminal contents in the colon due to the reabsorption of water. pH-sensitive delivery utilizes solubility of the drug carrier in the luminal content of the colon, while in bacteria dependant delivery, colonic bacteria are utilized to degrade the drug/cell carrier. In pulsatile release systems, a complete and rapid release follows lag time. They are generally designed according to the circadian rhythm of the body with an aim to deliver the active ingredient at the right site of action, at the right time and in the right amount. In the colon delivery, this approach is based on principle of delaying the time of release of about 5 hours.

3.1 Conventional topical dosage forms

Rectal installation is an established approach for the treatment of the disease distally located up to the sigmoid descending junction. It has the advantage of shortest distance to the colon; however, it is inconvenient and followed by difficulties in reaching the proximal colon (Table 3). In general, suppositories, foams and liquid enemas as dosage forms are used. The selection of the type of the rectal preparation depends on the proximal extent of inflammation, ease of insertion and patient preference. Suppositories or foams reach about 15 to 20 cm, while liquid enemas distribute to about 30 to 60 cm (to the splenic flexure) and sometimes as far as the ascending colon (Washington et al., 2001). So, suppositories are generally indicated for the disease located to the rectosigmoid junction, whereas foam enemas are usually distributed to the proximal sigmoid colon. In most patients, liquid enemas can deliver the drug as proximal as the splenic flexure. Foam and liquid enemas appear to be equally effective in treating patients with proximal UC, however, foam enemas are preferred because their administration is more easier and retention is more comfortable. Suppositories are usually better tolerated than enemas (Travis et al., 2008). Instilled volume and the viscosity of the enema are the most important variables defining proximal spreading of drugs. As large is the volume and the viscosity, more consistent is the proximal coating.

Rectal preparations of 5-ASA and corticosteroids are used as preferred treatment for mildly to moderately active left-sided or distal UC. The mechanism of action of 5-ASA is very complex and includes inhibition of cyclooxigenase and lypooxigenase, blocked production of leukotrienes and prostaglandins, inhibition of adenosine-induced secretion and bacterial peptide-induced neutrophil chemotaxis, scavenging of reactive oxygen metabolites and inhibition of activation of nuclear regulatory factor kappa B (Hemstreet & Diprio, 2008). Meta-analyses of clinical trials point to superior effect of rectal 5-ASA in comparison with placebo and conventional rectal corticosteroids in inducing remission of distal UC, which indicates the use of rectal steroids as reserves for 5-ASA when treatment with amino-salicylates failures or intolerance occurs (Marshall et al., 2010). When efficacy and convenience of administration of different rectal 5-ASA formulations were compared, no significant difference in efficacy was observed, while foams and gels were evaluated as the most convenient, producing less abdominal bloating. Considering adverse effects, reduced rate in respect to oral administration was reported (Sonu, 2010).

In colitis, corticosteroids are believed to modulate the immune response and inhibit production of cytokines and mediators being the benchmark therapy for moderate to severe UC and CD. Because of their adverse effects (Table 1), they should be used only in short term to induce remission in active UC, stopped once remission has been achieved and gradually discontinued. As selection criteria for rectal administration, corticosteroids with high efficacy and low systemic concentration are preferred, in order first-pass effect and adrenal suppression to be minimized and other adverse effects as well (Hanauer, 2002). Rectal formulations of prednisolone-metasulfobenzoate, budesonide, fluticasone, tixocortol pivalate and beclomethasone dipropionate are commercialized due to their lower interference with the adrenocortical function in comparison with hydrocortisone acetate and betamethasone (Gionchetti et al., 2004; Hanauer, 2002). Budesonide has been the corticosteroid of choice marketed as foams, liquid enemas and suppositories. It manifested efficacy in the induction and short-term maintenance of CD and induction of remission in collagenous and microscopic colitis (O'Donell, 2010). Comparison of the efficacy, tolerability, safety and patient's preference of budesonide foam *vs.* enema pointed to no significant difference in efficacy and safety and confirmed better tolerability and easier application of the foam formulations (Gross et al., 2006).

The use of immunosuppressant drugs is effective for long-term treatment of UC and CD. These agents are generally reserved for patients refractive to steroids and they are associated with serious adverse effects, which are potentiated with their relatively long-term use (Table 1). Rectal foams of azathioprine have been patented (Sandborn, 2002) and in one study in which healthy human subjects were included, pharmacokinetics of azathioprine after intravenous, oral, oral delayed release and rectal foam was compared. Rectal foams considerably reduced systemic 6-mercaptopurine bioavailability indicating the possibility for limited toxicity by local delivery of high doses of azathioprine (Van Os et al., 1996).

3.2 Advanced drug and cell delivery systems

Oral route is more convenient in the treatment of colitis. However, it is the longest one and associated by lot of obstacles for drug and cell stability and achieving high concentrations in the colon. Various strategies have been used to overcome these obstacles and to avoid high systemic bioavailability. These approaches utilize either formulation-specific or (pro)drug-specific design, while drug/cell targeting and modified release can be achieved by one or more of the well-established mechanisms: pH-sensitive, time-dependent, pressure-dependent and bacteria-dependent delivery (Table 3).

Principle	Advantages	Disadvantages
Conventional, topical delivery systems		
Deliver drugs by rectal instillation of liquid enemas, foams and suppositories	Deliver therapeutic drug concentrations to the distal regions of the colon Limited systemic toxicity Drug is protected from digestion	Difficulties in reaching the proximal colon Inconvenient administration and local irritation (e.g., leakage, problems with retention, burning sensation and bloating)

Principle	Advantages	Disadvantages
		Less compliance than optimal Not suitable when high doses are required
Advanced delivery		
pH–responsive delivery systems		
Release active ingredient in response to the change in pH throughout the GIT utilizing enteric polymers with high pH threshold	Provide uniform and prolonged release of the active ingredient throughout the intestinal region specifically at the diseased site Maintain physical and chemical integrity of the drugs in the GIT Preserve cell viability above therapeutic value during the passage through the stomach	Possibility for premature release of the active ingredient in the upper GIT and loss of therapeutic efficacy (e.g., rupture of the coating in the stomach, etc.) Failure of the enteric coating to dissolve at the desired site of action (e.g., formulation error, reduced colonic pH due to the presence of SCFAs, residue of bile acids, CO_2, etc.) Uncertainty of the location of the active ingredient release due to the variability in gut pH in colitis (e.g., reduced pH in UC, unknown pH in CD, etc.)
Bacteria-triggered delivery systems		
Release active ingredient in response to the specific enzymatic activity of the microflora present in the colon by biodegradation of the drug/cell carrier	Precise and direct effect at the diseased site of the colon (colon- targeted delivery) Maintain stability of drugs/ viability of cells in the upper GIT Control drug/cell release Lower the required dose and frequency of administration Have minimal effect/lower toxicity on the rest of the body Flexibility in design (e.g., prodrug design, CODES™, TARGIT®, COLAL™, etc.)	Risk of producing harmful substance as a product of carrier degradation (e.g. azo-polymer-based formulations) Difficulties in attaining desired rate of drug/cell release (e.g., rapid swelling in the upper GIT, fast disintegration or excessive slow enzymatic degradation of the delivery system) Inconsistency in drug/cell release due to the factors that might affect degradation of the delivery system (e.g. dietary fermentation pre-cursors, type of food consumed, co-administration of chemo-therapeutic agents, etc.) In a case of prodrug, new

Principle	Advantages	Disadvantages
		chemical entity needs additional evaluation before being used as a carrier
Time-dependent delivery systems		
Release active ingredient after a predetermined lag time (5-6 hours) utilizing enteric coating to withstand the variations in gastric emptying time and pH	Deliver drug at preselected time or pre-selected site of the GIT Delay or sustain drug release Maintain physical and chemical integrity of the drug in the stomach Lower the required dose and frequency of administration Reduce side-effects Integrate pH-sensitive and time-release functions into a single dosage form	Time-specific delivery cannot be accurately predicted due to the inter- and intra-individual variations in gastric emptying time, peristalsis or contraction in the stomach and type and amount of food consumed Delivery can be affected by the symptoms of colitis (e.g., accelerated transit time through different regions of colon due to diarrhea, etc.)
Osmotic-controlled delivery systems		
Release active ingredient utilizing osmotic pressure with a 3-4 hour post gastric delay	Release drug with pre-determined zero order rate Target drug locally to the colon Deliver drug independently of the physiological factors in the GIT Suitable for delivery of drugs with moderate water solubility Versatile designs deliver drug as short as 4 hours or provide constant release for up to 24 h Reduce side-effects Lower the required dose and frequency of administration	Delivery can be, to a certain degree, affected by administered food Delivery varies with the gastric motility Irritation or ulcer may occur due to release of saturated solution of drug More expensive treatment (because of multiple formulation steps and necessity of using special equipment for making an orifice in the system)
Pressure-controlled delivery systems		
Release active ingredient in response to the increased luminal pressure caused by the strong peristaltic waves in the colon	Colon-specific delivery Drug release mechanism is independent of pH Reduce side-effects Lower the required dose and frequency of administration	Limited understanding of the raised pressure phase in subjects with colitis Unpredictable delivery in the fed state because of the contractions in the stomach that may disintegrate the system in the stomach

Table 3. Characteristics of various approaches for drug and cell delivery in colitis

3.2.1 pH-dependent systems

Colonic formulations are very similar to conventional enteric-coated formulations, but consisted of enteric polymers with ability to withstand an environment ranging from low to neutral pH and stay intact for minimum 5 hours. In order to prevent premature drug release in the upper intestine, a combination of polymers with different solubility properties and water permeability/hydration rate and/or higher coating levels of enteric polymers are applied, thereby taking care coats not to rupture. The amount of coating depends on the solubility characteristics of both, the drug and the polymer(s), desired release profile and type of the final dosage form. Most commonly used coating polymers are derivatives of acrylic acid, methacrylic acid copolymers, known as Eudragit®S, Eudragit®L and Eudragit®S, copolymers of methacrylic acid and methyl methacrylate, Eudragit®L-100 and Eudragit®S-100, Eudragit FS, Eudragit P4135 F, and derivatives of cellulose in a form of salts, such as hydroxypropylmethyl-cellulose phthalate (HPMCP 50 and 55), cellulose acetate phthalate (CAP), etc., generally, with threshold pH above 4.8 to 7.0. In respect to formulation, coated dosage forms may be either single-unit or multi-particulate systems formulated as a single- or multi-layer product. The coating can be applied to a wide variety of solid core formulations such as (mini)tablets, capsules, pellets, granules, micro- and nano-particles. Most of them can be further filled into gelatin capsules or compressed as tablets, which can be additionally coated with the same or different suitable enteric polymer. The multi-particulate forms are less affected by the variations in the GIT, have larger surface, greater potential for homogenous spreading and reproducible drug release in the inflamed sites of the colon (Chourasia & Jain, 2003; Singh, 2007).

5-ASA tablets coated with Eudragit®L-100 are commercially available as Claversal™, Salofalak™, Mesasal®, Calitofalk® and Rowasa®, while sulfasalazine tablets coated with Eudragit® L-100-55 and CAP as Colo-pleon® and Azulfidine®, accordingly. They can effectively deliver 5-ASA to the terminal ileum and proximal colon in patients with IBD, with a delayed release which is achieved by a relatively thick coating. Clinical studies indentified a mean disintegration time of 3.2 h after gastric emptying and possibility the drug release to start at pH 6.6. In order 5-ASA release to be delayed and release to start at pH above 7.0, Eudragit®S-100 was used and the prepared delayed-release tablets were marketed as Asacol® (Schroeder et al., 1987). In January 2007, first 5-ASA formulation for once-a-day dosing was approved (Lialda™, Mezavant™). It uses a patented multi-matrix system, whereby the 5-ASA is incorporated into microparticles of a lipophilic matrix dispersed within a hydrophilic matrix. This is coated by a gastroresistant polymer which breaks down at pH of 7.0, allowing controlled release and delayed degradation of the 5-ASA in the colon. Multi-particulate forms of 5-ASA pellets coated with a combination of different Eudragits® (Eudragit® FS 30D, Eudragit® L-100, Eudragit® S-100) and Eudragits® with derivatives of cellulose (e.g. EC, microcrystalline cellulose, HPMC) were also prepared to achieve site specific release close to the ileocaecal valve. Rapid release at pH above 7.5 was observed, between 6.8 and 7.2 drug release was found to be zero order, while below 6.5 no release occurred (Cheng et al., 2004; Di Pretoro et al., 2010). Makham & Vakhshouri (2010) prepared and characterized methacrylic acid/perlite composites loaded with 5-ASA. In pH 7.4, with completed ionization, hydrolysis rate of the polymer was increased resulting in significant drug release.

For budesonide, similar pH-based systems, generally multi-particulate in a form of coated pellets or granules filled in gelatin capsule, are also commercially available (Budenofalk® and Entocort®EC) and patented (Beckert et al., 2005) In Budenofalk®, colon targeting and delayed release is accomplished by using ammonio methacrylate copolymer (Eudragit®RL), ammonio methacrylate copolymer (Eudragit®RS) and Eudragit®L-100 and Eudragit®S-100 for coating of granules with budesonide. In Entocort®EC, coating of the granules dissolves at pH>5.5 when they reach the duodenum. Thereafter, a matrix of EC with budesonide controls the release of the drug in a time-dependent manner. Budesonide was also efficiently entrapped in a micro-particulate system consisted of drug loaded acetate butyrate microspheres coated by Eudragit®S. No drug was released below pH 7 (Rodriguez et al., 1998). Similar results were obtained when budesonide-layered pellets were coated with an inner layer of a combination of Eudragit®RL PO and RS PO and an outer layer of Eudragit FS (Patel et al., 2010). Also, novel pH-sensitive budesonide loaded nanospheres designed for colon-specific delivery were prepared using polymeric mixtures of poly (lactic-co-glycolic) acid (PLGA) and methacrylate copolymer. They showed strongly pH-dependent drug release properties in acidic and neutral pH followed by a sustained release phase at pH 7.4. In addition, superior therapeutic effect in alleviating the conditions of induced colitis in animal model was observed (Makhlof et al., 2009).

Colon targeted drug delivery systems based on methacrylic resins and/or cellulose derivatives has also been described for prednisolone (Thomos et al., 1985), beclomethazone dipropionate (Levine et al., 1987), dexamethasone (Wang et al., 2010), cyclosporine (Kim et al., 2001), quinolones (Van Saene, 1986), metronidazole (Obite et al., 2010) and azathioprine (Kotagale et al., 2010). In the study of Kotagale et al. (2010), coated tablets with azathioprine exploiting different polymer combinations of Eudragit-S®, Eudragit-L® and CAP were prepared. Desired release pattern was achieved with only 9.75% drug release in the first 5 h. Tacrolimus has been also formulated in colon delivery system. Namely, PLGA nanoparticles containing the drug were entrapped into pH sensitive microspheres, showing strongly pH-sensitive release kinetics of both nanoparticles and the drug (Lamprecht et al., 2005).

3.2.2 Bacteria-dependent systems

Microbially controlled delivery is the most utilized and probably the most site-specific approach for colon targeting of drugs and cells because it relays on drug/cell carriers that are recalcitrant to the conditions of the stomach and upper intestine. When reaching the colon, these materials undergo degradation by enzyme or break down of the polymer back-bone, which leads to reduction in their molecular weight, loss of mechanical strength and subsequent drug/cell release with a rate that correlates with the biodegradation rate. For this type of drug/cell delivery, synthetic and natural polymers are used utilizing prodrug or multi-particulate approach. Multi-particulate approach has been utilized for oral delivery of sulfasalazine and betamethasone, based on microparticles of different synthetic biodegradable (co)polymers i.e. poly(epsilon-caprolactone), polylactic acid and PLGA (Lamprecht et al., 2000). However, the most of the multi-particulate systems, especially those carrying probiotic cells, utilize natural, generally regarded as safe (GRAS) polysaccharide polymers. Their fermentation by the bacterial enzymes results in formation of volatile SCFAs, such as lactic, acetic, propionic and butyric acids. Knowing that their deficiency causes UC, one can postulate that administering probiotics alone or with prebiotics, with complex carbohydrate structure, or embedded in polysaccharide carriers could be significantly beneficial in the treatment of colitis.

i. Polysaccharide-based systems

Lot of advantages promote the use of polysaccharides as drug carries for colon-targeted and controlled delivery, such as wide availability and inexpensiveness, variety of structures, simplicity for (bio)chemical modification, stability, safety, non-toxicity, mucoadhesivity, pH sensitive solubility and gel-forming properties. Of polysaccharides, guar gum, inulin, chitosan, chondroitin sulphate, alginates and dextran are the most used (Kumar et al., 2009). However, these materials are with certain limitations. Their hydrophilic nature makes them either soluble or prone to swelling in an aqueous environment and hence unsuitable as drug or cell carriers. So, when they are used alone, large quantities are needed to target the colon and control the drug release. To overcome these problems, cross-linking of soluble polysaccharides with poly- or di-valent cations or anions, accordingly, to form insoluble salts, or coating with mucoadhesive and oppositely charged pH sensitive polymers is applied. In this way, combined mechanisms for colon targeting, controlling drug release and increasing mean residence time in the colon are utilized.

For 5-ASA delivery, colon specificity has been achieved using a system based on amylose (COLAL™), which is susceptible to digestion by amylase-producing bacteria present in the colon. To control the swelling in the aqueous media and in that way, 5-ASA release rate, pellets were coated with amylose coating solution prepared along with the hydrophobic polymers Ethocel®, Eudragit RS/RL 30D and Aquacoat ECD30 (Milojevic et al., 1996). In addition, successful colon delivery of prednisolone metasulfobenzoate with COLAL™ system in patients with active UC was reported (Thompson et al., 2002). Similarly, dispersion of pectin in EC was used as the film former for coating of 5-ASA pellet cores. Negligible drug release during first 5 h in the simulated gastric and small intestinal conditions was observed. Osmotically driven release and formation of channels in the film caused by dissolution of pectin and activated by the presence of rat caecal contents was proposed as a drug release mechanism (Wei et al., 2008). Similar results have been obtained when a tablet systems based on swelling matrix core containing pectin, HPMC, microcrystalline cellulose and 5-ASA was developed in which drug release rate was controlled by pectinases (Talukder & Fasihi, 2008). The systems were designed based on GI time concept, assuming colon arrival time of 6 h.

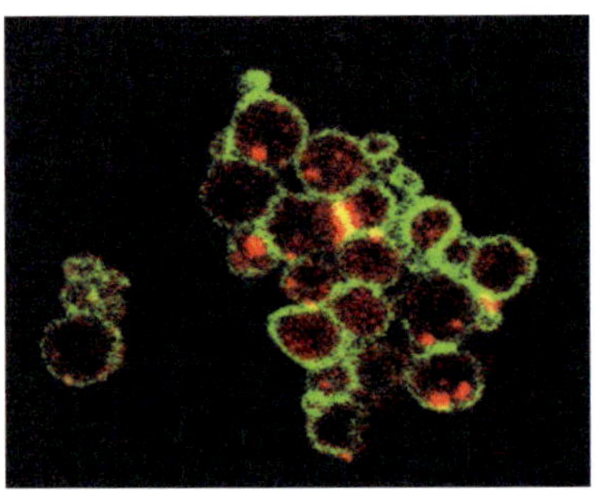

Fig. 1. Confocal laser scanning microscopy of 5-ASA loaded chitosan-Ca-alginate microparticles showing FITC-labeled chitosan (green) coating RBITC-labeled Ca-alginate matrix (red) (Mladenovska et al., 2007a,b).

Chitosan has also been extensively exploited as a 5-ASA carrier. For example, specific release of 5-ASA in the colon was achieved with chitosan capsules coated with HPMCP as enteric solvent material; efficacy in induced colitis in rats was confirmed as well as superiority in respect to the commercial 5-ASA products (Tozaki et al., 2002). 5-ASA loaded chitosan microspheres showing colon specific and controlled release were also prepared by Zambito & Di Colo (2003). In our studies (Mladenovska et al., 2007a,b), chitosan-Ca-alginate microparticles (Fig. 1) for colon-specific delivery and controlled release of 5-ASA after oral administration were prepared. *In vitro* drug release studies carried out in simulated *in vivo* conditions and biodistribution studies performed in colitic rats confirmed the potential of the particles to release the drug in the colon, with low systemic bioavailability. Similarly, beads containing 5-ASA, Eudragit FS 30D, Eudragit S-100 and chitosan were prepared (Iruin et al., 2005).

Corticosteroids were also incorporated in polysaccharide-based colon delivery systems. Multi-particulate system showing specific biodegradability and pH-dependent triamcinolone release were prepared based on chitosan, amidated pectin, HPMCP and CAP. Only 1% of drug was released in the acidic media after 2h (Oliveira et al., 2010). Novel colon delivery system COLAL-PRED has been developed by Alizyme for the treatment of UC as a combination of Alizyme's properitary colonic drug delivery system COLAL and prednisolone sodium metasulfobenzoate. The product has a coating that breaks down only in the colon by locally present bacteria, thus increasing local drug delivery without significant systemic side effects (Rangasamu, 2010). Budesonide was microencapsulated with dextran and the formulation was *in vitro/in vivo* characterized in induced colitis in rats. Colon targeting was confirmed and the macroscopic damage and total colitis scores were significantly reduced in comparison with the control group receiving 5-ASA and budesonide suspension (Varshosaz et al., 2011a). When budesonide release from directly compressed matrix tablets prepared of different molecular weights of dextran was evaluated, app. 10% of the drug was released in acidic pH and pH 7.4, while a very drastic increase was observed after exposure to pH 6.8 containing rat caecal contents (Ahmadi et al., 2011). Budesonide loaded chitosan-Ca-alginate microparticles coated with Eudragit S-100 were also prepared showing sustained release in pH 2.0 and 6.8 and efficient release in pH 7.4 controlled by the erosion and biodegradation rate of the polymer matrix. Clinical and histological evaluation in rat model of colitis showed that colitis severity was significantly suppressed (Crcarevska et al., 2009).

A multi-particulate system combining pH-sensitive property and specific biodegradability for colon-targeted delivery of metronidazole has been also investigated. The system was prepared by coating cross-linked chitosan microspheres with Eudragit L-100 and S-100. No release was observed at acidic pH, but in the presence of rat caecal contents, significant release was observed, indicating the susceptibility of chitosan matrix to colonic enzymes (Chourasia & Jain, 2004). Pectin microspheres were also prepared and coated with Eudragit® S-100 showing continuous release of metronidazole at colonic pH in the presence of rat caecal contents (Vaidya et al., 2009). In the studies of Nasra et al. (2007), pectin as a carrier of metronidazole was combined with chitosan in a form of coated tablets with ability to prevent premature drug release.

Azathioprine loaded Ca-gellan beads coated with Eudragit®S-100 were also prepared. The results suggest that gellan gum undergoes significant degradation in the presence of galactomannanase, which in turn facilitates the drug release from beads in the simulated colonic fluid (pH 7.4) in a controlled manner (Singh et al., 2004). In the work of Chaurasie et al. (2008), Ca-pectinate microspheres were prepared to deliver methotrexate in the colon. *In vitro* drug release studies in simulated gastric and intestinal fluids showed that app. 8% of the drug was released in 5 hours, whereas most of the loaded drug was released in simulated colonic fluid containing pectinase.

Polysaccharides have been also investigated as carriers for protection of the probiotics. Entrapment of cells in a gel matrix of alginates, chitosan, gellan, *k*-carageenan and starch or mixture of polysaccharide and protein is the most utilized approach. Cells are either compressed into a pellet, which is then encapsulated with the coating material by further compression, or encapsulated in an inner core surrounded by a semi-permeable, spherical, thin and strong membrane to form microcapsules or immobilized within or throughout a polymer matrix to form microspheres which can be subsequently filled into gelatin capsule. The coating of the microparticles, with a diameter from few microns to 1 mm, is designed to withstand acidic conditions and open in the lower intestine to release the cells by many different mechanisms, including fracture by heat, solvation, diffusion, pressure, erosion and biodegradation. The lower intestine provides right conditions for probiotic to survive, multiply and exert health beneficiary effects. With such a protection from acidity, molecular oxygen, hydrogen peroxide, digestive enzymes, bacteriophages and SCFAs, the viability of the probiotic after oral administration is significantly improved and targeted and controlled release achieved (Rokka & Rantamaki, 2010).

Literature data point to abundance researches related to microencapsulation of probiotics alone or with prebiotics in coated and non-coated alginate microparticles. As prebiotics, usually FOS or isomaltooligosaccharides are used, while as coating materials, other polysaccharides or proteins. When probiotic cells were compressed into pellets and encapsulated within alginate as the coating material, significant improvement in survival (104-105-fold) was observed after exposure to acidic pH. *In vitro* tests pointed to a cell release near the end of the ileum and beginning of the colon with a mechanism involving erosion of the alginate gel layer (Eng Seng & Zhang, 2005). Many other formulations of encapsulating materials for probiotic microparticles were optimized; all of them showed improved tolerance to gastric conditions and high survival of the probiotic in colonic conditions. Of probiotics, strains of *L. acidophilus, L. casei, B. bifidum* and *B. longum,* proved to show health effects in colitis, are among the most studied. For example, *L. casei* NCDC-298 loaded Ca-alginate microparticles showed better survival of the probiotic at low pH and high bile salt concentration. In colonic pH solution, the release of cells was increased, with a count above therapeutic minimum of 10^7–10^9 cfu g^{-1} (Mandal et al., 2006). Similarly, encapsulated *L. acidophilus* ATCC 43121 in Ca-alginate microparticles exhibited a significantly higher resistance to artificial intestinal juice than non-encapsulated samples (Kim et al., 2008). The beads made with alginate-pectin blends provided a significant better protection to the entrapped *L. casei* under all conditions tested (Sandovall-Castilla et al., 2010). Strains of *L. acidophilus* and *L. casei* were encapsulated into uncoated Ca-alginate beads and the same beads were coated with three types of material, chitosan, Na-alginate and poly-L-lysine in combination with alginate. Chitosan-coated alginate beads provided the best protection for the lactobacillus strains in simulated GI conditions (Krasaekoopt et al., 2004). Also, chitosan coated microspheres were produced to encapsulate *L. gasseri* and *B.*

bifidum, separately with the prebiotic quercetin, with an aim to keep them intact during exposure to the harsh conditions of the GIT. Resistance to simulated gastric conditions during 2 h and bile salt solution for 2 h was observed (Chavarri et al., 2010).

In our study, in which the probiotic *L. casei* was microencapsulated with FOS in chitosan-Ca-alginate beads, the optimal formulation of synbiotic microparticles was stable during exposure to simulated gastric and intestinal juices and release of viable cells above the therapeutic value in the simulated colonic pH was observed (Fig. 2) (Petreska et al., 2010, 2011). Similar results were obtained when *L. casei* was entrapped in whey protein-Ca-alginate microparticles (Smilkov et al., 2011a,b). The same combination of whey protein and alginate was used for microencapsulation of strains of *L. plantarium*; only bacteria in the coated beads survived in the simulated gastric and intestinal fluid (Gbassi et al., 2009). Other protein and polysaccharides mixtures were also used to microencapsulate probiotics. For e.g, alginate-coated gelatin microspheres were prepared to encapsulate strain of *B. adolescentis*; the alginate core prevented pepsin-induced degradation of the gelatin microspheres and thus, cell release in simulated gastric juice for 2 h (Annan et al., 2008).

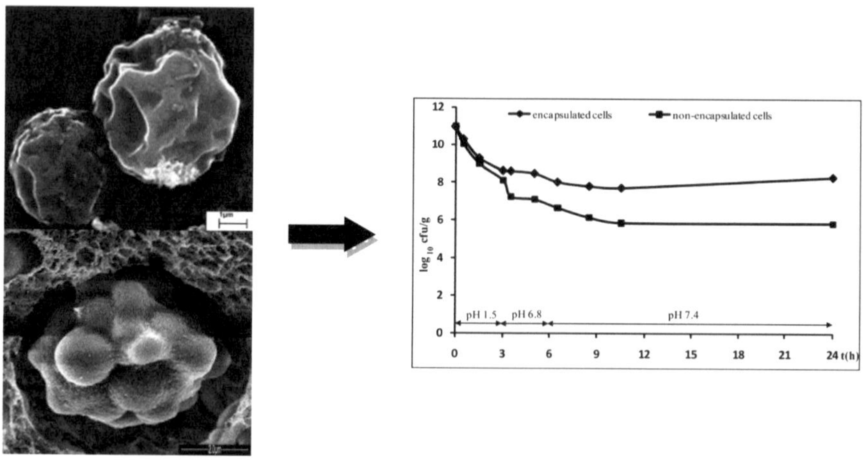

Fig. 2. Microstructure of (a) whole and (b) fractured *L. casei* loaded chitosan-Ca-alginate microparticles (left) and viability of non-encapsulated and encapsulated *L. casei* in simulated gastric conditions (0.08 M HCl; 0.2% NaCl; pH 1.5), bile salts solution (0.05 M KH_2PO_4; pH 6.8 with 1% bile salts) and colonic pH (0.1 M KH_2PO_4; pH 7.4) (right). The inner part of the particles is built of a mesh-like alginate network through which the bacteria groups are distributed and sequestered in voids.

ii. CODES™ delivery system

CODES™ is a specific polysaccharide based system exploiting specific biodegradability of the polymers by the colonic bacteria only in combination with pH-sensitive polymer coating (Fig. 3). It is consisted of a core tablet (consisted of drug, one or more polysaccharides and other necessary excipients) coated with three layers of polymers, acid-soluble polymer (e.g., Eudragit E®) around the core, outer layer of enteric polymer and a barrier between to prevent complexation of oppositely charged polymers (e.g., HPMC) (Pantel et al., 2008). The system remains intact in the stomach. Upon entry into the colon, the polysaccharides (e.g., FOS, mannitol, lactulose, etc.) dissolve and diffuse through the coating whereby they become subject to enzymatic degradation to organic acids. As colonic pH starts to decrease, the acidic-soluble polymer begins to dissolve, which is followed by subsequent drug release.

CODES, consisted of three components, a core containing lactulose and 5-ASA, an inner acid-soluble material layer and an outer layer of an enteric soluble material, was prepared and orally administered to fasting and fed dogs to evaluate the pharmacokinetic profiles of the drug. The results of the study confirmed that lactulose can act as a trigger for 5-ASA release in the colon (Katsuma et al., 2002). Recently, Varshosaz et al. (2011b) reported development of a novel budesonide pellets based on CODES™ technology. Pellet cores containing lactulose or manitol were coated with an acidic soluble polymer Eudragit E®100, HPMC and an enteric coat consisted of Eudragit® FS 30D. Absence of drug release in pH 1.2 and 7.4 was observed, while in medium with rat caecal contents (pH 6.8), controlled release occurred. Promising results in decreasing colitis score in animal model were also observed.

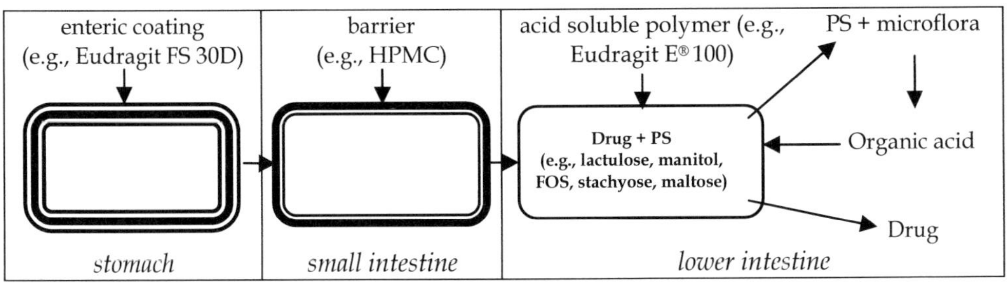

Fig. 3. Schematics of the CO(lon)DE(livery)S(ystem)™

iii. Prodrugs

Prodrug approach for colon targeting in colitis includes formation of a covalent linkage between the drug and a carrier, which upon oral administration of the drug remains intact in the acidic environment of the stomach and upper intestine and undergoes spontaneous or enzymatic transformation in the colon. This approach solves not only the problem of achieving high drug concentration at the diseased site, but also the problem of preserving chemical stability and avoiding high systemic bioavailability and thereby toxicity. There are three classes of prodrugs commercially available or under investigation: (i) anti-inflammatory agents (e.g. 5-ASA, SCFAs); (ii) immunomodulators (e.g. corticosteroids, azathioprine); and (iii) antioxidants (e.g. glutathione, cysteine, S-adenosyl-methionine) (Chourasia & Jain, 2003; Oz & Ebersole, 2008).

All available methods for covalent linking of 5-ASA molecule were used: linking via azo-bond to another 5-ASA molecule (in olsalazine) or inert carrier 4-amino-benzoyl-β-alanine (in balsalazine) or active carrier sulfapyridine (in sulfasalazine) and subsequent activation of the drug in the colon by the bacterial azoreductases as well as conjugation with amino acids or polymers as polymeric prodrug systems. Sulfasalazine releases 5-ASA specifically in the colon, however, a small quantity of the ingested dose is absorbed in the upper intestine resulting in serious adverse effects of sulfapyridine (Table 1). Olsalazine and balsalazine were formulated to overcome disadvantages of sulfapyridine. In the studies of Yokoe et al. (2003), a new prodrug was synthesized, salicylazosulfanyl acid. Azoreductases cleave it into 5-ASA and sulfanyl acid; owing to the high hidrophylicity of the carrier and thereby low absorption in the GIT, adverse effects observed with sulfapyridine were avoided. The use of β-cyclodextrins as 5-ASA carriers in a prodrug form was characterized by a relatively successful prevention of 5-ASA release in simulated gastric and intestinal medium and subsequent release mediated by the colonic microflora (Bonsignore, 2000). Jung et al. (1998) formulated stable dextrane conjugate of 5-ASA with delayed release. Lately, they focused their research towards conjugation of 5-ASA with amino acid derivatives where 5-aminosalicyl-L-aspartic acid and 5-aminosalicyl-L-glutamic acid were synthesized and their properties as colon-specific prodrugs of 5- ASA investigated in colitic rats (Jung et al., 2001). The most of 5-ASA-Asp was delivered to the large intestine and about half of the administered dose was activated to liberate 5-ASA. Recently, an amino acid (mutual) aza-prodrug of 5-ASA was synthesized by coupling L-tryptophan with salicylic acid (Nagpal et al., 2007). *In vitro* kinetic studies showed negligible release of 5-ASA in acidic medium, while *in vivo* studies pointed to equal attenuation of the colitis in rats as that of sulfasalazine without ulcerogenicity of 5-ASA. One more attempt was made to conjugate 5-ASA for colon delivery. Specificity includes conjugation with bile acids (chenodeoxycholic and ursodeoxycholic acid) (Goto et al., 2001). *In vivo* studies in guinea pigs showed that with lower doses, higher efficacy could be achieved. Polymeric prodrugs of 5-ASA were also formulated in which 5-ASA was linked with polyacrylic or polyamide polymers via degradable ester or amide bonds (Zou et al., 2005) as well as polymeric prodrugs in which 5-ASA was bond via azo-carrier to polyanhydride polymers and derivatives of dextrane and poly[(2-hydroxylethyl)aspartamine] (Cai et al., 2003). In the recent studies of Yadav & Mahatma (2011), acrylic type polymeric systems having degradable ester bonds linked to the 5-ASA were synthesized and evaluated for colon targeted drug delivery. *In vitro* drug release studies, conducted at pH 1.2, 7.4 and in rat fecal content, pointed to a burst release of app. 40% in the first 2 h followed by a sustained release over a period of 12 h. In general, most of the mentioned prodrugs and polymeric prodrugs release 5-ASA successfully in the colon, but the complex coupling processes and the fact that the 5-ASA content is app. 10% of the total mass made them inappropriate for oral administration because a very large amount would need to be taken orally (Chourasia & Jain, 2003).

Corticosteroids were also subject to prodrug design. Steroid glycosides, galactosides and cellobiosides were designed, from which dexamethasone, prednisolone, hydrocortisone and fludrocortisone were released in the colon with hydrolysis mediated by β-D-galactosidase, β-D-glucosidase, α-L-arabinofuranosidase, β-D-xylopyranosidase (Friend & Chang, 1985). *In vivo* researches involving rat stomach, proximal small intestine, distal small intestine and caecum pointed to the most rapidly hydrolysis in the caecal content followed by the distal small intestine. Conjugates of budesonide and dexamethasone and glucuronic acid and dextran, accordingly, were also synthesized, showing excellent efficacy in rats with induced UC and decreased toxicity, especially in respect to adrenal suppression (Nolen et al., 1997; Varshosaz et al., 2009). Also, dexamethasone 21-sulfate sodium as a colon specific prodrug of dexamethasone was prepared (Kim et al., 2006). The degree of prodrug hydrolysis and production of dexamethasone amounted to 70% of healthy rats when a prodrug was incubated with caecal contents collected from colitic rats. In comparison with prednisolone, hydrocortisone and cortisone, dexamethasone was stable against bioinactivation by the cecal contents. Anti-inflammatory effect and systemic side effects of prednisolone succinate/α-cyclodextrin ester conjugate were also studied in animal model of IBD (Yano et al., 2002). The side-effects were significantly alleviated due to the passage of the conjugate through the stomach and small intestine without significant degradation or absorption. Dextran ester prodrugs of dexamethasone and methylprednisolone, with a succinate linking the drug and dextran, were also synthesized and proved their preclinical efficacy and lower toxicity (Pang et al., 2002). Similarly, budesonide-succinate-dextran conjugate as a prodrug of budesonide showed huge improvement in macroscopic and histological scores of colitis in induced colitis in rats (Varshosaz et al., 2010). Polymeric prodrug colon delivery system of dexamethasone was also prepared, with poly-(L-aspartic acid) as a carrier with superior efficacy and lower toxicity in respect to oral dexamethasone (Leopold & Friend, 1995).

3.2.3 Time-dependent systems

In ideal time-controlled colon delivery system, drug release occurs after precisely determined lag phase of minimum 3±1 h necessary for the system to pass the stomach and small intestine. In fact, the system relays on the consistent small intestine transit time, while for the formulation to withstand the individual variations in gastric emptying time and pH, usually enteric coating is used. This prevents rapid swelling and disintegration in the upper GIT, while in the colon, drug release rate is controlled by the mechanisms of swelling, osmosis or diffusion, erosion or a combination of all (Singh, 2007). In general, it is very difficult colon specific and controlled release in a state of colitis and diarrhea with this type of delivery systems to achieve because the transit through different regions of the colon is accelerated and unpredictable.

Various structures and formulation designs were commercialized (Pulsincap®, Time Clock®) and described for this type of delivery systems, mostly adapted from the pulsatile delivery systems. They can be subdivided into reservoir and capsular formulations prepared in a form of single- or multiple-unit preparations (Iamartino et al., 1992; Takada, 1997; Ueda et al., 1989). Usually, in all designs, drug, one or more swellable hydrophilic excipients (e.g., sodium starch glycolate, CMC sodium, low substituted HPC) and water-insoluble enteric polymers (e.g., EC, Eudragit® RL) are present. Patent assigned to Hoffman-La Roche (Shah et al., 2000) contains also a plasticizer in an inner semi-permeable polymer membrane, which allows water influx but prevents the outward diffusion of the drug. An outer enteric-coating, which dissolves above pH 5.5, swells during the transit of the tablet through the small intestine and after a consistent period of minimum 4 h transit in the small intestine, the swollen core burst the semi-permeable membrane and the drug is released in the colon. In the erodible systems, the penetration of the GI fluids through the micropores of the outer layer causes swelling/expansion, dissolution and/or erosion of the swelling agent(s), which accordingly, pushes the drug out of the system or delays the drug release for a time determined with the selection of the coating polymer(s). In rupturable reservoirs, a time for release of the drug is programmed by the disruption of a semi-permeable membrane consisted of insoluble polymer(s). In the device of Ritschel & Agrawal (2002), for example, self-destruction of the semi-permeable membrane occurs and the drug goes out of the system though the orifice made by a specific press-coating. Concerning the capsular systems, the drug release occurs after dissolution of a protective polymer cap and subsequent removal of a matrix plug from a drug-containing insoluble capsule body; the time of ejection corresponds to the lag phase.

Time-dependent system for delivering 5-ASA to the colon was prepared in which the core tablet of 5-ASA was compression-coated with HPMC and then coated with Eudragit®L-100.

The results revealed that the lag time increases with the amount of HPMC (Patel et al., 2009). Combined time- and pH-dependent microparticulate system consisting of non-enzymatically degrading PLGA core for delivering budesonide specifically to the distal ileum and colon was also developed. Eudragit®S-100 was used to form a coating on the surface of the microparticles. Complete retardation of drug release in an acidic pH and controlled release in pH 7.4 and 6.8 was observed (Krishnamachar et al., 2007). In addition, Yehia et al. (2009) optimized a formulation of budesonide loaded compression-coated tablets where as time-dependent variable, cellulose acetate butyrate was used.

3.2.4 Osmotic-controlled systems

In general, in osmotic drug delivery systems, the delivery of the active agent(s) is delayed or pulsed, driven by an osmotic gradient and it is not dependent / affected by the physiological variables within the GIT. After administration, the water diffuses into the core of the osmotic system through a semi-permeable membrane increasing the hydrostatic pressure, which pumps the active agent containing solution out of the core through one or more orifices. The drug release follows zero order kinetics and the rate is controlled by the diffusion rate of the water into the system (Gupta et al., 2009).

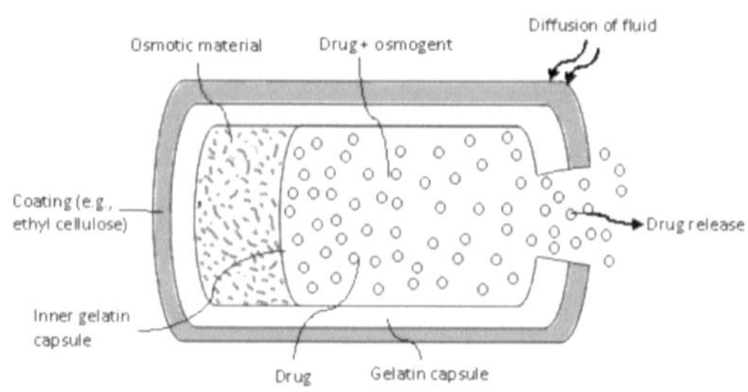

Fig. 4. Osmotic pump capsule structure

Lots of osmotic delivery systems, with membrane plug retention mechanism or with osmotic device in an osmotic device, have been patented, with a potential to carry the drugs for the treatment of different states of colitis. Therapeutic System Research Laboratory Arm Arbor (Michigan, USA) developed the Port system consisting of a capsule coated with a semi-permeable membrane. Inside the capsule is an insoluble plug consisting of osmotically active agent and the drug formulation (Fig. 4). Osmotic system OROS-CT was designed by Alza Corporation to target the active agent(s) to the colon. It is a system composed of a single or multiple (5-6) bi-layered osmotic units encapsulated within a hard gelatin capsule. Each layer, the push and drug layer, are surrounded by a semi-permeable membrane, while the orifice is drilled through the membrane next to the drug layer. Semi-permeable membrane, usually consisted of CA and cellulose acylate, is insoluble in body fluids, non-erodible, but permeable to the passage of fluids. Each unit is surrounded by enteric coating, usually phthalates, keratin, formalin-treated protein, oils and anionic polymers, which do not dissolve, disintegrate or change their structure in the stomach. The osmogents are either hydrophilic polymers (e.g., HPMC, poly(hydroxyalkyl-methacrylate), poly(vinyl-pyrrolidone), poly(vinyl alcohol), acidic carboxy-polymers or inorganic water-soluble agents (e.g., magnesium sulfate, sodium- and potassium chloride, sodium bicarbonate, etc.). In UC, drug release begins when the drug enters the colon, with 3-4 h post gastric delay. Then, a constant release follows which may last up to 24 h (Gupta et al., 2009; Patel et al., 2010).

Specifically, a new microbial-triggered colon targeted osmotic pump was developed for colon delivery of budesonide based on chitosan. Chitosan was used to produce osmotic pressure by swelling and with its degradation, *in situ* delivery pores were formed through which budesonide was released. CA along with chitosan was coated on a tablet as a semi-permeable membrane, while as entering coat, Eudragit®L-100-55 was used (Liu et al.; 2007).

3.2.5 Pressure-controlled systems

The rationale behind the design of the pressure-dependent colon delivery systems lies in the existence of strong peristaltic waves that move intestinal content from ascending to transverse colon, temporarily increasing the luminal pressure within the colon. Significantly higher viscosity of the colonic content is a reason for much higher luminal pressure in the colon in comparison with the one in the small intestine. So, the delivery system is formulated to withstand the pressure in the upper GIT and to collapse in the lower intestine.

So far, pressure-controlled colon delivery capsules (PCDCs) as a unique system were prepared by coating an inner surface of gelatin capsules with EC. By adjusting the coating thickness of the EC membrane, colon delivery of 5-ASA in beagle dogs was obtained. Namely, after administration, 5-ASA appeared into the systemic circulation after 3-5 h, which corresponds to the colon arrival time observed with sulfasalazine (Muraoka et al., 1998). Avoiding side effects of sulfapyridine is a great achievement with this type of colon delivery system. Furthermore, 5-ASA was loaded in microcapsules prepared of EC or Eudragit L-100 or S-100 and filled into PCDCs, which were prepared as fast release colon delivery system with 5-ASA powder suspended in a suppository base. The release rate of 5-ASA from the microcapsules was significantly prolonged as compared to 5-ASA powder with no significant differences in the release rates between the microcapsules. The first appearance time of 5-ASA into the systemic circulation after oral administration was 3 h for all the colon delivery preparations, while both EC microcapsules and Eudragit®S-100/RS-100 microcapsules in PCDCs showed longer mean residence time than Eudragit®L-100/RS-100 microcapsules, suggesting sustained release characteristics (Hu et al., 1999).

4. Conclusion and future perspectives

Undoubtedly, advanced colon drug delivery systems (CDDSs) offer significant advantages in respect to both efficacy and safety of drugs used for the treatment of colitis and considering probiotic cells, significantly increased survival and colonization rate. However, commercial products for oral administration based on the mentioned CDDSs for all the drugs needed for the treatment of colitis, especially for biologic drugs, are still not available. In this respect, multidisciplinary project was initiated by the research group from the University Medical Center Groningen to develop and evaluate oral formulations of infliximab, including formulation based on pH-responsive coating containing Eudragit®S-100. Similarly, formulation of infliximab loaded PLGA microspheres was developed by Foong et al. (2010) as a prospective novel treatment of CD fistulae showing controlled release under zero-order kinetics of the anti-TNF-α antibody and biological activity against

TNF-α. Also, to the present knowledge, no commercial pharmaceutical product containing microencapsulated probiotic cells exists.

Of all the primary above-mentioned approaches proposed for the CDDSs none is ideal when separately used and colon specificity and controlled delivery is more likely to be achieved with systems based on mucoadhesive natural materials that are degraded by the colonic bacterial enzymes. Considering the complexity of the CDDSs and the difficulties in establishing *in-vitro/in-vivo* correlation by actual dissolution methods, a validated dissolution method for their evaluation has to be developed, which considers the physiological characteristics of the colon and can be used routinely in an industry. In addition, novel approaches developed for colon-targeting and controlled release, as even more specific, have to be comprehensively explored and commercialized as drug/cell carriers in the treatment of colitis. Extensive clinical data showing promising efficacy in active colonic diseases, including IBD, are now available for TARGIT Technology (West Pharmaceutical services) designed for targeted release into the colonic region. The technology is based on application of pH-sensitive coatings onto injection-moulded starch capsules. Also, the ENTERION capsule has recently been developed (Phacton Research, UK) for targeted delivery of different drug formulations into any region of the gut. The round-ended capsule sealed by inserting a push-on cap fitted with a silicone O-ring can be loaded with either a liquid formulation or a particulate formulation (e.g., micro/nanoparticles, pellets, etc.). The bottom of the drug reservoir is the piston face which is held back against a compressed spring by a high tensile strength polymer filament. Once the capsule reaches the target location in the GIT, the drug is actively ejected by the external application of an oscillating magnetic field. Clinical application and converting this tool into a product-carrier of drugs for colitis treatment remains a big challenge. Therefore, a search for new delivery systems that can provide increased therapeutic benefits to the patients with colitis continues.

5. References

Ahmadi, F.; Varshosaz, J.; Emami, J.; Tavakoli, N.; Minaiyan, M.; Mahzouni, P. & Dorkoosh, F. (2011) Preparation and in vitro/in vivo evaluation of dextran matrix tablets of budesonide in experimental ulcerative colitis in rats. *Drug Deliv.* (Feb 2011), Vol. 18, No. 2, pp. 122-30, ISSN 1071-7544.

Annan, N. T.; Borza, A. D. & Hansen, L. T. (2008). Encapsulation of alginate-coated gelatin microspheres improves survival of the probiotic *Bifidobacterium adolescentis* 15703T during exposure to simulated gastro-intestinal conditions. *Food Res Int*, Vol. 41, No 2, (Jan 2008), pp. 184-193, ISSN 0963-9969.

Beckert, T.; Dressman, J.; Rudolph, M. (2005) Pharmaceutical formulation for the active ingredient budesonide. United States Patent Application 20050089571.

Bonsignore, L.; Loy, G.; Fadda, A. M. (2000). The cyclodextrin conjugation approach for the site-specific delivery of 5-ASA to colon. Proceeding to the 3rd World Meeting APV/APGI, ISBN 963 00 6467 7, Berlin, Apr 2000, pp. 223-224.

Cai, Q. X.; Zhu, K. J.; Chen, D. & Gao, L. P. (2003). Synthesis, characterization and in vitro release of 5-ASA and 5-acetyl aminosalycilic acid of polyanhydride P(CBFAS). *Eur J Pharm Biopharm*, Vol. 55, No. 2, (Mar 2003), pp. 203-208, ISSN 0939-6411.

Chaurasia, M.; Chourasia, M. K.; Jain, N. K.; Jain, A.; Soni, V.; Gupta, Y. & Jain, S. K. (2008). Methotrexate bearing Ca-pectinate microspheres: a platform to achieve colon-specific drug release. *Curr Drug Deliv*, Vol. 5, No. 3, (Jul 2008), pp. 215-219, ISSN: 1567-2018.

Chavarri, M.; Maranon, I.; Ares, R.; Ibanez, F.C.; Marzo, F. & Villaran, M. (2010). Microencapsulation of probiotic and prebiotic in alginate-chitosan capsules improves survival in simulated gastro-intestinal conditions. *Int J Food Microbiol*, Vol. 142, No. 1-2, (Aug 2010), pp. 185-189, ISSN 0168-1605.

Cheng, G.; An, F.; Zou, M. J.; Sun, J.; Hao, X. H. & He, Y. X. (2004). Time- and pH-dependent colon-specific drug delivery for orally administered diclofenac sodium and 5-ASA. *World J Gastroenterol*, Vol. 10, No. 12, (Jun 2004), pp. 1769-74, ISSN 1007-9327.

Chourasia, M. & Jain, S. K. (2003). Pharmaceutical approaches to colon targeted drug delivery systems. *J Pharm Pharm Sci*, Vol. 6, No. 1, (Jan 2003), pp. 33-66, ISSN 1482-1826.

Chourasia, M. K. & Jain, S. K. (2004). Design and development of multiparticulate system for targeted drug delivery to colon. *Drug Deliv*, Vol. 11, No. 3, (May 2004), pp. 201-7, ISSN 1071-7544.

Crcarevska, M. S.; Dodov, M. G.; Petrusevska, G.; Gjorgoski, I. & Goracinova, K. (2009). Bioefficacy of budesonide loaded crosslinked polyelectrolyte microparticles in rat model of induced colitis. *J Drug Target*, Vol. 17, No. 10, (Dec 2009), pp. 788-802, ISSN 1061-186X.

Di Pretoro, G.; Zema, L.; Gazzaniga, A.; Rough, S. L. & Wilson, D. I. (2010). Extrusion-spheronisation of highly loaded 5-ASA multiparticulate dosage forms. *Int J Pharm*, Vol. 402, No. 1-2, (Dec 2010), pp. 153-64, ISSN: 0378-5173.

Eng Seng, C. & Zhang. Z. (2005). Bioencapsulation by compression coating of probiotic bacteria for their protection in an acidic medium. *Process Biochemistry*, Vol. 40, No. 10, (Oct 2005), pp. 3346-3351, ISSN 1359-5113

Foong, K. S.; Patel, R.; Forbes, A. & Day, R. M. (2010). Anti-tumor necrosis factor-alpha-loaded microspheres as a prospective novel treatment for Crohn's disease fistulae. *Tissue Eng Part C Methods*, Vol. 16, No. 5 (Oct 2010), pp. 855-64, ISSN 1937-3384.

Ford, A. C.; Bernstein, C. N.; Khan, K. J.; Abreu, M. T.; Marshall, J. K.; Talley, N. J. & Moayyedi, P. (2011). Glucocorticosteroid therapy in inflammatory bowel disease: systematic review and meta-analysis. *Am J Gastroenterol*, Vol. 106, No. 4, (Apr 2011), pp. 590-9, ISSN: 0002-9270.

Friend, D. R. & Chang, G. W. (1992). Drug glycosides: potential prodrugs for colon-specific drug delivery. *J Med Chem*, Vol. 28, No. 1 (Jan 1985), pp. 51-7, ISSN 1520-4804.

Gbassi, G. K.; Vandamme, T.; Ennahar, S. & Marchioni, E. (2009). Microencapsulation of *Lactobacillus planatrum* spp in an alginate matrix coated with whey proteins. *Int J Food Microbiol*, Vol. 129, No. 1, (Jan 2009), pp. 103-105, ISSN: 1687-918X.

Geier, M. S.; Butler, R. N. & Howarth, G. S. (2007). Inflammatory bowel disease: Current insights into pathogenesis and new therapeutic options; probiotics, prebiotics and synbiotics. *Int J Food Microbiol*, Vol. 115, No. 1, (Apr 2007), pp. 1-11, ISSN 0168-1605.

Gibson, G. R. & Roberfroid, M. B. (1995). Dietary modulation of the human colonic microbiota: introducing the concept of prebiotics. *J Nutr,* Vol. 125, No. 6, (Jun 1995), pp. 1401-12, ISSN 0022-3166.

Gionchetti, P.; Rizzello, F.; Morselli, C. & Campieri, M. (2004). Review article: problematic proctitis and distal colitis. *Aliment Pharmacol Ther* (Sept 2004), Vol. 20, Suppl. 4, pp. 93–96. ISSN 1365-2036.

Gisbert, J. P.; Linares, P. M.; McNicholl, A. G.; Mate, J. & Gomollon, F. (2009). Meta-analysis: the efficacy of azathioprine and mercaptopurine in ulcerative colitis. *Aliment Pharmacol Ther* Vol. 1, No. 2, (Jul 2009), pp. 126-37, ISSN 1365-2036.

Goto, M.; Okamoto, Y.; Yamamaoto, M. & Aki, H. (2001). Aniti-inflammatory effect of 5-ASA conjugates with chenodeoxycholic acid and ursodeoxycholic acid on carageenan-induced colitis in guinea pigs. *J Pharm Pharmacol,* Vol. 53, No. 12, (2001), pp. 1711-20, ISSN 0022-3573.

Gross, V.; Bar-Meir, S.; Lavy, A.; Mickisch, O.; Tulassay, M.; Pronai, L.; Kupicinskas, L.; Kiudelis, G.; Pokretnieks, J.; Kovacs, A.; Faszczyk, M.; Razbadauskas, A.; Margus, B.; Stolte, M.; Muller, R. & Grienwald, R. (2006). Budesonide foam versus budesonide enema in active ulcerative proctitis and proctosigmoiditis. *Aliment Pharmacol Ther,* Vol. 23, No. 2, (Jul 2006), pp. 303–312. ISSN 1365-2036.

Gupta, R. N.; Gupta, R.; Basniwal, P. K.; Rathore, G. S. (2009). Osmotically controlled oral drug delivery system: a review. (2009). *Int J Ph Sci,* Vol. 1, No. 2, (Sept 2009), pp. 269-275, ISSN 0975-4725.

Hanauer, S. B. (2002). New steroids for IBD: progress report. *Gut,* Vol. 51, No. 2, (Aug 2002), pp. 182-183. ISSN 1468-3288.

Hemstreet, B. A. & Dipiro, J. T. (2008). Chapter 36: Inflammatory bowel diseases, In: *Pharmacotherapy; Pathophysiological approach.* Dipiro Joseph T., Robert L. Talbert, Yee C. Gary, Matzke R. Garry, Wells G. Barbara, Posey L. Michael, pp. 589-605, McGrow Hill Companies, ISBN 0-07-164325-7, New York.

Hu, Z.; Kimura, G.; Ito, Y.; Mawatari, S.; Shimokawa, T.; Yoshikawa, H.; Yoshikawa, Y. & Takada, K. J. (1999). Technology to obtain sustained release characteristics of drugs after delivered to the colon. *J Drug Target,* Vol. 6, No. 6, (1999), pp. 439-48, ISSN 1061-186X.

Iamartiono, P., Maffione, G. & Pontello, L. (1992). US5171580.

Iruin, A.; Fernandez-Arevalo, M.; Alvarez-Fuentes, J.; Fini, A. & Holgado, M. A. (2005). Elaboration and "in vitro" characterization of 5-ASA beads. *Drug Dev Ind Pharm,* Vol. 31, No. 2, (Jan 2005), pp. 231-239, ISSN 0363-9045.

Jung, J. Y.; Lee, S. J.; Kim M. Y.; (2001). Colon-specific prodrugs of 5-ASA: synthesis and *in vitro/in vivo* properties of acidic amino acid derivatives of 5-ASA. *J Pharm Sci,* Vol. 90, No. 11, (Nov 2001), pp. 1767-1775, ISSN 0022-3549.

Jung, J. Y.; Lee, S. J.; Kim, H. H.; Kim, Y. T. & Kim, Y. M. (1998). Synthesis and properties of dextran-5-ASA ester as a potential colon specific prodrug of 5-ASA. *Arch Pharm Res,* Vol. 21, No. 2, (Apr 1998), pp. 179-186, ISSN 0253-6269.

Katsuma, M.; Watanabe, S.; Kawai, H.; Takemura, S.; Masuda, Y. & Fukui, M. (2002). Studies on lactulose formulations for colon-specific drug delivery. *Int J Pharm,* Vol. 5, No. 1-2, (Dec 2002), pp. 33-43, ISSN 0378-5173.

Khan K. J.; Ullman, T. A.; Ford, A. C.; Abreu, M. T.; Abadir, A.; Marshall, J. K.; Talley, N. J. & Moayyedi, P. (2011). Antibiotic therapy in inflammatory bowel disease: a systematic review and meta-analysis. *Am J Gastroenterol*, Vol. 106, No. 4, (Apr 2011), pp. 661-73. ISSN 0002-9270.

Kim I. H.; Kong H. S.; Choi B. I.; Kim Y. S.; Kim H. J.; Yang Y. W.; Jung Y. J. & Kim Y. M. (2006). Synthesis and in vitro properties of dexamethasone 21-sulfate sodium as a colon-specific prodrug of dexamethasone. *Drug Dev Ind Pharm*, (Mar 2006), Vol. 32, No. 3, pp. 389-97, ISSN 0363-9045.

Kim, C. K.; Shin, H. J.; Yang, S. G.; kim, J. H. & Oh, Y. (2001). Once a day oral dosing regimen of cyclosporine A: Combined therapy of cyclosporine a premicroemulsion concentrates and enteric coated solid-state premicroemulsion concentrates. *Pharm Res*, Vol. 18, No. 4, (Apr 2001), pp. 454-459, ISSN: 0724-8741.

Kim, S-J.; Cho, S. Y.; Kim, S. H.; Song, O-J.; Shin, II-S.; Cha D. S. & Park, H. J. (2008). Effect of microencapsulation on viability and other characteristics in *L. acidophilus* ATCC 43121. *LWT-Food Sci Technol*, Vol. 41, No. 3, (Apr 2008), pp. 493-500, ISSN 0023-6438.

Kotagale, N.; Maniyar, M.; Somvanshi, S.; Umekar, M. & Patel, C. J. (2010). Eudragit-S, Eudragit-L and cellulose acetate phthalate coated polysaccharide tablets for colonic targeted delivery of azathioprine. *Pharm Dev Technol*, Vol. 15, No. 4, (Jul 2010), pp 431-437, ISSN 1083-7450.

Koutroubakis, J. E. (2008). Spectrum of non-inflammatory bowel diseases and non-infectious colitis. *World J Gastroenter*, Vol. 14, No. 48, (Dec 2008), pp. 7277-7279, ISSN 1007-9327.

Krasaekoopt, W.; Bhandari, B. & Deeth, H. (2004). The influence of coating materials on some properties of alginate beads and survivability of microencapsulated probiotic bacteria. *Int Dairy J*, Vol. 14, No. 8, (Aug 2004), pp. 737-743, ISSN 0958-6946.

Krishnamachari, Y.; Madan, P. & Lin, S. (2007). Development of pH- and time-dependent oral microparticles to optimize budesonide delivery to ileum and colon. *Int J Pharm*, Vol. 338, No. 1-2, (Jun 2007), pp. 238-47, ISSN 0378-5173.

Kumar, R.; Patil, M. B.; Patil, S. R. & Paschapur, M. S. (2009). Polysaccharides based colon specific drug delivery: review. *Int J Pharm Tech Res*, Vol. 1, No. 2, (Apr 2009), pp. 334-346, ISSN 0974-4304.

Lamprecht, A.; Rodero Torres H.; Schafer, U. & Lehr, C. M. Biodegradable microparticles as a two-drug controlled release formulation: a potential treatment of inflammatory bowel disease. *J Control Rel*, Vol. 69, No. 3, (Dec 2000), pp. 445-54, ISSN 0168-3659.

Lamprecht, A.; Yamamoto, H.; Takeuchi, H. & Kawashima, P. A (2005). pH-sensitive microsphere system for the colon delivery of tacrolimus containing nanoparticles. *J Control Rel*, Vol. 104, No 2, (May 2005), pp 337-346, ISSN 0168-3659.

Leopold, C. S. & Friend, D. R. (1995). In vivo pharamcokinetics study for the assessment of poly(L-aspartic acid) as a drug carrier for colon specific drug delivery. *J Pharmacokinet Biopharm*, Vol. 23, No. 4, (Aug 1995), pp. 397-406, ISSN 0090-466X.

Levine, D. S.; Raisys, V. A. & Ainardi, V. (1987). Coating of oral beclomethasone dipropionate capsules with cellulose acetate phthalate enhances delivery of topically active anti-inflammatory drug to the terminal ileum. *Gastroenterology*, Vol. 92, No. 4 (Apr 1987), pp. 1037-1044, ISSN 0016-5085.

Linares, V.; Alonso, V. & Domingo, J. L. (2011). Oxidative stress as a mechanism underlying sulfasalazine-induced toxicity. *Expert Opin Drug Saf*, Vol. 10, No. 2, (Mar 2011), pp. 253-63, ISSN 1474-0338.

Liu, H.; Yang, X-G.; Nie, S-F.; Wei, L-L.; Zhou, L-L.; Liu, H.; Tang, R. & Pan, W-S. (2007). Chitosan-based controlled porosity osmotic pump for colon-specific delivery system: screening of formulation variables and *in vitro* investigation. *Int J Pharm*, Vol. 332, No. 1-2, (Mar 2007), pp. 115–124, ISSN 0378-5173.

Mahkam, M. & Vakhshouri, L. (2010). Colon-specific behavior of pH-responsive PMAA/ perlite composite. *Int J Mol Sci*, Vol. 11, No. 4, (Apr 2010), pp. 1546-1556, ISSN 1422-0067.

Makhlof, A.; Tozuka, Y. & Takeuchi H. (2009). pH-Sensitive nanospheres for colon-specific drug delivery in experimentally induced colitis rat model. *Eur J Pharm Biopharm*, Vol. 72, No 1, (May 2009), pp 1-8, ISSN 0939-6411.

Mandal, S.; Puniya, A. K. & Singh, K. (2006). Effect of alginate concentrations on survival of microencapsulated *L. casei* NCDC-298. *Int Dairy J*, Vol. 16, No, 10 (Oct 2006), pp. 1190-1195, ISSN 0958-6946.

Marshall, J. K.; Thabane, M.; Steinhart, A. H.; Newman, J. R.; Anand, A. & Irvine, E. J. (2010). Rectal 5-aminosalicylic acid for induction of remission in ulcerative colitis. *Cochrane Database Syst Rev*, No. 1, ISSN 1469-493X.

Milojevic, S.; Newton, J. M., Cummings, J. H.; Gibson, G. R., Botham, R. L.; Ring, S. G.; Stockham, M. & Allwood, M. C. (1996). Amylose as a coating for drug delivery to the colon: Preparation and in vitro evaluation using 5-ASA pellets. *J Control Rel*, Vol. 38 No. 1, (Jan 1996), pp. 85-94, ISSN 0168-3659.

Mladenovska, K.; Cruaud, O.; Richomme, P.; Belamie, E.; Raicki, R. S.; Venier-Julienne, M-C.; Popovski, E.; Benoit, J. p. & Goracinova, K. (2007). 5-ASA loaded chitosan–Ca–alginate microparticles: Preparation and physicochemical characterization. *Int J Pharm*, Vol. 345, No. 1-2, (Dec 2007), pp. 59-69, ISSN 0378-5173.

Mladenovska, K.; Raicki, R. S.; Janevik, E.I.; Ristoski, T.; Pavlova, M. J.; Kavrakovski, Z.; Dodov, M. G. & Goracinova K. (2007). Colon-specific delivery of 5-aminosalicylic acid from chitosan-Ca-alginate microparticles. *Int J Pharm*, Vol 342, No. 1-2, (Sept 2007), pp. 124-136, ISSN 0378-5173.

Muraoka, M.; Kimura, G.; Zhaopeng, H. & Takada K. (1998). Ulcerative colitis-colon delivery of 5-ASA. *Nippon Rinsho*, Vol. 56, No. 3, (Mar 1998), pp. 788-94, ISSN 0047-1852.

Nagpal, D.; Singh, R.; Gairola, N.; Bodhankar, S. L. & Dhaneshwar, S. S. (2006). Mutual azo-prodrug of 5-ASA for colon targeted drug delivery: synthesis, kinetic studies and pharmacological evaluation. *Indian J Pharm Sci*, Vol. 68, No. 2, (Jun 2006), pp. 171-178, ISSN 0250-474X.

Nasra, M. A.; El-Massik, M. A. & Naggar, V. F. (2007). Development of metronidazole colon-specififc delivery systems. *Asian J Pharm Sci*, Vol. 2, No. 1, (Apr 2007), pp. 18-28, ISSN 1818-0876.

Nolen, H. W.; Fedorak, R. N. & Friend, D. R. (1997). Steady-state pharmacokinetic of corticosteroids delivery from glucuronide prodrugs in normal and colitic rats. *Biopharm Drug Dispos*, Vol. 18, No. 8, (Nov 1997), pp. 681-695, ISSN 0142-2782.

Novaneethan U. & Giannella, R. A. (2011). Infectious colitis. *Current Opinion in Gastroenterology*, Vol. 27, No. 1, (Jan 2011), pp. 66-71. ISSN 0267-1379.

Nugent, S. G., Kumar, D., Rampton, D. S. & Evans, D. F. (2001). Intestinal luminal pH in inflammatory bowel diseases: possible determinants and implications for therapy with aminosalicylates and other drugs. *Gut*, Vol. 48, No .4, (Apr 2001), pp. 571-7, ISSN 0017-5749.

Obitte, N.C.; Chukwu, A.; Onyishi, I. V. (2010). The use of a pH-dependent and non pH-dependent natural hydrophobic biopolymer (*Landolphia owariensis* latex) as capsule coating agents in *in vitro* controlled release of metronidazole for possible colon targeted delivery. *International Journal of Applied Research in Natural Products.* Vol. 3, No. 1, (Mar 2010), pp. 1-17, ISSN 1940-6223.

O'Donnell, S. (2010) Therapeutic benefits of budesonide in gastroenterology. *Therapeutic Advances in Chronic Disease* (Nov 2010) Vol. 1, No. 4, pp. 177-186, ISSN 2040-6223.

Oliveira, G. F.; Ferrari, P. C.; Carvalho, L. Q. & Evangelista, R. C. Chitosan–pectin multiparticulate systems associated with enteric polymers for colonic drug delivery. *Carbohydrate Polymers*, Vol. 82, No. 3 (Oct 2010), pp. 1004-1009, ISSN 0144-8617.

Oz, H. S. & Ebersole, J. L. (2008). Application of prodrugs to inflammatory diseases of the gut. *Molecules*, Vol. 13, No. 2, (Feb 2008), pp. 452-74, ISSN 1420-3049.

Pang, Y-N.; Zhang, Y. & Zhang, Z-R. (2002). Synthesis of an enzyme-dependent prodrug and evaluation of its potential for colon targeting. *World J Gastroenterol*, Vol. 8, No. 5, (Oct 2002), pp. 913-917, ISSN 1007-9327.

Pantel, N.; Patel, J.; Gandhi, T.; Soni, T. & Shah, S. (2008). Novel pharmaceutical approach for colon-specific drug delivery: an overview. *J Pharm Res*, Vol. 1, No. 1 (Jul 2008), pp. 2-10, ISSN: 0974-6943.

Patel, D. B.; Patel, D. M.; Parikh, B. N.; Prajapati, S. T. & Patel, C. N. (2010). A review on time-dependent systems foro colonic delivery. *Journal of Global Pharma Technology*, Vol. 2, No. 1, (Jan 2010), pp. 65-71, ISSN 0975-8542.

Patel, M. M.; Shah, T. J.; Amin, A. F. & Shah, N, N. (2009). Design, development and optimization of a novel time and pH-dependent colon targeted drug delivery system. *Pharm Dev Technol*, Vol. 14, No.1, (Feb 2009), pp. 62-9, ISSN: 1083-7450.

Peran,L.; Camuesco, D.; Comalada, M.; Bailon, E.; Henriksson, A.; Xaus, J.; Zarzuelo, A. & Galvez, J. (2007). A comparative study of the preventative effects exerted by three probiotics, *B. lactis*, *L. casei* and *L. acidophilus*, in the TNBS model od rat colitis. *J Appl Microbiol*, Vol. 103, No. 4, (Oct 2007), pp. 836-844, ISSN 1364-5072.

Petreska Ivanovska, T.; Petrusevska-Tozi, L.; Smilkov, K.; Popovski, E.; Stafilov, T.; Grozdanov, A.; Geskovski, N.; Petkovska R. & Mladenovska, K. (2011) Influence of formulation variables on survival of *L. casei* loaded in chitosan-Ca-alginate microparticles prepared by spray-drying, *Eur J Pharm Sci*, Vol. 44, Suppl. 1, (Sept 2011), pp. 119-120, ISSN: 0928-0987.

Petreska Ivanovska, T.; Dabevska-Kostoska, M.; Geskovski, N.; Smilkov, K.; Popovski, E.; Petrusevska-Tozi, L. & Mladenovska, K. (2010) Viability of *L. casei* during microencapsulation in chitosan-calcium-alginate microparticles and in simulated *in vivo* conditions. *Arh Farm.*, Vol. 60, No. 5 (Oct 2010), pp. 748-749, ISSN: 004-1963.

Prakash, S. & Urbanska, M. A. (2008). Colon-targeted delivery of live bacterial cell biotherapeutics including microencapsulated live bacterial cells. *Biologics: Targets & Therapy,* Vol. 2, No. 3, (Sept 2008), pp. 355-378, ISSN 1177-5475.

Rangasamy, M. (2010). Colon targeted drug delivery systems: a review. *International Journal of Drug Formulation & Research,* Vol. 1, No. II, (Oct 2010), pp. 30-54, ISSN 2229-5054.

Ritschel, W. A. & Agrawal, M. A. (2002). US20026365185.

Rodriguez, M.; Vila-Jato, J. L. & Torres, D. (1998). Design of a new multiparticulate system for potential site-specific and controlled drug delivery to the colonic region. *J Control Rel,* Vol. 55, No. 1, (Oct 1998), pp. 67-77, ISSN 0168-3659.

Rokka, S. & Rantamaki, P. (2010). Protecting probiotic bacteria by microencapsulation: challenges for industrial applications. *Eur Food Res Technol,* Vol. 231, No. 1, (Feb 2010), pp. 1-12, ISSN 1438-2385.

Sandborn, W J. (2002). Enema and enterically-coated oral dosage forms of azathioprine. Patent No. 6432967; 5905081.

Sandoval-Castilla, O.; Lobato-Calleros, C.; Garcia-Galindo, H. S.; Alvarez-Ramirez, J. & Vernon-Carter E.J. (2010). Textural properties of alginate-pectin beads and survival of entrapped Lb. Casei in siumlated gastrointetsinal conditions and in yoghurt. *Food Res Int,* Vol. 43, No 1, (Jan 2010), pp. 111-117, ISSN 0963-9969.

Schroeder, K. W.; Tremaine, W. J. & Ilstrup, D. M. (1987). Coated oral 5-aminosalicylic acid therapy for mildly to moderately active ulcerative colitis. A randomized study. *N Engl J Med,* Vol. 317, No. 26, (Dec 1987), pp. 1625-9, ISSN 0028-4793.

Shah, N. H.; Railkar, A. M. & Phuapradit W. (2000). US20006039975.

Singh, B. M. (2007). Modified-release solid formulations for colonic delivery. Recent Patents on Drug Delivery & *Formulation,* Vol. 1, No. 1, (Jan 2007), pp. 53-63, ISSN 1872-2113.

Singh, B. N.; Trombetta, L. D.; Kim, K. H. (2004). Biodegradation behavior of gellan gum in simulated colonic media. *Pharm Dev Technol,* Vol. 9, No. 4, (Nov 2004) pp. 399-407, ISSN 1083-7450.

Smilkov, K.; Petrusevska-Tozi, L.; Petreska Ivanovska, T.; Dodov Glavas, M.; Baceva, K.; Dimitrovski, D.; Geskovski, N.; Petkovska, R. & Mladenovska, K. (2011). Effects of formulation variables on viability of *L. casei* loaded in whey protein-Ca-alginate microparticles in simulated *in vivo* conditions. *Eur J Pharm Sci,* Vol. 44, Suppl. 1, (Sept 2011), pp. 128-129, ISSN: 0928-0987.

Smilkov, K.; Petreska Ivanovska, T.; Petrusevska-Tozi, L.; Grozdanov, A.; Dodov Glavas, M.; Geskovski, N.; Petkovska, R. & Mladenovska, K. (2011). Effects of formulation variables on the particle size and viability of *L. casei* loaded in whey protein- Ca-alginate microparticles. *Mac Pharm Bull,* 2011, Vol. 57, Suppl. 1 (Sept, 2011), pp. 285-287, ISSN 1409-8695.

Sonu, I.; Lin, M. V.; Blonski, W. & Lichtenstein, G. R. (2010) Clinical Pharmacology of 5-ASA Compounds in Inflammatory Bowel Disease. *Gastroenterology Clinics of North America*, Vol. 39, No 3, (Sept 2010), pp. 559-599, ISSN: 0889-8553.

Strugala, V.; Dettmar, P. W. & Pearson, J. P. (2008). Thickness and continuity of the adherent colonic mucus barrier in active and quiescent ulcerative colitis and Crohn's disease. *Int J Clin Pract,* Vol. 62, No. 5, (May 2008), pp. 762-769, ISSN 1742-1241.

Takada, K. (1997). US5637319.

Talley , N. J.; Abreu, M. T.; Achkar, J-P.; Bernstein, C. N.; Dubinsky, M. C.; Hanauer, S. B.; Sunanda V. Kane, S. V.; Sandborn, W. J.; Ullman, T. A. & Moayyedi, P. (2011). An Evidence-Based Systematic Review on Medical Therapies for Inflammatory Bowel Disease. *Am J Gastroenterol,* Vol. 106, Suppl. No 1, (Apr 2011) pp. S2-S25, ISSN 0002-9270.

Talukder, R. M. & Fassihi, R. (2008). Development and in-vitro evaluation of a colon-specific controlled release drug delivery system. *J Pharm Pharmacol,* Vol. 60, No. 10, (Oct 2008), pp. 1297-1303, ISSN 0022-3573.

Thomos, P.; Richards, D. & Richards, A. (1985). Absorption of delayed release prednisolone in ulcerative colitis and Crohn's disease. *J Pharm Pharmacol,* Vol. 37, No. 10, (Oct 1985), pp. 757-758, ISSN 0022-3573.

Thompson, R. P. H.; Bloor, J. R.; Ede, R. J.; Hawkey, C.; Hawtorne, B.; Muller, F. A. & Palmer, R. M. J. (2002) Preserved collagenous cortisol levels during treatment of ulcerative colitis with COLAL-PRED™, a novel oral system consistently delivering prednisolone metasulhobenzoate to the colon. *Gastroenterology,* Vol. 122, Suppl. 1, T1, 207, ISSN 0016-5085.

Tozaki, H.; Odoriba, T.; Okada, N.; Fujita, T.; Terabe, A.; Suzuki, T.; Okabe, S.; Muranishi, S. & Yamamoto, A. (2002). Chitosan capsules for colon-specific drug delivery: enhanced localization of 5-ASA in the large intestine accelerates healing of TNBS-induced colitis in rats. *J Control Release*, Vol. 82, No. 1, (Jul 2002), pp. 51-61, ISSN 0168-3659.

Travis, S. P.; Stange, E. F.; Lemann, M.; Oresland, T.; Bemelman, W. A.; Chowers, Y.; Colombel, J. F.; D'Haens, G.; Ghosh, S.; Marteau, P.; Kruis, W.; Mortensen, N. J.; Penninckx, F. & Gassull, M. (2008). European evidence-based Consensus on the management of ulcerative colitis: Current management. *Journal of Crohn's and Colitis,* Vol. 2, No. 1, (March 2008), pp. 24-62, ISSN 1876-4479.

Tursi, A.; Elisei, W.; Brandimarte, G.; Giorgetti, G.; Penna, A. & Castrignano, V. (2010). Safety and effectiveness of infliximab for inflammatory bowel diseases in clinical practice. *Eur Rev Med Pharmacol Sci,* Vol. 14, No. 1, (Jan 2010), pp. 47-55, ISSN 1128-3602.

Ueda, Y.; Hata, T.; Yamaguchi, H.; Ueda, S. & Kodani, M. (1989). US4871549.

Vaidya, A.; Jain, A.; Khare, P.; Agrawal, R. K. & Jain, S. K. (2009) Metronidazole loaded pectin microspheres for colon targeting. *J Pharm Sci,* Vol. 98, No. 11, (Nov 2009), pp. 4229-36, ISSN 0250-474X.

Van Os, E. C.; Zins, B. J.; Sandborn, W. J.; Mays, D. C.; Tremaine, W. J.; Mahoney, D. W.; Zinsmeister, A. R. & Lipsky, J. J. (1996). Azathioprine pharmacokinetics after intravenous, oral, delayed release oral and rectal foam administration. *Gut*, Vol. 39, No. 1, (Jul 1996), pp. 63-68, ISSN 0017-5749.

Van Saene, J. J. M.; Van Saene, H. F. K.; Geitz, J. N.; Tarko-Smit, N. J. P. & Lerk, C. F. (1986). Quinolones and colonization resistance in human volunteers, *Pharm Weekbl Sci Ed*, Vol. 8, No. 1, (Feb 1986), pp. 67-71, ISSN 0149-6395.

Varshosaz J.; Ahmadi, F.; Emami, J.; Tavakoli, N.; Minaiyan, M.; Mahzouni, P. & Dorkoosh, F. (2011a). Microencapsulation of budesonide with dextran by spray drying technique for colon-targeted delivery: an in vitro/in vivo evaluation in induced colitis in rat. *J Microencapsul*, Vol. 28, No. 1, (Feb 2011), pp. 62-73, ISSN 0265-2048.

Varshosaz J.; Emami J.; Tavakoli N.; Fassihi A.; Minaiyan M.; Ahmadi F. & Dorkoosh F. (2009). Synthesis and evaluation of dextran-budesonide conjugates as colon specific prodrugs for treatment of ulcerative colitis. *Int J Pharm*, Vol. 365, No. 1-2, (Jan 2009), pp. 69-76, ISSN 0378-5173.

Varshosaz, J.; Emami, J.; Fassihi, A.; Tavakoli, N.; Minaiyan, M.; Ahmadi, F.; Mahzouni, P. & Dorkoosh, F. (2010). Effectiveness of budesonide-succinate-dextran conjugate as a novel prodrug of budesonide against acetic acid-induced colitis in rats. *Int J Colorectal Dis*, Vol. 25, No. 10, (Oct 2010), pp. 1159-65, ISSN 0179-1958.

Varshosaz, J.; Emami, J.; Tavakoli, N.; Minaiyan, M.; Rahmani, N.; Dorkoosh, F. & Mahzouni, P. (2011b). Development of novel budesonide pellets based on CODES™ technology: *in vitro/in vivo* evaluation in induced colitis in rats. *DARU*, Vol. 19, No. 2, (May 2011), pp. 107-117, ISSN 1560-8115.

Wahed, M.; Louis-Auguste, J. R.; Baxter, L. M.; Limdi, J. K.; McCartney, S. A.; Lindsay, J. O. & Bloom, S. L. Efficacy of methotrexate in Crohn's disease and ulcerative colitis patients unresponsive or intolerant to azathioprine /mercaptopurine. *Aliment Pharmacol Ther*, Vol. 30, No. 6, pp. (Sept 2009), pp. 614-20, ISSN 0269-2813.

Wang, K.; Xu, X.; Wang, YJ.; Yan, X.; Guo, G.; Huang, M.; Luo, F.; Zhao, X. Wei,YQ. & Qian, ZY. (2010). Synthesis and characterization of poly(methoxyl ethylene glycol-caprolactone-*co*-methacrylic acid-*co*-poly(ethylene glycol) methyl ether methacrylate) pH-sensitive hydrogel for delivery of dexamethasone *Int J Pharm*, Vol. 389, No 1-2, (Apr 2010), pp 130-138, ISSN 0378-5173.

Washington, N.; Washington, C. & Wilson, C. G. (2001). Chapter 7: Drug delivery to the large intestine and rectum, In: *Physiological pharmaceutics; Barriers to drug absorption*, pp. 143-180, Taylor & Francis, ISBN 0-748-406010-7, London and New York.

Wei, H.; Qing, D.; De-Ying, C.; Li-Fang, F. & Bai, X. (2008). Selective drug delivery to the colon using pectin-coated pellets. *PDA Journal of Pharmaceutical Science and Technology*, Vol. 62, No. 4, (Jul 2008), pp. 264-272, ISSN 1079-7440.

Yadav, R. & Mahatma, O. P. (2011). Ester Prodrug of 5-Aminosalicylic Acid for Colon Specific Drug Delivery: Synthesis, Kinetics, Hydrolysis and Stabilities studies. *J. Pharm. Sci. & Res*, Vol. 3, No. 1, (Jan 2011), pp. 966-972, ISSN 0975-1459.

Yano, H.; Hirayama, F.; Kamada, M.; Arima, H. & Uekama, K. (2002). Colon-specific delivery of prednisolone-appended α-cyclodextrin conjugate: alleviation of systemic side effect after oral administration. *J Control Rel*, Vol. 79, No. 1-3, (Feb 2002), pp. 103-112, ISSN 0168-3659.

Yehia, S. A.; Elshafeey, A. H.; Sayed, I. & Shehata, A. H. (2009). Optimization of budesonide compression-coated tablets for colonic delivery. *AAPS PharmSciTech*, Vol. 10, No. 1, (Feb 2009), pp. 147-57, ISSN 1530-9932.

Yokoe, J.; Iwasaki, N.; Haruta, S.; Kadono, K.; Ogawara, K.; Higaki, K. & Kimura T. (2003). Analysis and prediction of absorption behavior of colon-targeted prodrug in rats by GI-transit-absorption model. *J Control Release*, Vol. 86, No. 2-3, (Jan 2003), pp. 305-13, ISSN 0168-3659.

Zambito, Y. & Di Colo, G. (2003). Preparation and in vitro evaluation of chitosan matrices for colonic controlled drug delivery. *J Pharm Pharm Sci*, Vol. 6, No. 2, (May 2003), pp. 274-81, ISSN 1482-1826.

Zou, M.; Okamoto, H.; Cheng, G.; Hao, X.; Sun, J.; Cui, F. & Danjo, K. (2005). Synthesis and properties of polysaccharide prodrugs of 5-ASA as potential colon-specific delivery systems. *Eur J Pharm Biopharm*, Vol. 59, No. 1, (Jan 2005), pp. 155-60, ISSN 0939-6411.

8

Protective Effects of Japanese Black Vinegar "*Kurozu*" and Its Sediment "*Kurozu Moromimatsu*" on Dextran Sulfate Sodium-induced Experimental Colitis

Toru Shizuma, Chiharu Tanaka, Hidezo Mori and Naoto Fukuyama
Department of Physiology, School of Medicine, Tokai University, Japan

1. Introduction

Kurozu is a traditional Japanese black vinegar that is used in the preparation of foods. It is manufactured, mainly in Kagoshima prefecture in Japan, by fermentation of unpolished rice with lactobacillus and *Koji* bacillus in earthenware jars for more than one year, during which time it gradually becomes black. The supernatant is known as *Kurozu*, and the solid sediment, which is rich in organic materials, minerals, amino acids and so on, is known as *Kurozu Moromimatsu* (*Kurozu-M*). Many products containing *Kurozu* and *Kurozu-M* are available in Japan as health foods or supplements.

As reported by Murooka et al. (Murooka Y & Yamashita M, 2008), *Kurozu* has ameliorating effects on hyperlipemia and hypertension, as well as anti-cancer activity against colon cancer in vitro and in vivo (Nanda K et al., 2004; Shimoji Y et al., 2003; Shimoji Y et al., 2004). Further, we reported that *Kurozu-M* treatment reduced the activity of gelatinases (metalloproteinase-2, -9) in tumor tissues, inhibited the growth of human colon cancer cells, LoVo, in an animal model (Fukuyama N et al., 2007), and inhibited the growth of hepatocellular carcinoma in a diethylnitrosamine-induced animal model (Shizuma T et al., 2011). *Kurozu* has also been reported to have free radical-scavenging activity (Murooka Y & Yamashita M, 2008). Since active oxygen species or radicals are related to inflammation and tissue injury, *Kurozu* and *Kurozu-M* may be potential functional foods with preventive or therapeutic effects against inflammatory diseases.

Ulcerative colitis (UC) is an obstinate inflammatory bowel disease (IBD). The causes of UC are not well-established, but multiple genetic factors (van Lierop et al., 2009), immune responses of the colon (Hong SK et al., 2010) intestinal flora, and inflammatory cytokines (Polińska B et al., 2009; Ghosh N et al., 2010) have been suggested to be involved. Moreover, oxidative stress is thought to influence the severity of UC (Beckman JS et al., 1990; Babbs CF, 1992; Grudziński IP & Frankiewicz-Jóźko A, 2001; Hong SK et al., 2010). Enhanced release of reactive oxygen species (ROS), such as superoxide and hydroxyl radical, and reactive nitrogen species (RNS), such as peroxynitrite generated from nitric oxide (NO), is associated with aggravation of both clinical UC and dextran sulfate sodium (DSS)-induced colitis in an animal model (Elson CO et al., 1995).

Therefore, we decided to examine the protective effects of *Kurozu* and *Kurozu-M* in a rodent model of DSS-induced colitis, focusing on the possible role of anti-oxidative and anti-nitration effects.

2. Main body

2.1 Materials and methods

The experimental procedures were approved by the Animal Experimentation Committee, School of Medicine, Tokai University, Japan.

2.1.1 Experimental model

A solution of 3.5% DSS was given orally for 12 days to forty C57black6 female mice (CLEA Japan Inc., Tokyo, Japan). The mice were divided into 4 groups: the control group received the standard CE-2 rodent diet (CLEA Japan Inc., Tokyo, Japan) (n=10), the *Kurozu* group received CE-2 diet containing 3.2% solution of *Kurozu* (n=10), the *Kurozu-M* group received CE-2 diet including 2% *Kurozu-M* (n=10), and the acetic acid group received CE-2 diet including 0.3% solution of acetic acid (n=10). The amounts of *Kurozu*, *Kurozu-M* and acetic acid were based on volumes typically ingested by humans, adjusted for body weight. All mice were bred under specific pathogen-free conditions, because clinical UC is influenced by intestinal flora. CE-2 is a standard rodent diet, and includes soybean or white fish meal as source of protein, soybean oil or germ as source of lipids, rice bran or alfalfa as a source of carbohydrate, vegetable fiber, several vitamins, and minerals.

The three rodent diets other than the standard CE-2 diet were supplied by Sakamoto Kurozu Inc. (Kagoshima, Japan). The standard CE-2 and the three special diets were started a week before the initiation of oral DSS administration.

2.1.2 Experimental procedures

After initial DSS administration, changes of body weight and bloody stool frequency were monitored every 2 days for 12 days in all mice. Then, the mice were sacrificed and the proximal colon was resected. Microscopic examination (hematoxylin-eosin (H.E.) staining) was performed in all groups, and myeloperoxidase (MPO) staining, as a marker of leukocyte activation, was performed for all groups except the acetic acid group. Moreover, histological findings in the colon were evaluated and scored in the 4 groups according to the reported grading system (Tomita T et al., 2008), as follows. Mucosal damage: 0, normal; 1, 3–10 intraepithelial cells (IEL)/high power field (HPF) and focal damage; 2, >10 IEL/HPF and rare crypt abscesses; 3, >10 IEL/HPF, multiple crypt abscesses and erosion/ulceration. Submucosal damage: 0, normal or widely scattered leukocytes; 1, focal aggregates of leukocytes; 2, diffuse leukocyte infiltration with expansion of submucosa; 3, diffuse leukocyte infiltration. Muscularis damage: 0, normal or widely scattered leukocytes; 1, widely scattered leukocyte aggregates between muscle layers; 2, leukocyte infiltration with focal effacement of the muscularis; 3, extensive leukocyte infiltration with transmural effacement of the muscularis.

Moreover, enzyme-linked immunosorbent assay (ELISA) of serum tumor necrosis factor (TNF)-α and interleukin (IL)-2 as pro-inflammatory cytokines was carried out in the control and *Kurozu* groups. ELISA measurement of nitrotyrosine levels of resected colonic tissues at 12 days after initial DSS administration, as a marker of oxidative or nitration stress, was performed in all groups except the acetic acid group. Moreover, urinary excretion/day (during 11-12 days after initial DSS administration) of nitrite and nitrate (NOx) as a parameter of the bioavailability of NO was measured by means of the Griess method (Griess reagent kit; Invitrogen Japan K.K, Tokyo, Japan) in the (DSS-induced) control group, the *Kurozu* group, and the group given standard CE-2 diet without administration of DSS (each group: n=10).

2.1.3 Statistical analysis

The significance of differences of body weight, serum cytokines (TNF-α and IL-2), histological scores, and nitrotyrosine and NOx levels among the groups was examined by one-way analysis of variance (ANOVA) and Tukey's multiple comparison post-hoc test. The significance of differences in bloody stool frequency was examined by contingency table analysis. The criterion of significance was $p<0.05$.

Body weight after DSS administration is given as a percentage of basal body weight before DSS administration, taken as 100%. Levels of serum cytokines (TNF-α and IL-2) and histological scores, nitrotyrosine in colonic tissues, and NOx in urine, are presented as mean and standard deviation (SD). The frequency of mice with bloody stool after DSS administration is given as a percentage of the number of animals in each group.

2.2 Results

2.2.1 Change of body weight

There were no significant differences of diet or water intake among the four groups throughout the 12 days (data not shown).

The *Kurozu* group showed a significantly reduced body weight loss in the period of 6-12 days after initial DSS administration compared with the control group ($p<0.001$) and in the period of 8-12 days after initial DSS administration compared with the acetic acid group ($p<0.001$). The *Kurozu-M* group showed a significantly reduced body weight loss in the period of 6-8 days after initial DSS administration compared with the control group ($p<0.05$) and at 8 and 12 days after initial DSS administration compared with the acetic acid group ($p<0.05$). The acetic acid group showed a significantly reduced body weight loss only at 6 days after initial DSS administration compared with the control group ($p<0.01$). The results are summarized in Table 1.

2.2.2 Frequency of bloody stool

The appearance of bloody stool was noted in all mice of the control and acetic acid groups in the period of 4-12 days after initial DSS administration. In contrast, bloody stool was rarely noted in the *Kurozu* group: the frequency was 0% (0/10) during 2-8 days after initial DSS administration and only 20% (2/10) at 12 days after initial DSS administration. Similarly, in the *Kurozu-M* group, bloody stool was not noted during 2-8 days after initial DSS administration and the frequency was only 30% (3/10) at 12 days (Table 2).

	2	4	6	8	10	12 (days)*
control group	97.1 ±1.2	95.9 ±3.3	90.6 ±3.3	80.8 ±2.2	73.4 ±2.1	71.1 ±1.6
Kurozu group	99.2 ±2.2	98.2 ±1.8	97.8 ±1.3	89.4 ±2.9	87.2 ±2.9	81.6 ±2.4
Kurozu-M group	97.6 ±3.1	97.2 ±1.9	96.2 ±3.6	86.1 ±3.6	76.8 ±2.9	74.4 ±3.9
acetic acid group	99.2 ±2.3	97.8 ±1.9	96.6 ±2.1	80.1 ±2.3	72.0 ±3.5	69.1 ±3.1

[a] $p<0.001$; [b] $p<0.01$; [c] $p<0.05$; *days after initial administration of DSS
Body weight after DSS administration is given as a percentage of the basal body weight before DSS administration, taken as 100% (mean ±SD). (Shizuma T et al., 2011)

Table 1. Changes of body weight after initial adminsitration of DSS

	2	4	6	8	10	12 (days)†
control group	9/10 (90%)	10/10 (100%)	10/10 (100%)	10/10 (100%)	10/10 (100%)	10/10 (100%)
Kurozu group	0/10 (0%)	0/10 (0%)	0/10 (0%)	0/10 (0%)	1/10 (10%)	2/10 (20%)
Kurozu-M group	0/10 (0%)	0/10 (0%)	0/10 (0%)	0/10 (0%)	2/10 (20%)	3/10 (30%)
acetic acid group	7/10 (70%)	10/10 (100%)	10/10 (100%)	10/10 (100%)	10/10 (100%)	10/10 (100%)

*$p<0.01$; †days after initial administration of DSS
The bloody stool frequency in mice after initial DSS administration is given as a percentage of the number of animals in each group. (Shizuma T et al., 2011)

Table 2. Frequencies of bloody stool after initial administration of DSS

2.2.3 Histology

H.E. staining revealed epithelial abrasions, cryptal disturbance, hemorrhage and inflammatory cell invasion, and thickening of layers in the mucosa and submucosa of the colon in the control group, but these changes were minimal in the *Kurozu* and *Kurozu-M* groups. There was no marked difference between the control group and the acetic acid group (Fig.1a~d). Moreover, the *Kurozu* and the *Kurozu-M* groups showed fewer MPO-positive cells than the control group (Fig. 2a~c).

Histological scores (Tomita T et al., 2008) were as follows: control group, 5.88±0.33; *Kurozu* group, 0.50±0.50; *Kurozu-M* group, 0.88±0.33; acetic acid group, 4.38±0.48. In the *Kurozu* group and *Kurozu-M* groups, the scores were significantly ($p<0.001$) reduced compared with the control and acetic acid groups. Moreover, there was no significant difference between the control group and acetic acid group.

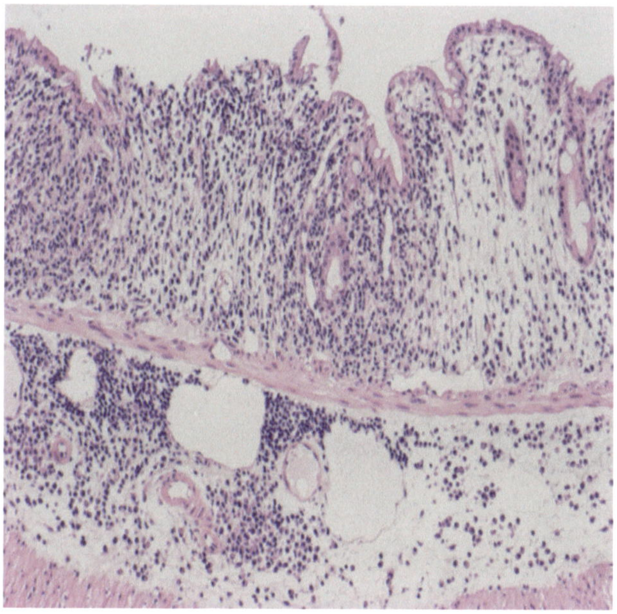

(a) control group

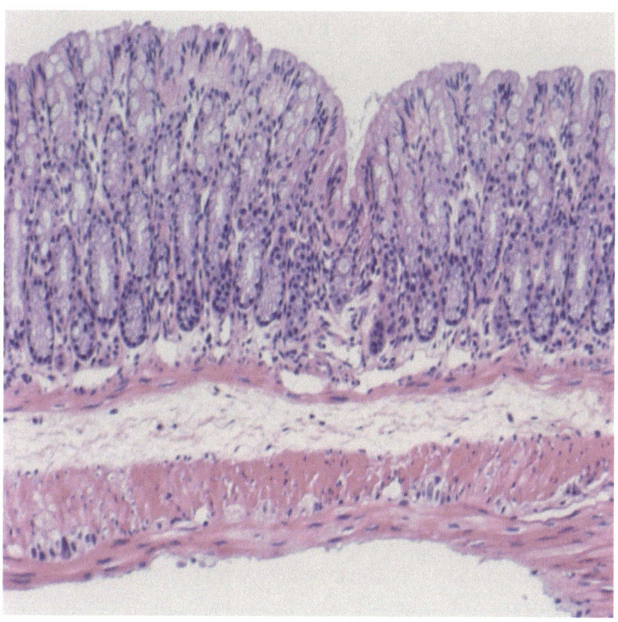

(b) *Kurozu* group

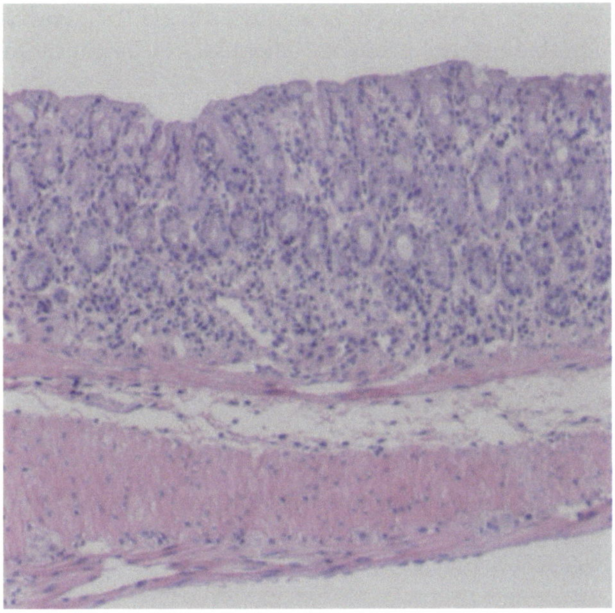

(c) *Kurozu-M* group

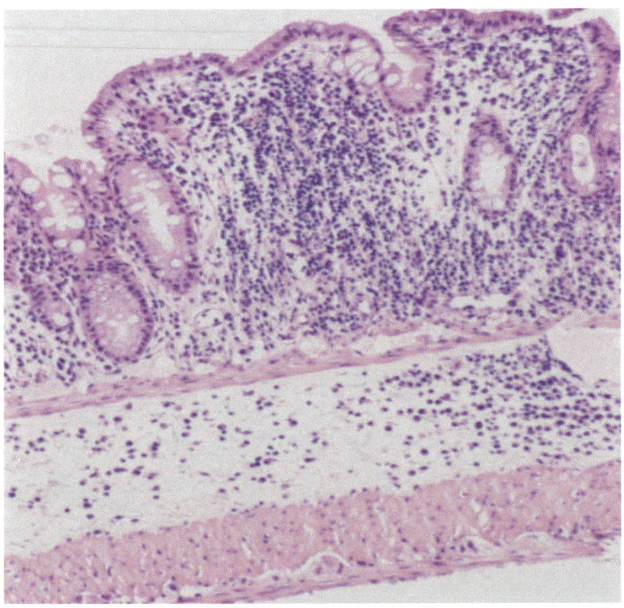

(d) acetic acid group

H.E. staining of resected colon revealed abrasions of epithelium, cryptal disturbance, and inflammatory cell infitration in mucosa and submucosal areas of colon in the control group. *Kurozu* and *Kurozu-M* treatment remarkably attenuated these changes in comparison to the control group. The acetic acid group showed no marked attenuation of colitis compared with the control group (a, the control group; b, the *Kurozu* group; c, the *Kurozu-M* group; d, the acetic acid group).

Fig. 1 Histological findings of resected colon

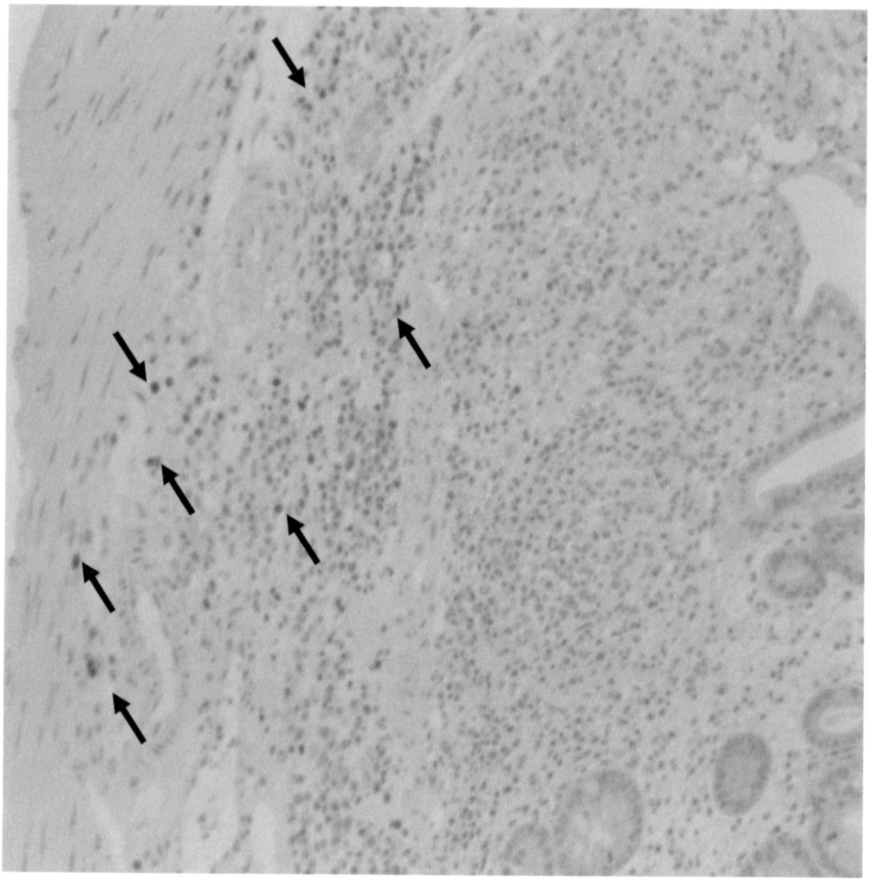

(a) Control group

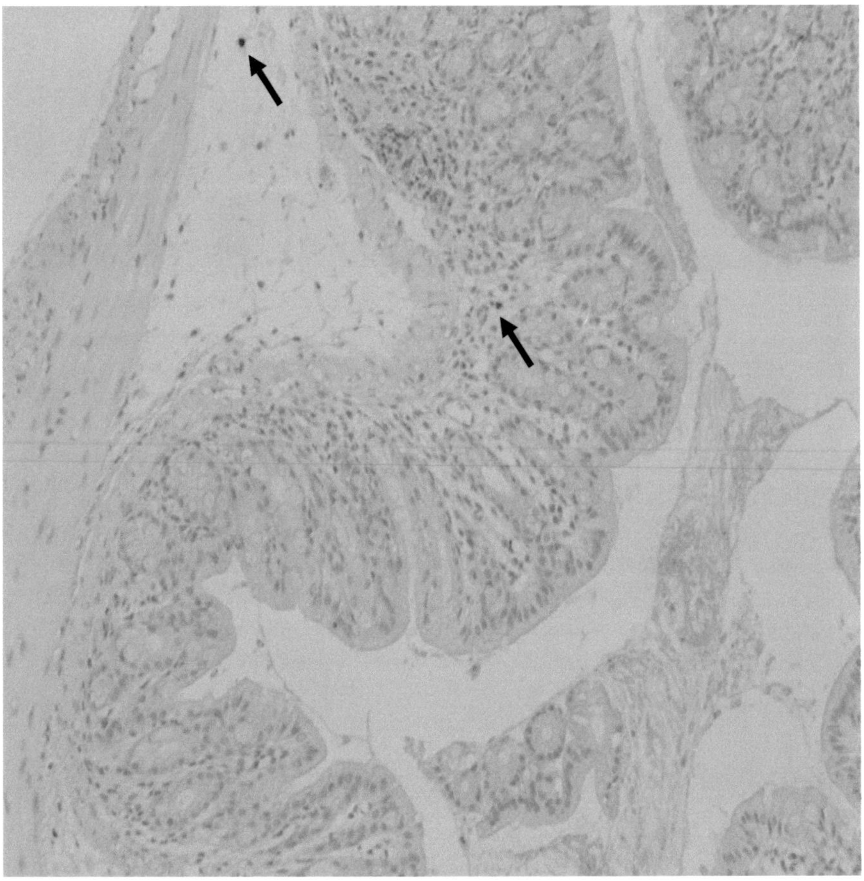

(b) *Kurozu* group

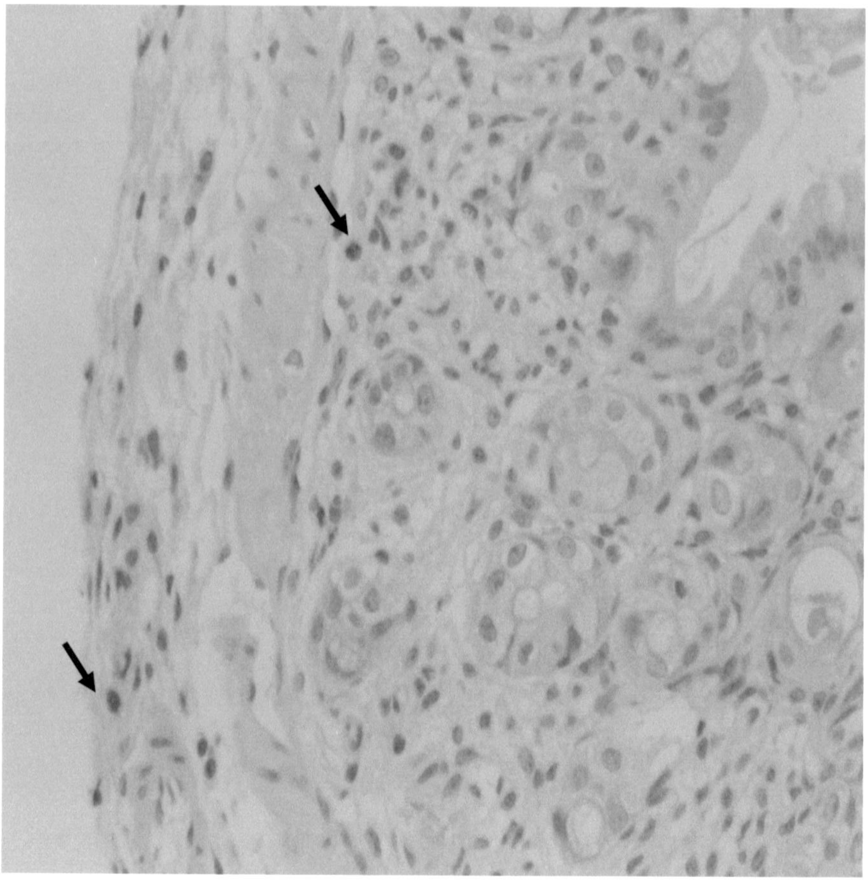

(c) *Kurozu-M* group

MPO-positive cells are indicated by ↗ and ↘ (a, control group; b, *Kurozu* group; c, *Kurozu-M* group). The *Kurozu* and the *Kurozu-M* groups showed fewer MPO-positive cells than the control group.

Fig. 2. MPO staining in colonic tissuse

2.2.4 Levels of cytokines

The levels of TNF-α (pg/ml) were 17.2±3.25 in the control group with administration of DSS and 15.9±5.77 in the *Kurozu* group (normal range: 0.6~2.8). Levels of IL-2 (U/ml) were 1.23±0.37 in the control group with administration of DSS and 1.13±0.39 in the *Kurozu* group (normal range: below 0.8). There were no significant differences in the levels of either of the cytokines between the two groups.

2.2.5 Level of nitrotyrosine in colonic tissue

The *Kurozu* group showed a significantly reduced nitrotyrosine level (53.1±7.1 ng/g protein) in resected colonic tissue compared with the control group (86.9±11.7 ng/g protein, $p<0.001$). However, the difference from the control was not significant in the *Kurozu-M* group (74.2±15.1 ng/g protein) (Fig. 3).

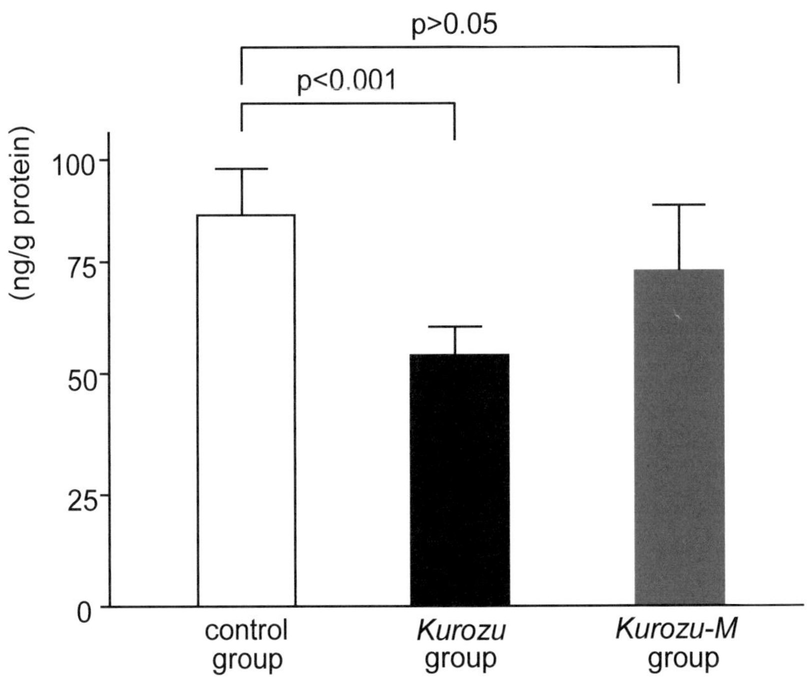

Kurozu treatment significantly ($p<0.001$) reduced the nitrotyrosine level in resected colonic tissue, in comparison to the control group. On the other hand, the difference from the control was not significant in the *Kurozu-M* group.

Fig. 3. Nitrotyrosine levels in resected colonic tissue

2.2.6 Level of NOx in urine

NOx levels in urine (μM) in the (DSS-induced) control group (807±172) and the *Kurozu* group (723±196) were significantly increased compared with the group that did not receive DSS administration (517±87). However, there were no significant difference between the (DSS-induced) control group and the *Kurozu* group (Fig. 4).

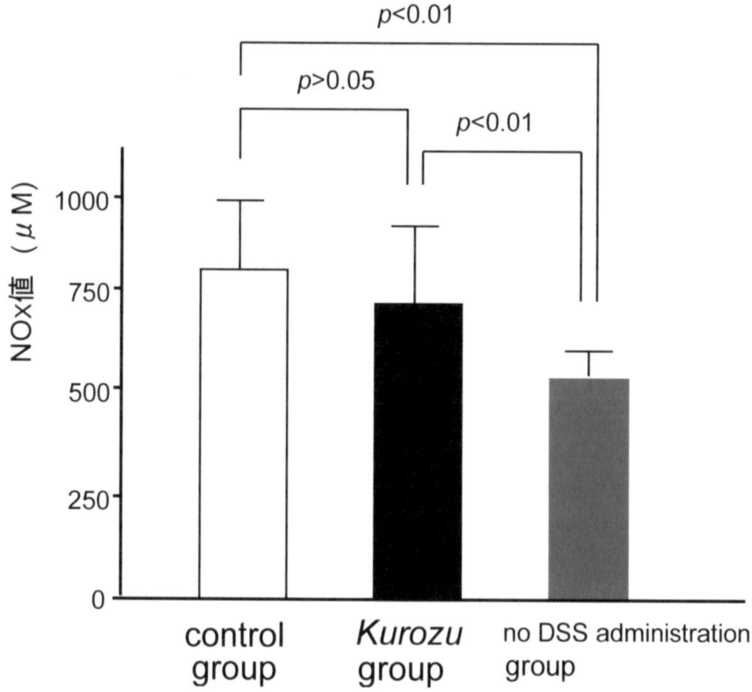

NOx levels in urine (μM) in the (DSS-induced) control group and the *Kurozu* group were significantly increased compared with the control group without DSS administration. However, there was no significant difference between the (DSS-induced) control group and the *Kurozu* group.

Fig. 4. NOx levels among the three groups

2.3 Discussion

Our results indicate that *Kurozu* and *Kurozu-M* exert protective effects against DSS-induced colitis in mice. *Kurozu* and *Kurozu-M* both reduced the bloody stool frequency and attenuated inflammatory changes of colon tissue, as well as inhibiting body weight loss.

Further, *Kurozu* and *Kurozu-M* decreased the number of MPO-positive cells. Since MPO is a marker of activation of leukocytes (Schindhelm RK., 2009), both *Kurozu* and *Kurozu-M* treatments appear to have anti-inflammatory effects in our model. Moreover, *Kurozu*, but not *Kurozu-M*, significantly reduced the nitrotyrosine level in colonic tissues in comparison with the control, although there was no significant difference in NOx level between the control and *Kurozu* groups. Nitrotyrosine is produced via at least two pathways, reaction of superoxide and NO, and reaction of nitrite and MPO (Beckman JS et al., 1990; Radi R, 2009). Therefore, *Kurozu* may suppress either of these pathways, or both. On the other hand, NOx is a good index of generation of NO by NO synthase (NOS) (Akuta T et al., 2006; Yang GY et al., 2009). Since no significant reduction of NOx level by *Kurozu* treatment was found in this study, suppression of NO and nitrite formation can be ruled out as a mechanism of reduction of nitrotyrosine generation. Therefore, *Kurozu* may reduce nitrotyrosine formation by suppressing the generation of superoxide or the activity of MPO.

In inflammatory states, including UC, generation of superoxide and NO is generally accelerated (Cross RK & Wilson KT, 2003). Superoxide itself is cytotoxic and is associated with tissue damage in many diseases. Moreover, superoxide and NO rapidly react with each other to form highly reactive peroxynitrite, leading to severe tissue damage via nitration of protein tyrosine residues to form nitrotyrosine, which is consequently considered to be a marker of oxidative and nitration stress. Therefore, peroxynitrite may have played a key role in the induction of colitis in this study.

Regarding the MPO pathway, MPO is mainly released from activated neutrophils. Since it is possible that *Kurozu* may block MPO release from neutrophils in the colonic tissues, we can not rule out the possibility that *Kurozu* suppresses the reaction of MPO and nitrite, thereby leading to a reduction of nitrotyrosine formation. However, *Kurozu-M* treatment did not reduce the generation of nitrotyrosine significantly, although infiltration of MPO-positive cells was remarkably suppressed. Moreover, the cytotoxity of MPO itself is unclear; our previous study demonstrated that MPO was protective against tissue injury in MPO knock-out mice, although in that case, we examined brain tissue (Takizawa S et al., 2002). However, at present, we have no evidence that the reduction of nitrotyrosine level in the *Kurozu* group involves suppression of MPO. Rather, our findings indicate that the mechanism predominantly mediating the anti-colitis effect of *Kurozu* is suppression of superoxide production, leading to decreased generation of peroxynitrite, which is strongly cytotoxic, or other ROS and RNS, although at this stage we can not rule out the possibility that suppression of MPO also contributes.

Overall, our results indicate that *Kurozu* and *Kurozu-M* both have an anti-colitis effect in the DSS-induced mouse colitis model, though *Kurozu* is more potent. This, in turn, suggests that the active materials are predominantly soluble compounds, because *Kurozu-M* is the precipitate formed during the manufacture of *Kurozu*.

Kurozu contains acetic acid, free amino acids, peptides, minerals, water-soluble vitamins, organic compounds including bacterial fermentation products, lipids and saccharides. Its main component is acetic acid, but we found here that acetic acid did not affect body weight loss, bloody stool frequency, or pathological findings in DSS-induced mice, compared with the control. Further, acetic acid is not present in *Kurozu-M*. Therefore, acetic acid is not one of the major protective components against colitis.

Amino acids seem to be good candidates for the anti-colitis agents in *Kurozu* and *Kurozu-M*. For example, glutamine has a protective effect on gut function, and has been suggested to have an anti-colitis effect in an animal model (Ameho CK et al., 1997). Other amino acids or their metabolites or degradation products, including arginine, asparagine, cysteine, serine (Faure M et al., 2006), methionine, and tryptophan, are known to have anti-oxidative effects (Wu G, 2009). Moreover, cysteine (Kim CJ et al., 2009), serine and tryptophan (Kim CJ et al., 2010) were found to have protective effects in animal models of colitis. Therefore, free amino acids or peptides may be among the active agents present in *Kurozu* and *Kurozu-M*.

Other organic materials, including lactic acid and products of lactobacillus or *Koji* bacillus fermentation, are also candidate protective agents. *Kurozu* is fermented with lactobacillus or *Koji* bacillus for several years in earthenware jars, and lactobacillus is well known as a beneficial component of human intestinal flora. Moreover, clinically significant anti-colitis effects of administration of probiotics (Sartor RB, 2004) or synbiotics (Kanauchi O et al.,

2009) have been reported in patients with mild UC. Further, anti-oxidative effects and protective effects against animal colitis were reported for *Koji* bacillus (Fukuda Y et al., 2006;Lee IH et al.,2008). Therefore, many components of *Kurozu* and *Kurozu-M*, including amino acids and oligopeptides, as well as other organic materials, may contribute to the anti-colitis effects observed here.

At present, UC is generally treated with anti-inflammatory agents, such as 5-aminosalicylic acid (5-ASA) and prednisolone (Rogler G, 2009). However, administration of these drugs is sometimes accompanied with severe side effects. Therefore, a dietary therapy would be desirable, particularly from the viewpoints of safety and long-term effectiveness.

In order to further examine the mechanism of action of *Kurozu*, additional study will be needed to evaluate the quantitative changes of pro-inflammatory cytokines in resected colonic tissues, for example, measurement of mRNA expression levels in tissues of the DSS-induced control and *Kurozu* groups, because there was no difference in the serum levels of pro-inflammatory cytokines. It could not be determined in this study whether *Kurozu* has a direct anti-oxidant effect, because the absorption, distribution, metabolism and excretion characteristics of *Kurozu* and its constituents in the mouse remain to be determined. This question might be addressed by means of in vitro experiments on colonic cell lines or rectal application of *Kurozu* in an animal model.

For the practical use of *Kurozu* in the management of colitis patients, it will be necessary to identify optimum dosages and administration schedules. Many products containing *Kurozu* are available in Japan as health foods or supplements, and in this study, the amounts of *Kurozu* used were based on volumes typically ingested by humans, adjusted for body weight. The next step will be a clinical trial to examine the anti-colitis effects of *Kurozu* as an oral supplement in patients with mild ulcerative colitis, focusing initially on typical dose and administration schedules recommended for existing health foods and supplements.

3. Conclusion

Our results indicate that *Kurozu* exerts a protective effect against DSS-induced colitis in mice, and one of the mechanisms involved may be an anti-oxidative or anti-nitration stress activity.

4. Acknowledgement

This work was supported by grants in 2009 Tokai University, School of Medicine Research Aid, 2009 and 2010 Grant-in-Aid for Scientific Research in Japan Society for the Promotion of Science (No. 21659295 and No.22659106) and 2009 Grant-in-Aid for Japanese Society for Parenteral and Enteral Nutrition.

5. References

Akuta, T.,; Zaki, MH.,; Yoshitake, J.,; Okamoto, T. & Akaike, T. (2006). Nitrative stress through formation of 8-nitroguanosine: insights into microbial pathogenesis. *Nitric Oxide*, vol.14:101-108

Ameho, CK.,; Adjei, AA.,; Harrison, EK.,; Takeshita, K.,; Morioka, T.,; Arakaki, Y.,; Ito, E.,; Suzuki, I.,; Kulkarni, AD.,; Kawajiri, A. & Yamamoto, S. (1997). Prophylactic effect of dietary glutamine supplementation on interleukin 8 and tumor necrosis factor alpha production in trinitrobenzene sulphonic acid induced colitis. *Gut*, vol.41:487-493

Babbs, CF. (1992). Oxygen radicals in ulcerative colitis. *Free Radic Biol Med*, vol.13:169-181

Beckman, JS.,; Beckman, TW.,; Chen, J.,; Marshall, PA. & Freeman, BA. (1990). Apparent hydroxyl radical production by peroxynitrite: implications for endothelial injury from nitric oxide and superoxide. *Proc Natl Acad Sci USA*, vol.87:1620-1624

Cross, RK. & Wilson, KT. (2003). Nitric oxide in inflammatory bowel disease. *Inflamm Bowel Dis*, vol.9:179-189

Elson, CO.,; Sartor, RB.,; Tennyson, GS. & Riddell, RH. (1995). Experimental models of inflammatory bowel disease. *Gastroenterology*, vol.109:1344-1367

Faure, M.,; Mettraux, C.,; Moennoz, D.,; Godin, JP.,; Vuichoud, J.,; Rochat, F.,; Breuillé, D.,; Obled, C. & Corthésy-Theulaz, I. (2006). Specific amino acids increase mucin synthesis and microbiota in dextran sulfate sodium-treated rats. *J Nutr*, vol.136:1558-1564

Fukuda, Y.,; Tao, Y.,; Tomita, T.,; Hori, K.,; Fukunaga, K.,; Noguchi, T.,; Hayashi, T.,; Shimoyama, T. & Tahahashi, R. (2006). A traditional Japanese medicine mitigates TNBS-induced colitis in rats. *Scand J Gastroenterol*, vol.41:1183-1189

Fukuyama, N.,; Jujo, S.,; Ito, I.,; Shizuma, T.,; Myojin, K.,; Ishiwata, K.,; Nagano, M.,; Nakazawa, H. & Mori, H. (2007). Kurozu moromimatsu inhibits tumor growth of LoVo cells in a mouse model in vivo. *Nutrition*, vol.23:81-86

Ghosh, N.,; Chaki, R.,; Mandal, V.,; Lin, GD. & Mandal, SC. (2010). Mechanisms and efficacy of immunobiologic therapies for inflammatory bowel diseases. *Int Rev Immunol*, vol.29:4-37

Grudziński, IP. & Frankiewicz-Jóźko, A. (2001). Nitric oxide synthase inhibitors reduced lipid peroxidation in N-nitrosodiethylamine-treated rats. *Rocz Panstw Zaki Hig*, vol.52:89-95

Hong, SK.,; Chaturvedi, R.,; Piazuelo, MB.,; Coburn, LA.,; Williams, CS.,; Delgado, AG.,; Casero, RA Jr.,; Schwartz, DA. & Wilson, KT. (2010). Increased expression and cellular localization of spermine oxidase in ulcerative colitis and relationship to disease activity. *Inflamm Bowel Dis*, vol.16:1557-1566

Kanauchi, O.,; Mitsuyama, K. & Andoh, A. (2009). The therapeutic impact of manipulating microbiota in inflammatory bowel disease. *Curr Pharm Des*, vol.15:2074-2086

Kim, CJ.,; Kovacs-Nolan, JA.,; Yang, C.,; Archbold, T.,; Fan, MZ. & Mine, Y. (2009). L-cysteine supplementation attenuates local inflammation and restores gut homeostasis in a porcine model of colitis. *Biochim Biophys Acta*, vol.1790:1161-1169

Kim, CJ.,; Kovacs-Nolan, JA.,; Yang, C.,; Archbold, T.,; Fan, MZ. & Mine, Y. (2010). l-Tryptophan exhibits therapeutic function in a porcine model of dextran sodium sulfate (DSS)-induced colitis. *J Nutr Biochem*, vol.21:468-475

Lee, IH.,; Hung, YH. & Chou, CC. (2008). Solid-state fermentation with fungi to enhance the antioxidative activity, total phenolic and anthocyanin contents of black bean. *Int J Food Microbiol*, vol.121:150-156

Murooka, Y. & Yamashita, M. (2008). Traditional healthful fermented products of Japan. *J Ind Microbiol Biotechnol*, vol.35:791-798

Nanda, K.,; Miyoshi, N.,; Nakamura, Y.,; Shimoji, Y.,; Tamura, Y.,; Nishikawa, Y.,; Uenakai, K.,; Kohno, H. & Tanaka, T. (2004). Extract of vinegar "Kurosu" from unpolished rice inhibits the proliferation of human cancer cells. *J Exp Clin Cancer Res*, vol.23:69-75.

Polińska, B.,;Matowicka-Karna, J. & Kemona, H. (2009). The cytokines in inflammatory bowel disease. *Postepy Hig Med Dosw*, vol.63:389-394

Radi, R. (2009). Peroxynitrite and reactive nitrogen species: the contribution of ABB in two decades of research. *Arch Biochem Biophys*, vol. 484:111-113

Rogler, G. (2009). Medical management of ulcerative colitis. *Dig Dis*, vol.27:542-549

Sartor, RB. (2004). Therapeutic manipulation of the enteric microflora in inflammatory bowel diseases: antibiotics, probiotics, and prebiotics. *Gastroenterology*, vol.126:1620-1633

Schindhelm, RK.,; van der Zwan, LP.,; Teerlink, T. & Scheffer, PG. (2009). Myeloperoxidase: a useful biomarker for cardiovascular disease risk stratification?. *Clin Chem*, vol.55:1462-1470

Shimoji, Y.,; Sugie, S.,; Kohno, H.,; Tanaka, T.,; Nanda, K.,; Tamura, Y.,; Nishikawa, Y.,; Hayashi, R.,; Uenakai, K. & Ohigashi, H. (2003). Extract of vinegar "Kurosu" from unpolished rice inhibits the development of colonic aberrant crypt foci induced by azoxymethane. *J Exp Clin Cancer Res*, vol.22:591-597

Shimoji, Y.,; Kohno, H.,; Nanda, K.,; Nishikawa, Y.,; Ohigashi, H.,; Uenakai, K. & Tanaka, T. (2004). Extract of Kurosu, a vinegar from unpolished rice, inhibits azoxymethane-induced colon carcinogenesis in male F344 rats. *Nutr Cancer*, vol.49:170-173

Shizuma, T.,; Ishiwata, K.,; Nagano, M.,; Mori, H. & Fukuyama, N. (2011). Protective effects of Kurozu and Kurozu Moromimatsu on dextran sulfate sodium-induced experimental colitis. *Dig Dis Sci*, vol.56:1387-1392

Shizuma, T.,; Ishiwata, K.,; Nagano, M.,; Mori, H. & Fukuyama, N. (2011). Protective effects of fermented rice vinegar sediment (*Kurozu Moromimatsu*) in a diethylnitrosamine-induced hepatocellular carcinoma animal model. *J Clin Biochem Nutr*, vol.49:31-35

Takizawa, S.,; Aratani, Y.,; Fukuyama, N.,; Maeda, N.,; Hirabayashi, H.,; Koyama, H.,; Shinohara, Y. & Nakazawa, H. (2002). Deficiency of myeloperoxidase increases infarct volume and nitrotyrosine formation in mouse brain. *J Cereb Blood Flow Metab*, vol.22:50-54

Tomita, T.,; Kanai, T.,; Fujii, T.,; Nemoto, Y.,; Okamoto, R.,; Tsuchiya, K.,; Totsuka, T.,; Sakamoto, N.,; Akira, S. & Watanabe, M. (2008). MyD88-dependent pathway in T cells directly modulates the expansion of colitogenic CD4+T cells in chronic colitis. *J Immunol*, vol.180:5291-5299

van Lierop, PP.,; Samsom, JN.,; Escher, JC. & Nieuwenhuis, EE. (2009). Role of the innate immune system in the pathogenesis of inflammatory bowel disease. *J Pediatr Gastroenterol Nutr*, vol.48:142-151

Wu, G. (2009). Amino acids: metabolism, functions, and nutrition. *Amino Acids*, vol.37:1-17

Yang, GY.,; Taboada, S. & Liao, J. (2009). Induced nitric oxide synthase as a major player in the oncogenic transformation of inflamed tissue. *Methods Mol Biol*, vol.512 :119-156

9

Innate Immunity: A Potent Target for Management of Inflammatory Bowel Disease

Masayuki Fukata
Division of Gastroenterology, Department of Medicine, University of Miami Miller School of Medicine, Miami, Florida, USA

1. Introduction

The gastrointestinal tract is a unique organ that cooperates with commensal flora to maintain physiological homeostasis. A layer of mucosa forms the interface between the host and the luminal contents where an elaborate immune system allows co-existence of diverse microorganisms and dietary antigens. The mucosal immunity regulates tolerance to commensal microorganisms while inducing effector immunity to pathogens through a fine interplay between innate and adaptive immune responses. In this process, innate immunity is responsible for recognition of microorganisms and initiation of effector and/or regulatory adaptive immune responses. Therefore, innate immunity is crucial for regulation of luminal microorganisms to maintain mucosal homeostasis.

Within the gastrointestinal mucosa, the effector and regulatory immune responses to commensal microorganisms are normally induced simultaneously, and constantly maintain mucosal immune homeostasis. Loss of this balance may cause uncontrolled mucosal inflammation, the state often seen in inflammatory bowel disease (IBD). IBD is a group of chronic inflammatory disorders in the gastrointestinal tract mainly classified into two types: ulcerative colitis and Crohn's disease. Although the etiology of IBD remains obscure and thus a curative therapy has not been established, genetic and immunological studies have provided cues for therapeutic targets of IBD based on the molecular pathogenesis of the disease. Because the central pathogenesis of IBD lies in abnormal mucosal immune responses to commensal flora, elucidation of immune regulation in gastrointestinal mucosa will help establish more effective strategies for treatment of IBD.

The initial step of the innate immunity is sensing pathogen-associated molecular patterns (PAMP)s through pathogen recognition receptors (PRRs), which induces a variety of gene expression via distinct intracellular signaling pathways. Different types of PRRs induce distinct sets of signaling pathways in response to the pathogens. Because different PRRs within a host cell can simultaneously recognize several molecular patterns of a pathogen, each pathogen triggers a unique combination of signaling pathways. In addition, different cell types may induce different responses to a pathogen, which increases host capacity to establish organized immune responses to a variety of pathogens. Diverse pathogen patterns are precisely recognized by TLRs, nucleotide-binding oligomerization domain (NOD)s and other PRRs including RIG-like helicases and C-type lectins (Table. 1). TLRs are expressed on the plasma membrane or endosomes, and NODs are expressed within the cytosol of the most cell types in intestinal mucosa (Abreu *et al.*, 2005; Inohara *et al.*, 2005; Kawai and Akira, 2006). Interestingly, several reports have demonstrated up-regulation or down-regulation of certain TLR expression in intestinal epithelial cells and mucosal antigen-presenting cells in patients with IBD (Cario and Podolsky, 2000; Hausmann *et al.*, 2002). Genome-wide association studies have also linked mutations within the genes encoding NODs and TLRs with development of IBD (Franchimont *et al.*, 2004; Hugot *et al.*, 2001; Ogura *et al.*, 2001; Pierik *et al.*, 2006). These findings suggest that signaling of NODs and TLRs may be potent targets for the treatment of IBD.

PRRs		Ligands	Sauces
TLRs	TLR1	Triacyl Lipoproteins	Mycobacteria
	TLR2	Peptidoglycan, Lipoteichoic acid	Gram-positive bacteria
	TLR3	Double Stranded RNA, poly I:C	Viruses
	TLR4	Lipopolysaccharide	Gram-negative bacteria
	TLR5	Flagellin	Bacteria
	TLR6	Diacyl LipopeptidesZymosan	MycobacteriaFungi
	TLR7	Single Stranded RNA	Viruses
	TLR8	Single Stranded RNA	Viruses
	TLR9	CpG-ODN	Bacteria and viruses
	TLR10	Unknown	Bacteria and Fungi
	TLR11	Uropathogenic bacteria	Uropathogenic Escherichia coli
	TLR12	Unknown	Unknown
	TLR13	Unknown	Unknown
NLRs	NOD1	meso-lanthionine, meso-DAP	Bacteria
	NOD2	Muramyldipeptide	Bacteria
	NLRCs	Flagellin. etc.	Bacteria
	NALPs	Muramyldipeptide, Bacterial RNA, crystals	Bacteria, Viruses, Uric acid crystals Maitotoxin
RNA helicases	RIG-1	Cytoplasmic dsRNA	Viruses
	MDR5	Cytoplasmic dsRNA	Viruses
Other	C-type lectins	Various	Bacteria, Viruses, and Fungi

Table 1. **PRRs and their respective ligands.**

Several TLR agonists and antagonists have been developed. Some TLR and NOD2 agonists have been shown to ameliorate murine IBD (Cario *et al.*, 2007; Fort *et al.*, 2005; Krieg *et al.*, 1995; Vijay-Kumar *et al.*, 2007a; Watanabe *et al.*, 2008). Defective immune responses to the NOD2 ligand have been reported in individuals homozygous for the major Crohn's disease-associated NOD2 mutation (Girardin *et al.*, 2003; Inohara *et al.*, 2003). Decreased mucosal expression of TLR3 has been observed in patients with Crohn's disease (Cario and Podolsky, 2000). Restoring the respective innate immune pathways may be a therapeutic strategy for patients carrying these innate immune defects. By contrast, blocking certain TLR signaling may be another possibility for treating IBD since some TLRs are up-regulated in IBD mucosa. Therefore, combination strategies of agonists and antagonists that target individual innate immune signaling may need to be considered for future treatment to obtain more effective therapeutic strategies.

2. Role of innate immunity in the pathogenesis of IBD – clinical findings.

The innate and adaptive immunities are the two major immune systems of our body. Innate immunity confers an immediate response to microbial pathogens, which is antigen non-specific and normally completed within several hours (Mahida and Rolfe, 2004). In this process, PRRs play a crucial role in recognition of pathogens and initiation of respective signaling pathways (Figure. 1).

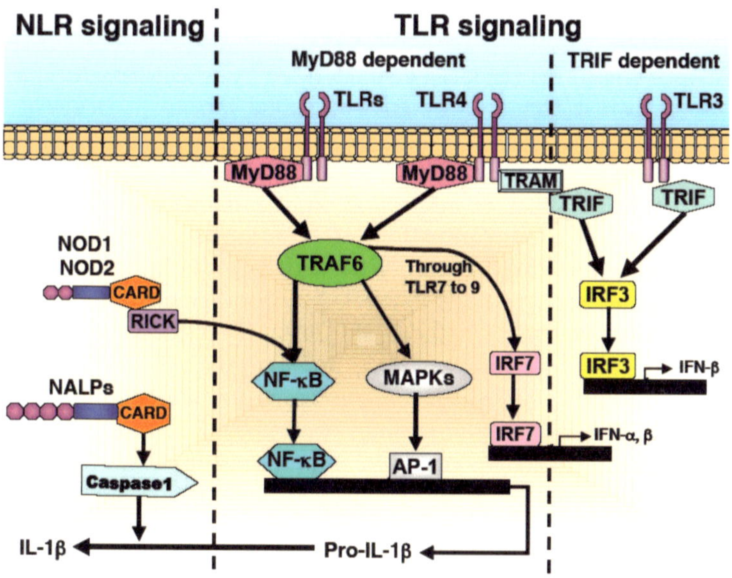

TLR signaling is initiated through the interaction of Toll/Interleukin-1 receptor (TIR) domains of the TLRs and recruited adaptor molecules. Depending on the adaptor molecule, TLR signaling may induce one of the two major downstream pathways, i.e., the MyD88-dependent and TRIF-dependent pathways. Most TLRs induce the MyD88-dependent pathway except for TLR3. In the MyD88-dependent pathway, tumour-necrosis-factor-receptor-associated factor 6 (TRAF6) is recruited and activated by phosphorylation and ubiquitylation to induce sequential phosphorylations of MAP kinases and IκB. These cascades lead to the activation of the transcriptional factors AP-1 and NF-κB, respectively. Activated AP-1 and NF-κB translocate to the nucleus and induce the expression of multiple pro-inflammatory genes including pro-IL-1β. The MyD88-dependent pathway may also induce Type I interferons (IFNs) through transcriptional factor IRF7 activation, when it is induced by TLR7, TLR8 or TLR9. The TRIF-dependent pathway can be induced directly by TLR3 and indirectly by TLR4 via recruitment of an adapter molecule TRAM (TRIF-related adaptor molecule), which results in the expression of the type I IFNs through activation of IRF3. NLRs induce signaling pathways through interaction of their Caspase recruitment domains (CARD)s with other CARD-containing molecules in the cytoplasm. NOD1 and NOD2 recruit a CARD-containing RICK resulting in NF-κB activation. NALPs form a complex of CARD-containing molecules called inflammasome, which activates Caspase-1. Activated Caspase-1 processes pro-IL-1β into mature IL-1β.

Fig. 1. Pathogen recognition receptors and their signaling pathways.

2.1 Innate immune function in the intestine

The rapid response of innate immunity to pathogens induces the production of antimicrobial peptides, phagocytic microbial killing and expression of cytokines, chemokines, and reactive oxygen species, leading to the recruitment of acute inflammatory cells to establish localized inflammation. Therefore, a defect in innate immunity may result in increased susceptibility of the host to pathogenic invasion even to commensals. In addition, proper induction of innate immunity is important to initiate an adaptive immune response that is antigen-specific and has an ability to temper ongoing inflammation through induction of regulatory immune properties. Abnormal innate immune signaling thus leads to inadequate induction of adaptive immunity that may result in disorganized immune responses to luminal pathogens.

2.2 Innate immune abnormalities in the pathogenesis of IBD

Clinical and basic science studies have indicated that etiology of IBD is associated with a disregulated adaptive immune response characterized by an aggressive T cell response to commensal flora, which is triggered by environmental factors particularly in genetically susceptible individuals (Packey and Sartor, 2008). Both environmental factors and the genetic alterations seen in patients with IBD vary, further making identification of exact etiology of IBD difficult. What is interesting in the pathogenesis of IBD is that any combination of environmental triggers and genetic alterations still result in aggressive T cell response to commensal flora forming chronic inflammation in gastrointestinal mucosa. On the other hand, several reports have demonstrated abnormal innate immune functions as an important pathogenesis of IBD (Latella *et al.*, 2010). The expression of mucosal TLRs, especially in epithelial cells and lamina propria antigen-presenting cells, is normally down-regulated, presumably to avoid inducing an excessive immune response to commensals (Melmed *et al.*, 2003; Otte *et al.*, 2004; Smythies *et al.*, 2005). However, several reports have shown increased expression of TLR4 and TLR2 in intestinal epithelial cells as well as lamina propria antigen-presenting cells in patients with both Crohn's disease and ulcerative colitis (Cario and Podolsky, 2000; Frolova *et al.*, 2008; Hausmann *et al.*, 2002; Szebeni *et al.*, 2008). Increased expression and *in vitro* cytokine responses of TLR2, TLR4, and TLR9 in peripheral blood mononuclear cells or dendritic cells have also been reported in IBD patients (Baumgart *et al.*, 2005; Baumgart *et al.*, 2009; Canto *et al.*, 2006; Jyonouchi *et al.*, 2010). Although increased TLR expression in peripheral blood cells has been found even in IBD patients in remission, up-regulation of these TLRs might not be a primary event in the pathogenesis of IBD, because expression of TLR4 and TLR2 is transcriptionally induced by inflammatory cytokines such as IFN-γ (Abreu *et al.*, 2002; Lin *et al.*, 2000; Rehli *et al.*, 2000). Similarly, NOD2 expression in intestinal epithelial cells is induced by inflammatory cytokines and increased in patients with IBD (Hisamatsu *et al.*, 2003; Rosenstiel *et al.*, 2003). Nevertheless, these findings strongly suggest a substantial involvement of innate immune abnormalities in the pathogenesis of IBD.

2.3 Genetic links between innate immunity and IBD pathogenesis.

Genome-wide association studies have demonstrated that most genetic alterations associated with IBD susceptibility relate to host mucosal barrier or anti-microbial functions, especially those involved in innate immune responses (Abraham and Medzhitov, 2011;

Vermeire *et al.*, 2011). For example, variants of the genes involving mucosal permeation and clearance of bacterial toxins such as mucin gene 19 (MUC19), organic cation transporter (OCTN) 1/2, multidrug resistance-1 (MDR1), have been reported to be associated with IBD (Barrett *et al.*, 2008; Ho *et al.*, 2005; Russell *et al.*, 2006; Waller *et al.*, 2006). Crohn's disease susceptibility genes NOD2, autophagy related protein 16-like 1 (ATG16), and immunity-related GTPase family M (IRGM) are involved in production of anti-microbial peptides and intracellular bactericidal functions (Hampe *et al.*, 2007; Hisamatsu *et al.*, 2003; McCarroll *et al.*, 2008; Rioux *et al.*, 2007; Wehkamp *et al.*, 2005). Moreover, TLR4 gene variants have been associated with both Crohn's disease and ulcerative colitis (Browning *et al.*, 2007; Franchimont *et al.*, 2004; Ouburg *et al.*, 2005; Torok *et al.*, 2004b). Polymorphisms in TLR1, 2, and 6 (TLR2 forms heteromeric receptor complexes with TLR1 or TLR6 to induce signal transduction) have been associated with greater disease extension in both ulcerative colitis and Crohn's disease (Pierik *et al.*, 2006). Polymorphisms in regulatory gene elements of TLR5 (stop codon) and TLR9 (promoter region) have also been associated with Crohn's disease (Hawn *et al.*, 2003; Torok *et al.*, 2004a).

Most of the IBD associated gene variants are loss-of-function type alterations. Therefore, in the pathogenesis of IBD, chronic inflammation due to aggressive T cell responses to commensal flora may be a result from the host's defective ability to maintain burdens of commensals and/or elimination of invading microbes and microbial toxins, rather than T cell function itself.

3. Role of innate immunity in the pathogenesis of colitis – animal studies

Mouse models of colitis are invaluable tools to determine the involvement of individual molecules in the pathogenesis of colitis. Gene recombination technology has provided ways to investigate the roles of individual PRRs in the pathogenesis of IBD by applying targeted gene knockout mice to animal models of IBD. Although none of the current murine models of IBD perfectly reproduce the human disease, each model has distinctive advantages to investigate a particular aspect of IBD pathogenesis. Most murine models of IBD require commensal flora to develop colitis, indicating that host response to commensal flora may play an important role in initiation of intestinal inflammation. However, the dextran sulfate sodium (DSS)-induced colitis, which is one of the well-established murine models of IBD, demonstrates more severe manifestations of colitis when depleted with the commensal flora (Kitajima *et al.*, 2001; Rakoff-Nahoum *et al.*, 2004). Since the underlying mechanism of DSS-induced colitis is associated with chemical damage of mucosal epithelium, this finding suggests a possible contribution of commensal flora to the protection of mucosa from damages induced by the noxious stimuli. This section details the roles played by the individual PRRs in induction and/or resolution of colitis based on knowledge obtained through studies in murine models of IBD.

3.1 Spontaneous colitis observed in PRR-deficient mice

Many knockout mice have been generated by targeting individual PRRs. Among them, only TLR5 and retinoid acid-inducible gene-I (RIG-I: a RNA helicase that recognizes intracellular RNA viruses) deficient mice develop spontaneous colitis, suggesting their regulatory roles in mucosal inflammation in the context of host-microbial interactions. Despite their importance in host defense against pathogens, most other PRR knockout mice do not develop spontaneous colitis in the presence of commensal flora. Therefore, some compensatory mechanisms may exist involving both host and microbial factors. For instances, many pathogens carry multiple PAMPs. Host antigen-presenting cells can recognize surface PAMPs of a bacterial pathogen by TLR2 (and TLR1 or TLR6), TLR4, or TLR5, and the same pathogen can be recognized by TLR9 or Nod-like receptors after being digested in the cytoplasm. Importantly, these PRRs share several key innate immune signaling pathways including NF-κB and MAP-kinases. This redundancy of the pathogen recognition system may be reasonable to reduce the risks of outbreaks of pathogens that acquire evolutional changes to evade host immune responses. Cross regulations between PRRs exist as TLR4 deficiency protects TLR5-/- mice from developing spontaneous colitis (Vijay-Kumar *et al.*, 2007a). What we need to take into account is that the roles of PRRs during mucosal damage or inflammation may differ from their roles in homeostatic maintenance of mucosal integrity. Therefore, the lack of intestinal spontaneous phenotypes in the PRR knockout animals does not simply negate their contribution to the pathogenesis of IBD.

3.2 Role of PRRs in acute murine colitis

Consistent with the finding in germ-free mice, most TLR knockout mice demonstrate increased susceptibility to DSS-induced acute colitis. For example, deficiency in TLR2, TLR4, TLR5, and TLR9 has been individually associated with the increased susceptibility to DSS-induced colitis (Fukata *et al.*, 2005; Ivison *et al.*, 2010; Lee *et al.*, 2006; Rakoff-Nahoum *et al.*, 2004). Mice deficient in MyD88, a major downstream molecule of most TLRs except for TLR3, also demonstrated more severe disease than WT mice in this colitis model suggesting the importance of MyD88-dependent TLR signaling in protection against chemically induced mucosal damage (Fukata *et al.*, 2005; Rakoff-Nahoum *et al.*, 2004).

3.3 Role of PRRs in chronic murine colitis

TLR signaling may act differently during chronic colitis where sustained inflammation exists. Unlike their increased susceptibility to the acute DSS model, most TLR-deficient mice are protected in the chronic models of colitis. For example, TLR9-deficient mice demonstrate less severe manifestations of chronic colitis induced by four cycles of DSS treatments compared to WT mice (Obermeier *et al.*, 2005). As I mentioned earlier, TLR9-deficient mice should be more susceptible to each cycle of DSS treatment than WT mice, while mechanism inducing chronic inflammation may differ from acute mucosal damage in this model. MyD88 deficiency protects mice from development of chronic colitis in several IBD models including the IL-10-/- model (Rakoff-Nahoum *et al.*, 2006). IL-10-/- mice are known to develop spontaneous colitis due to uncontrolled pro-inflammatory cytokine production in the presence of commnesal flora (Berg *et al.*, 1996; Kuhn *et al.*, 1993).

There are conflicting data in IL-10 x TLR4 double knockout mice demonstrating either increased or reduced colitis compared to IL-10-/- mice depending on the facilities (Biswas *et al.*, 2011; Gonzalez-Navajas *et al.*, 2010). In the presence of *Helicobacter hepaticus*, IL-10 x TLR4 double knockout mice generate atypical regulatory T cells which possess pro-inflammatory properties (Matharu *et al.*, 2009). Therefore, TLR4 deficiency may be colitogenic or protective in the IL-10-/- model depending on the presence or absence of *H. hepaticus*. Regulatory T cells are indispensable for termination of ongoing inflammation, and TLR4 has been suggested to foster the recruitment and/or proliferation of regulatory T cells in the intestine during colitis (Heimesaat *et al.*, 2007).

3.4 Compartmental specificities of the role of PRRs in intestinal inflammation

Since TLRs are expressed by most cell types in intestinal mucosa, the complexity of their function during chronic colitis may be due to the distinct roles played by TLR signaling in different cell types in the pathogenesis of chronic colitis. Compartmental differences of the role of TLR signaling in chronic colitis have been examined mainly in the MyD88 pathway (Asquith *et al.*, 2010; Fukata *et al.*, 2008; Gong *et al.*, 2010). Intestinal inflammation induced by *H. hepaticus* infection has been shown to be myeloid cell MyD88 dependent. In this infectious model, RAG2 x MyD88 double knockout mice as well as RAG2-/- chimeric mice that carry MyD88-deficient bone marrow demonstrate no intestinal inflammation but succumb to the infection, while MyD88 sufficient RAG2-/- counterparts show chronic colitis with splenomegaly but are protected from mortality (Asquith *et al.*, 2010). On the other hand, epithelial specific deletion of MyD88 results in spontaneous chronic inflammation in the small intestine (Gong *et al.*, 2010). These findings indicate that the MyD88 pathway in the myeloid compartment is necessary to induce intestinal inflammation against luminal pathogens and sufficient to block invasion of *H. hepaticus* at the mucosal interface.

Although there is a conflicting report, we and others have shown a defective colitogenic function of MyD88-/- T cells in an adoptive T cell transfer model of colitis, in which MyD88-/- naïve T cells have less ability to induce chronic colitis compared to MyD88 sufficient T cells after transfer to RAG-/- mice (Fukata *et al.*, 2008; Tomita *et al.*, 2008). In addition, we have shown that MyD88-/- regulatory T cells are unable to sufficiently suppress T cell mediated colitis, indicating that TLR signaling in T cells is important to elicit the full suppressive activities of regulatory T cells (Fukata *et al.*, 2008).

Ligation with TLR2 in combination with T cell receptor stimulation has also been reported to expand regulatory T cells in a MyD88-dependent manner, while it induces transient loss of their suppressive function (Sutmuller *et al.*, 2006). Therefore, TLR signaling in T cells seems to act as a co-stimulatory factor. Although antigen-presenting cells are thought to be a major cell type expressing TLRs, their TLR signaling is normally down regulated in the intestine (Rescigno and Matteoli, 2008; Smith *et al.*, 2005). Nevertheless, There unique roles for TLRs in individual cell types in intestinal inflammation may be revealed with future exploration.

3.5 Animal studies of phenotypic testing of disease susceptibility genes in human IBD

Testing the phenotype of individual susceptibility genes in IBD using mouse models is one of the priorities in the field of IBD research. Most IBD susceptible genes carry loss-of-function mutation, but by now we have not seen spontaneous intestinal inflammation in any mouse models that carry a functional deletion of the disease candidate gene. NOD2 deficient mice and those with an insertion of the human disease-associated mutation 3020insC do not demonstrate spontaneous intestinal inflammation but are more susceptible to DSS-induced colitis (Kobayashi *et al.*, 2005; Maeda *et al.*, 2005). ATG16L1 hypomorphic mice have abnormal Paneth cell granules and defective cryptdin production similar to Crohn's disease patients with ATG16L1 mutation, but these mice do not develop spontaneous colitis

(Cadwell *et al.*, 2008). The phenotypic discrepancies in these IBD susceptibility genes between human and mouse may be due to differences of species, but these results remind us the fact that the pathogenesis of IBD is complex of abnormalities of genetic, immunological, and environmental factors.

4. Challenges manipulating innate immunity (stimulate or suppress)

Manipulation of a particular immune pathway especially within a targeted organ is challenging. In this regard, manipulating an innate immune response as a therapeutic target of IBD has some advantages and disadvantages. The major advantage includes the non-specific nature of the innate immune responses, which provides broader effects than targeting adaptive immune responses which are antigen-specific. The rapid responses in both induction and resolution of innate immune signaling imply that exogenous control may be relatively easy. On the other hand, the multiple effects that can be induced by activation of a PRR may be a difficult point to enhance or suppress a specific function of the innate immune responses. In this section, possible targets in the innate immunity that may be utilized to treat or prevent intestinal inflammation and their potential pitfalls will be discussed through reviewing previously reported challenges in murine models of IBD (Table 2).

PRRs	**Agonist / Antagonist**	**Model of IBD used**	**Major effect**
TLR2	Agonist (Pam3CSK4)	Acute DSS colitis Chronic MDR1α-/-	Prevention and treatment. Strengthen epithelial barrier. Increase TFF3.
TLR3	Agonist (poly I:C)	Acute DSS colitis	Prevention. Involvement of Type I IFN?
TLR4	Antagonist (1A6) Antagonist (CRX-526)	Acute DSS colitis Chronic MDR1α-/-T cell transfer colitis	Prevention. Blocking acute inflammatory infiltrate. Blocking cytokine responses.
TLR5	Agonist (flagellin)	Acute DSS colitis	Prevention if it is administered intraperitoneally.
TLR9	Agonist (CpG-ODN) Antagonist (AV-ODN)	Acute DSS colitis TNBS colitis Chronic DSS colitis IL-10-/-, T cell transfer colitis	Prevention. Anti-apoptotic effect. Immuno-modulatory effect. Induction of tolerance. Blocking host response to luminal bacterial CpG.
NOD2	Agonist (MDP)	Acute DSS colitis TNBS colitis	Down-regulation of multiple TLR responses.

Table 2. Therapeutic challenges of PRR manipulation for murine models of IBD.

4.1 TLR2

Oral administration of a TLR2 agonist Pam3CSK4 has been suggested to have therapeutic potential in DSS-induced colitis (Cario *et al.*, 2007). The protective effect of the TLR2 agonist is associated with preservation of epithelial tight junctions and reduced apoptosis, and largely depends on the expression of the gap-junctional protein Connexin 43 in epithelial cells (Cario *et al.*, 2007; Ey *et al.*, 2009; Podolsky *et al.*, 2009). TLR2 stimulation also increases the colonic production of trefoil factor (TFF) 3 that facilitates wound healing and blocks apoptotic signaling (Podolsky *et al.*, 2009). Moreover, oral TLR2 agonist has been shown to delay induction of spontaneous colitis in MDR1α-/- mice (Ey *et al.*, 2009). The central pathogenesis of MDR1α-/- colitis is an impaired epithelial barrier function (Collett *et al.*, 2008). Therefore, the TLR2 agonist can be a cytoprotective rather than immunomodulatory strategy for acute as well as chronic phases of colitis. TLR2 agonists have not yet entered clinical trials for human diseases. Conversely, a TLR2 antagonist (OPN-305) has been developed, but its effects have not been tested on murine colitis (Hennessy *et al.*, 2010).

4.2 TLR3

Interesting data has been reported regarding the preventive effect of a TLR3 agonist on murine models of IBD (Vijay-Kumar *et al.*, 2007b). Pre-treatment of mice with a synthetic TLR3 ligand, polyinosinic:polycytidylic acid (poly I:C) protected mice from development of DSS-induced acute colitis (Vijay-Kumar *et al.*, 2007b). Similar effects of poly I:C treatment were observed in IL-10-/- mice. In this report, poly I:C was subcutaneously injected and the oral application did not show any protective effect on the colitis probably due to degradation of poly I:C by abundant RNAse in the gastrointestinal lumen. Although the exact mechanism underlying poly I:C-mediated preventive effect on colitis has been obscure, type I interferons which are predominantly induced by TLR3 signaling may have an immuno-regulatory capacity. Since intraperitoneal administration of high dose poly I:C (about ten times more than the dose in the former report) has been reported to cause mucosal destruction in the small intestine, we have to adjust the dose and route of poly I:C administration before clinical application (Zhou *et al.*, 2007a; Zhou *et al.*, 2007b). Because TLR3 expression has been shown to be significantly down regulated in the inflamed and non-inflamed mucosa of Crohn's disease as well as the mucosa of ileal pouches in patients with ulcerative colitis, stimulating TLR3 may restore an immunological defect caused by its down regulation (Cario and Podolsky, 2000; Heuschen *et al.*, 2007; Toiyama *et al.*, 2006). The existence of clinically tested poly I:C analogue (poly I:C_{12}U: Ampligen) is advantageous for the development of a TLR3 stimulation strategy (Nicodemus and Berek, 2010). Ampligen has been proven to have less toxicity than poly I:C and completed a phase III clinical trial for chronic fatigue syndrome (Nicodemus and Berek, 2010). Several antagonists for TLR3 signaling has been reported, but have not been developed as a therapeutic strategy for colitis (Bunting *et al.*, 2011; Cheng *et al.*, 2011).

4.3 TLR4

TLR4 is one of the most studied PRRs as a therapeutic target of IBD. A TLR4 antagonist (CRX-526; a synthetic lipid A mimetic molecule) has been shown to prevent the development of acute (DSS-induced) and chronic (MDR1α-/-) colitis (Fort *et al.*, 2005). We have further detailed the effect of a specific TLR4 antagonist monoclonal antibody on induction and resolution of acute DSS-induced colitis (Ungaro *et al.*, 2009). Consistent with the former report, our TLR4 antagonist antibody suppressed induction of acute inflammatory infiltrate by blocking the expression of several chemokines in the large intestine when administered prior to DSS treatment (Ungaro *et al.*, 2009). However, blocking TLR4 signaling after colitis was established delayed mucosal healing from the DSS-induced injury (Ungaro *et al.*, 2009). These results indicate that there are multiple roles of TLR4 signaling in the pathogenesis of DSS-induced colitis; it is responsible for acute inflammatory infiltrate through induction of chemokines during induction of colitis, but also contributes to mucosal repair during resolution of colitis. The mechanism underlying the contribution of TLR4 to mucosal repair is associated with TLR4-dependent induction of cyclooxygenase 2 and following production of prostaglandin E_2 in response to mucosal damage (Fukata *et al.*, 2006). In addition, the therapeutic effect of the TLR4 antagonist antibody was not found in chronic model of T cell transfer colitis (Ungaro *et al.*, 2009). Therefore, blocking TLR4 may be beneficial in interfering with a particular aspect of colitis pathogenesis i.e., acute inflammatory infiltration, and thus combination therapies with cytoprotective agents may be required to proceed to the clinical stage using this strategy to treat colitis patients.

4.4 TLR5

Since deficiency of TLR5 results in spontaneous development of colitis, the targeting strategy of TLR5 has been focused on stimulating TLR5 signaling for treatment of colitis. There are conflicting data on the use of the TLR5 agonist flagellin as a therapeutic agent of acute DSS-induced colitis. Intraperitoneal injection of purified flagellin has been reported to be protective in acute DSS-induced colitis (Vijay-Kumar *et al.*, 2008). By contrast, rectal administration of flagellin has been reported to aggravate DSS-induced colitis (Rhee *et al.*, 2005). The discrepancy of the flagellin effect may be due to administration route (systemic vs. topical), but a recent report has suggested that flagellin-mediated aggravation of colitis is independent of TLR5 signaling as the exacerbation of DSS colitis by flagellin is also observed in TLR5-deficient mice (Ivison *et al.*, 2010). TLR5 agonist has been under pre-clinical stage, but further screening of its efficacy and adverse effects using different mouse models of colitis may be required in addition to clarifying the effector component of flagellin and optimization of their administration route.

4.5 TLR9

Augmentation and suppression of TLR9 signaling have been challenged in multiple mouse models of colitis. Unmethylated cytosin-guanosin dinucleotide (CpG) dinucleotides, the immunostimulatory components of bacterial DNA, are known to be a TLR9 ligand (Bauer and Wagner, 2002; Krieg *et al.*, 1995). Administration of CpG oligodeoxynucleotides (CpG-ODNs) has been shown to prevent the induction of DSS-induced colitis, but this treatment aggravates colitis when CpG-ODNs are administered after the onset of DSS colitis (Obermeier *et al.*, 2002; Obermeier *et al.*, 2003; Rachmilewitz *et al.*, 2002). The mechanism of these opposing effects of CpG-ODNs is associated with an anti-apoptotic effect and immunostimulatory effect of CpG-ODNs, respectively. Since abundant bacterial ODNs naturally exist in the colorectal lumen that play a part of inflammatory stimuli in the setting of mucosal damage, pretreatment with CpG-ODNs has been suggested to induce host immune tolerance against endogenous bacterial ODNs (Obermeier *et al.*, 2003). Preventive effect of CpG-ODNs on induction of colitis has also been shown in other models such as 2,4,6-trinitrobenzene sulfonic acid (TNBS) colitis and can be achieved by oral administration, making this strategy further relevant (Rachmilewitz *et al.*, 2002). Although CpG-ODNs are generally thought as immunostimulative, CpG-ODN stimulation suppresses TNF-α and IL-1β expression in *ex vivo* colonic mucosa taken from active UC patients (Rachmilewitz *et al.*, 2006). A subset of patients with ulcerative colitis responds to Type I INF therapy through a yet unknown mechanism (Jacobs *et al.*, 2000; Madsen *et al.*, 2001; Nikolaus *et al.*, 2003). Since TLR9 signaling may induce Type I interferons which may act as immunomodulatory property during intestinal inflammation, emphasizing this aspect of TLR9 signaling may be another therapeutic target in the management of IBD (Katakura *et al.*, 2005).

Suppression of TLR9 signaling has also been beneficial for treating chronic murine colitis. Intraperitoneal as well as oral administration of adenoviral-ODN (AV-ODN) known to block the effect of bacterial CpG-ODN effectively suppressed intestinal inflammation during chronic DSS colitis (Obermeier *et al.*, 2005). The protective effect of AV-ODN was also observed in other chronic colitis models such as IL-10-/- and T cell transfer colitis models (Obermeier *et al.*, 2005). The protective effect of blocking TLR9 signaling during chronic colitis is consistent with the fact that TLR9-deficient mice have reduced severity of chronic colitis (Obermeier *et al.*, 2005). These results indicate that bacterial CpG-ODN abundantly existing in colorectal lumen is one of the indispensable factors inducing intestinal inflammation during chronic colitis.

4.6 NOD2

NOD2 signaling is a plausible therapeutic target as NOD2 mutations are associated with susceptibility to Crohn's disease. The mutations are known to be loss-of-function type mutations and thus the backup of this signaling is a reasonable idea. The use of NOD2 knockout models is consistent with the human disease setting. NOD2 transgenic mice are resistant to TNBS colitis (Yang *et al.*, 2007). In addition, intraperitoneal injection of a NOD2 ligand MDP protected mice from induction of acute colitis in DSS and TNBS models (Watanabe *et al.*, 2008). The mechanism underlying MDP-mediated protection is associated with down regulation of multiple TLR responses by NOD2 stimulation, as pretreatment of dendritic cells with MDP has been shown to inhibit cytokine responses induced by TLR stimulation. One concern is that the NOD2-deficient mice introduced NOD2 construct with a CARD15 frame-shift mutation were not protected from colitis by MDP (Watanabe *et al.*, 2008). Nevertheless, development of NOD2-stimulation strategy is advantageous because MDP has already been applied to several clinical trials of cancer treatments (Meyers *et al.*, 2008).

5. Conclusion and future direction

We discussed the unique aspects of innate immunity in the context of intestinal homeostasis and the pathogenesis of colitis. It is important to understand intestinal-specific innate immune functions as host interactions with commensal flora are a crucial part of intestinal homeostasis. PRRs recognize microorganisms and thus play major roles in the regulation of the intestinal-specific innate immune functions. Since abnormal host immune responses to commensal microorganisms is thought to be a center of the pathogenesis of IBD, PRRs can be potent targets of therapeutic intervention. Despite our high excitement, recent studies in murine models of IBD have demonstrated the complexity of intestinal PRR signaling as therapeutic target of IBD. Much of the complexity lies in the fact that signaling of PRRs is not only involved in the induction of intestinal inflammation but also it is indispensable for maintenance of mucosal homeostasis. For instance, PRR signaling that contributes to the induction of colitis may be required for the mucosal repair process during resolution of inflammation; blocking a particular PRR signaling may suppress intestinal inflammation but may delay mucosal healing. The involvement of individual PRRs may also differ in different phases of colitis. Therefore, we may need to select phases of colitis to manipulate the selective PRRs to achieve more effective strategies. For example, TLR4 antagonists and TLR9 agonists appear to prevent intestinal inflammation if given prior to induction of colitis. By contract, TLR2 agonists and TLR9 antagonists may be more beneficial if they are given after the induction of or during the chronic phase of colitis. Nucleotide sensing PRRs may have a specific application in IBD therapy because of their potential immunomodulatory properties through induction of type I IFNs. Understanding of cell-type specific differences of PRR expression and responses and targeting their individual signaling pathways in intestinal mucosa may provide more practical strategies to utilize PRR signaling for the treatment of IBD.

6. References

Abraham C, Medzhitov R (2011). Interactions between the host innate immune system and microbes in inflammatory bowel disease. *Gastroenterology* 140: 1729-37.

Abreu MT, Arnold ET, Thomas LS, Gonsky R, Zhou Y, Hu B, Arditi M (2002). TLR4 and MD-2 expression is regulated by immune-mediated signals in human intestinal epithelial cells. *J Biol Chem* 277: 20431-7.

Abreu MT, Fukata M, Arditi M (2005). TLR signaling in the gut in health and disease. *J Immunol* 174: 4453-60.

Asquith MJ, Boulard O, Powrie F, Maloy KJ (2010). Pathogenic and protective roles of MyD88 in leukocytes and epithelial cells in mouse models of inflammatory bowel disease. *Gastroenterology* 139: 519-29, 529 e1-2.

Barrett JC, Hansoul S, Nicolae DL, Cho JH, Duerr RH, Rioux JD, Brant SR, Silverberg MS, Taylor KD, Barmada MM, Bitton A, Dassopoulos T, Datta LW, Green T, Griffiths AM, Kistner EO, Murtha MT, Regueiro MD, Rotter JI, Schumm LP, Steinhart AH, Targan SR, Xavier RJ, Libioulle C, Sandor C, Lathrop M, Belaiche J, Dewit O, Gut I, Heath S, Laukens D, Mni M, Rutgeerts P, Van Gossum A, Zelenika D, Franchimont D, Hugot JP, de Vos M, Vermeire S, Louis E, Cardon LR, Anderson CA, Drummond H, Nimmo E, Ahmad T, Prescott NJ, Onnie CM, Fisher SA, Marchini J, Ghori J, Bumpstead S, Gwilliam R, Tremelling M, Deloukas P, Mansfield J, Jewell D, Satsangi J, Mathew CG, Parkes M, Georges M, Daly MJ (2008). Genome-wide association defines more than 30 distinct susceptibility loci for Crohn's disease. *Nat Genet* 40: 955-62.

Bauer S, Wagner H (2002). Bacterial CpG-DNA licenses TLR9. *Curr Top Microbiol Immunol* 270: 145-54.

Baumgart DC, Metzke D, Schmitz J, Scheffold A, Sturm A, Wiedenmann B, Dignass AU (2005). Patients with active inflammatory bowel disease lack immature peripheral blood plasmacytoid and myeloid dendritic cells. *Gut* 54: 228-36.

Baumgart DC, Thomas S, Przesdzing I, Metzke D, Bielecki C, Lehmann SM, Lehnardt S, Dorffel Y, Sturm A, Scheffold A, Schmitz J, Radbruch A (2009). Exaggerated inflammatory response of primary human myeloid dendritic cells to lipopolysaccharide in patients with inflammatory bowel disease. *Clin Exp Immunol* 157: 423-36.

Berg DJ, Davidson N, Kuhn R, Muller W, Menon S, Holland G, Thompson-Snipes L, Leach MW, Rennick D (1996). Enterocolitis and colon cancer in interleukin-10-deficient mice are associated with aberrant cytokine production and CD4(+) TH1-like responses. *J Clin Invest* 98: 1010-20.

Biswas A, Wilmanski J, Forsman H, Hrncir T, Hao L, Tlaskalova-Hogenova H, Kobayashi KS (2011). Negative regulation of Toll-like receptor signaling plays an essential role in homeostasis of the intestine. *Eur J Immunol* 41: 182-94.

Browning BL, Huebner C, Petermann I, Gearry RB, Barclay ML, Shelling AN, Ferguson LR (2007). Has toll-like receptor 4 been prematurely dismissed as an inflammatory bowel disease gene? Association study combined with meta-analysis shows strong evidence for association. *Am J Gastroenterol* 102: 2504-12.

Bunting RA, Duffy KE, Lamb RJ, San Mateo LR, Smalley K, Raymond H, Liu X, Petley T, Fisher J, Beck H, Flavell RA, Alexopoulou L, Ward CK (2011). Novel antagonist antibody to TLR3 blocks poly(I:C)-induced inflammation in vivo and in vitro. *Cell Immunol* 267: 9-16.

Cadwell K, Liu JY, Brown SL, Miyoshi H, Loh J, Lennerz JK, Kishi C, Kc W, Carrero JA, Hunt S, Stone CD, Brunt EM, Xavier RJ, Sleckman BP, Li E, Mizushima N, Stappenbeck TS, Virgin HWt (2008). A key role for autophagy and the autophagy gene Atg16l1 in mouse and human intestinal Paneth cells. *Nature* 456: 259-63.

Canto E, Ricart E, Monfort D, Gonzalez-Juan D, Balanzo J, Rodriguez-Sanchez JL, Vidal S (2006). TNF alpha production to TLR2 ligands in active IBD patients. *Clin Immunol* 119: 156-65.

Cario E, Gerken G, Podolsky DK (2007). Toll-like receptor 2 controls mucosal inflammation by regulating epithelial barrier function. *Gastroenterology* 132: 1359-74.

Cario E, Podolsky DK (2000). Differential alteration in intestinal epithelial cell expression of toll-like receptor 3 (TLR3) and TLR4 in inflammatory bowel disease. *Infect Immun* 68: 7010-7.

Cheng K, Wang X, Yin H (2011). Small-molecule inhibitors of the TLR3/dsRNA complex. *J Am Chem Soc* 133: 3764-7.

Collett A, Higgs NB, Gironella M, Zeef LA, Hayes A, Salmo E, Haboubi N, Iovanna JL, Carlson GL, Warhurst G (2008). Early molecular and functional changes in colonic epithelium that precede increased gut permeability during colitis development in mdr1α(-/-) mice. *Inflamm Bowel Dis* 14: 620-31.

Ey B, Eyking A, Gerken G, Podolsky DK, Cario E (2009). TLR2 mediates gap junctional intercellular communication through connexin-43 in intestinal epithelial barrier injury. *J Biol Chem* 284: 22332-43.

Fort MM, Mozaffarian A, Stover AG, Correia Jda S, Johnson DA, Crane RT, Ulevitch RJ, Persing DH, Bielefeldt-Ohmann H, Probst P, Jeffery E, Fling SP, Hershberg RM (2005). A synthetic TLR4 antagonist has anti-inflammatory effects in two murine models of inflammatory bowel disease. *J Immunol* 174: 6416-23.

Franchimont D, Vermeire S, El Housni H, Pierik M, Van Steen K, Gustot T, Quertinmont E, Abramowicz M, Van Gossum A, Deviere J, Rutgeerts P (2004). Deficient host-bacteria interactions in inflammatory bowel disease? The toll-like receptor (TLR)-4 Asp299gly polymorphism is associated with Crohn's disease and ulcerative colitis. *Gut* 53: 987-92.

Frolova L, Drastich P, Rossmann P, Klimesova K, Tlaskalova-Hogenova H (2008). Expression of Toll-like receptor 2 (TLR2), TLR4, and CD14 in biopsy samples of patients with inflammatory bowel diseases: upregulated expression of TLR2 in terminal ileum of patients with ulcerative colitis. *J Histochem Cytochem* 56: 267-74.

Fukata M, Breglio K, Chen A, Vamadevan AS, Goo T, Hsu D, Conduah D, Xu R, Abreu MT (2008). The myeloid differentiation factor 88 (MyD88) is required for CD4+ T cell effector function in a murine model of inflammatory bowel disease. *J Immunol* 180: 1886-94.

Fukata M, Chen A, Klepper A, Krishnareddy S, Vamadevan AS, Thomas LS, Xu R, Inoue H, Arditi M, Dannenberg AJ, Abreu MT (2006). Cox-2 is regulated by Toll-like receptor-4 (TLR4) signaling: Role in proliferation and apoptosis in the intestine. *Gastroenterology* 131: 862-77.

Fukata M, Michelsen KS, Eri R, Thomas LS, Hu B, Lukasek K, Nast CC, Lechago J, Xu R, Naiki Y, Soliman A, Arditi M, Abreu MT (2005). Toll-like receptor-4 is required for intestinal response to epithelial injury and limiting bacterial translocation in a murine model of acute colitis. *Am J Physiol Gastrointest Liver Physiol* 288: G1055-65.

Girardin SE, Boneca IG, Viala J, Chamaillard M, Labigne A, Thomas G, Philpott DJ, Sansonetti PJ (2003). Nod2 is a general sensor of peptidoglycan through muramyl dipeptide (MDP) detection. *J Biol Chem* 278: 8869-72.

Gong J, Xu J, Zhu W, Gao X, Li N, Li J (2010). Epithelial-specific blockade of MyD88-dependent pathway causes spontaneous small intestinal inflammation. *Clin Immunol* 136: 245-56.

Gonzalez-Navajas JM, Fine S, Law J, Datta SK, Nguyen KP, Yu M, Corr M, Katakura K, Eckman L, Lee J, Raz E (2010). TLR4 signaling in effector CD4+ T cells regulates TCR activation and experimental colitis in mice. *J Clin Invest* 120: 570-81.

Hampe J, Franke A, Rosenstiel P, Till A, Teuber M, Huse K, Albrecht M, Mayr G, De La Vega FM, Briggs J, Gunther S, Prescott NJ, Onnie CM, Hasler R, Sipos B, Folsch UR, Lengauer T, Platzer M, Mathew CG, Krawczak M, Schreiber S (2007). A genome-wide association scan of nonsynonymous SNPs identifies a susceptibility variant for Crohn disease in ATG16L1. *Nat Genet* 39: 207-11.

Hausmann M, Kiessling S, Mestermann S, Webb G, Spottl T, Andus T, Scholmerich J, Herfarth H, Ray K, Falk W, Rogler G (2002). Toll-like receptors 2 and 4 are up-regulated during intestinal inflammation. *Gastroenterology* 122: 1987-2000.

Hawn TR, Verbon A, Lettinga KD, Zhao LP, Li SS, Laws RJ, Skerrett SJ, Beutler B, Schroeder L, Nachman A, Ozinsky A, Smith KD, Aderem A (2003). A common dominant TLR5 stop codon polymorphism abolishes flagellin signaling and is associated with susceptibility to legionnaires' disease. *J Exp Med* 198: 1563-72.

Heimesaat MM, Fischer A, Siegmund B, Kupz A, Niebergall J, Fuchs D, Jahn HK, Freudenberg M, Loddenkemper C, Batra A, Lehr HA, Liesenfeld O, Blaut M, Gobel UB, Schumann RR, Bereswill S (2007). Shift towards pro-inflammatory intestinal bacteria aggravates acute murine colitis via Toll-like receptors 2 and 4. *PLoS One* 2: e662.

Hennessy EJ, Parker AE, O'Neill LA (2010). Targeting Toll-like receptors: emerging therapeutics? *Nat Rev Drug Discov* 9: 293-307.

Heuschen G, Leowardi C, Hinz U, Autschbach F, Stallmach A, Herfarth C, Heuschen UA (2007). Differential expression of toll-like receptor 3 and 5 in ileal pouch mucosa of ulcerative colitis patients. *Int J Colorectal Dis* 22: 293-301.

Hisamatsu T, Suzuki M, Reinecker HC, Nadeau WJ, McCormick BA, Podolsky DK (2003). CARD15/NOD2 functions as an antibacterial factor in human intestinal epithelial cells. *Gastroenterology* 124: 993-1000.

Ho GT, Nimmo ER, Tenesa A, Fennell J, Drummond H, Mowat C, Arnott ID, Satsangi J (2005). Allelic variations of the multidrug resistance gene determine susceptibility and disease behavior in ulcerative colitis. *Gastroenterology* 128: 288-96.

Hugot JP, Chamaillard M, Zouali H, Lesage S, Cezard JP, Belaiche J, Almer S, Tysk C, O'Morain CA, Gassull M, Binder V, Finkel Y, Cortot A, Modigliani R, Laurent-Puig P, Gower-Rousseau C, Macry J, Colombel JF, Sahbatou M, Thomas G (2001). Association of NOD2 leucine-rich repeat variants with susceptibility to Crohn's disease. *Nature* 411: 599-603.

Inohara, Chamaillard, McDonald C, Nunez G (2005). NOD-LRR proteins: role in host-microbial interactions and inflammatory disease. *Annu Rev Biochem* 74: 355-83.

Inohara N, Ogura Y, Fontalba A, Gutierrez O, Pons F, Crespo J, Fukase K, Inamura S, Kusumoto S, Hashimoto M, Foster SJ, Moran AP, Fernandez-Luna JL, Nunez G (2003). Host recognition of bacterial muramyl dipeptide mediated through NOD2. Implications for Crohn's disease. *J Biol Chem* 278: 5509-12.

Ivison SM, Himmel ME, Hardenberg G, Wark PA, Kifayet A, Levings MK, Steiner TS (2010). TLR5 is not required for flagellin-mediated exacerbation of DSS colitis. *Inflamm Bowel Dis* 16: 401-9.

Jacobs LD, Beck RW, Simon JH, Kinkel RP, Brownscheidle CM, Murray TJ, Simonian NA, Slasor PJ, Sandrock AW (2000). Intramuscular interferon beta-1a therapy initiated during a first demyelinating event in multiple sclerosis. CHAMPS Study Group. *N Engl J Med* 343: 898-904.

Jyonouchi H, Geng L, Cushing-Ruby A, Monteiro IM (2010). Aberrant responses to TLR agonists in pediatric IBD patients; the possible association with increased production of Th1/Th17 cytokines in response to candida, a luminal antigen. *Pediatr Allergy Immunol* 21: e747-55.

Katakura K, Lee J, Rachmilewitz D, Li G, Eckmann L, Raz E (2005). Toll-like receptor 9-induced type I IFN protects mice from experimental colitis. *J Clin Invest* 115: 695-702.

Kawai T, Akira S (2006). TLR signaling. *Cell Death Differ* 13: 816-25.

Kitajima S, Morimoto M, Sagara E, Shimizu C, Ikeda Y (2001). Dextran sodium sulfate-induced colitis in germ-free IQI/Jic mice. *Exp Anim* 50: 387-95.

Kobayashi KS, Chamaillard M, Ogura Y, Henegariu O, Inohara N, Nunez G, Flavell RA (2005). Nod2-dependent regulation of innate and adaptive immunity in the intestinal tract. *Science* 307: 731-4.

Krieg AM, Yi AK, Matson S, Waldschmidt TJ, Bishop GA, Teasdale R, Koretzky GA, Klinman DM (1995). CpG motifs in bacterial DNA trigger direct B-cell activation. *Nature* 374: 546-9.

Kuhn R, Lohler J, Rennick D, Rajewsky K, Muller W (1993). Interleukin-10-deficient mice develop chronic enterocolitis. *Cell* 75: 263-74.

Latella G, Fiocchi C, Caprili R (2010). News from the "5th International Meeting on Inflammatory Bowel Diseases" CAPRI 2010. *J Crohns Colitis* 4: 690-702.

Lee J, Mo JH, Katakura K, Alkalay I, Rucker AN, Liu YT, Lee HK, Shen C, Cojocaru G, Shenouda S, Kagnoff M, Eckmann L, Ben-Neriah Y, Raz E (2006). Maintenance of colonic homeostasis by distinctive apical TLR9 signalling in intestinal epithelial cells. *Nat Cell Biol* 8: 1327-36.

Lin Y, Lee H, Berg AH, Lisanti MP, Shapiro L, Scherer PE (2000). The lipopolysaccharide-activated toll-like receptor (TLR)-4 induces synthesis of the closely related receptor TLR-2 in adipocytes. *J Biol Chem* 275: 24255-63.

Madsen SM, Schlichting P, Davidsen B, Nielsen OH, Federspiel B, Riis P, Munkholm P (2001). An open-labeled, randomized study comparing systemic interferon-alpha-2A and prednisolone enemas in the treatment of left-sided ulcerative colitis. *Am J Gastroenterol* 96: 1807-15.

Maeda S, Hsu LC, Liu H, Bankston LA, Iimura M, Kagnoff MF, Eckmann L, Karin M (2005). Nod2 mutation in Crohn's disease potentiates NF-kappaB activity and IL-1beta processing. *Science* 307: 734-8.

Mahida YR, Rolfe VE (2004). Host-bacterial interactions in inflammatory bowel disease. *Clin Sci (Lond)* 107: 331-41.

Matharu KS, Mizoguchi E, Cotoner CA, Nguyen DD, Mingle B, Iweala OI, McBee ME, Stefka AT, Prioult G, Haigis KM, Bhan AK, Snapper SB, Murakami H, Schauer DB, Reinecker HC, Mizoguchi A, Nagler CR (2009). Toll-like receptor 4-mediated regulation of spontaneous Helicobacter-dependent colitis in IL-10-deficient mice. *Gastroenterology* 137: 1380-90 e1-3.

McCarroll SA, Huett A, Kuballa P, Chilewski SD, Landry A, Goyette P, Zody MC, Hall JL, Brant SR, Cho JH, Duerr RH, Silverberg MS, Taylor KD, Rioux JD, Altshuler D,

Daly MJ, Xavier RJ (2008). Deletion polymorphism upstream of IRGM associated with altered IRGM expression and Crohn's disease. *Nat Genet* 40: 1107-12.

Melmed G, Thomas LS, Lee N, Tesfay SY, Lukasek K, Michelsen KS, Zhou Y, Hu B, Arditi M, Abreu MT (2003). Human intestinal epithelial cells are broadly unresponsive to Toll-like receptor 2-dependent bacterial ligands: implications for host-microbial interactions in the gut. *J Immunol* 170: 1406-15.

Meyers PA, Schwartz CL, Krailo MD, Healey JH, Bernstein ML, Betcher D, Ferguson WS, Gebhardt MC, Goorin AM, Harris M, Kleinerman E, Link MP, Nadel H, Nieder M, Siegal GP, Weiner MA, Wells RJ, Womer RB, Grier HE (2008). Osteosarcoma: the addition of muramyl tripeptide to chemotherapy improves overall survival--a report from the Children's Oncology Group. *J Clin Oncol* 26: 633-8.

Nicodemus CF, Berek JS (2010). TLR3 agonists as immunotherapeutic agents. *Immunotherapy* 2: 137-40.

Nikolaus S, Rutgeerts P, Fedorak R, Steinhart AH, Wild GE, Theuer D, Mohrle J, Schreiber S (2003). Interferon beta-1a in ulcerative colitis: a placebo controlled, randomised, dose escalating study. *Gut* 52: 1286-90.

Obermeier F, Dunger N, Deml L, Herfarth H, Scholmerich J, Falk W (2002). CpG motifs of bacterial DNA exacerbate colitis of dextran sulfate sodium-treated mice. *Eur J Immunol* 32: 2084-92.

Obermeier F, Dunger N, Strauch UG, Grunwald N, Herfarth H, Scholmerich J, Falk W (2003). Contrasting activity of cytosin-guanosin dinucleotide oligonucleotides in mice with experimental colitis. *Clin Exp Immunol* 134: 217-24.

Obermeier F, Dunger N, Strauch UG, Hofmann C, Bleich A, Grunwald N, Hedrich HJ, Aschenbrenner E, Schlegelberger B, Rogler G, Scholmerich J, Falk W (2005). CpG motifs of bacterial DNA essentially contribute to the perpetuation of chronic intestinal inflammation. *Gastroenterology* 129: 913-27.

Ogura Y, Bonen DK, Inohara N, Nicolae DL, Chen FF, Ramos R, Britton H, Moran T, Karaliuskas R, Duerr RH, Achkar JP, Brant SR, Bayless TM, Kirschner BS, Hanauer SB, Nunez G, Cho JH (2001). A frameshift mutation in NOD2 associated with susceptibility to Crohn's disease. *Nature* 411: 603-6.

Otte JM, Cario E, Podolsky DK (2004). Mechanisms of cross hyporesponsiveness to Toll-like receptor bacterial ligands in intestinal epithelial cells. *Gastroenterology* 126: 1054-70.

Ouburg S, Mallant-Hent R, Crusius JB, van Bodegraven AA, Mulder CJ, Linskens R, Pena AS, Morre SA (2005). The toll-like receptor 4 (TLR4) Asp299Gly polymorphism is associated with colonic localisation of Crohn's disease without a major role for the Saccharomyces cerevisiae mannan-LBP-CD14-TLR4 pathway. *Gut* 54: 439-40.

Packey CD, Sartor RB (2008). Interplay of commensal and pathogenic bacteria, genetic mutations, and immunoregulatory defects in the pathogenesis of inflammatory bowel diseases. *J Intern Med* 263: 597-606.

Pierik M, Joossens S, Van Steen K, Van Schuerbeek N, Vlietinck R, Rutgeerts P, Vermeire S (2006). Toll-like receptor-1, -2, and -6 polymorphisms influence disease extension in inflammatory bowel diseases. *Inflamm Bowel Dis* 12: 1-8.

Podolsky DK, Gerken G, Eyking A, Cario E (2009). Colitis-associated variant of TLR2 causes impaired mucosal repair because of TFF3 deficiency. *Gastroenterology* 137: 209-20.

Rachmilewitz D, Karmeli F, Shteingart S, Lee J, Takabayashi K, Raz E (2006). Immunostimulatory oligonucleotides inhibit colonic proinflammatory cytokine production in ulcerative colitis. *Inflamm Bowel Dis* 12: 339-45.

Rachmilewitz D, Karmeli F, Takabayashi K, Hayashi T, Leider-Trejo L, Lee J, Leoni LM, Raz E (2002). Immunostimulatory DNA ameliorates experimental and spontaneous murine colitis. *Gastroenterology* 122: 1428-41.

Rakoff-Nahoum S, Hao L, Medzhitov R (2006). Role of toll-like receptors in spontaneous commensal-dependent colitis. *Immunity* 25: 319-29.

Rakoff-Nahoum S, Paglino J, Eslami-Varzaneh F, Edberg S, Medzhitov R (2004). Recognition of commensal microflora by toll-like receptors is required for intestinal homeostasis. *Cell* 118: 229-41.

Rehli M, Poltorak A, Schwarzfischer L, Krause SW, Andreesen R, Beutler B (2000). PU.1 and interferon consensus sequence-binding protein regulate the myeloid expression of the human Toll-like receptor 4 gene. *J Biol Chem* 275: 9773-81.

Rescigno M, Matteoli G (2008). Lamina propria dendritic cells: for whom the bell TOLLs? *Eur J Immunol* 38: 1483-6.

Rhee SH, Im E, Riegler M, Kokkotou E, O'Brien M, Pothoulakis C (2005). Pathophysiological role of Toll-like receptor 5 engagement by bacterial flagellin in colonic inflammation. *Proc Natl Acad Sci U S A* 102: 13610-5.

Rioux JD, Xavier RJ, Taylor KD, Silverberg MS, Goyette P, Huett A, Green T, Kuballa P, Barmada MM, Datta LW, Shugart YY, Griffiths AM, Targan SR, Ippoliti AF, Bernard EJ, Mei L, Nicolae DL, Regueiro M, Schumm LP, Steinhart AH, Rotter JI, Duerr RH, Cho JH, Daly MJ, Brant SR (2007). Genome-wide association study identifies new susceptibility loci for Crohn disease and implicates autophagy in disease pathogenesis. *Nat Genet* 39: 596-604.

Rosenstiel P, Fantini M, Brautigam K, Kuhbacher T, Waetzig GH, Seegert D, Schreiber S (2003). TNF-alpha and IFN-gamma regulate the expression of the NOD2 (CARD15) gene in human intestinal epithelial cells. *Gastroenterology* 124: 1001-9.

Russell RK, Drummond HE, Nimmo ER, Anderson NH, Noble CL, Wilson DC, Gillett PM, McGrogan P, Hassan K, Weaver LT, Bisset WM, Mahdi G, Satsangi J (2006). Analysis of the influence of OCTN1/2 variants within the IBD5 locus on disease susceptibility and growth indices in early onset inflammatory bowel disease. *Gut* 55: 1114-23.

Smith PD, Ochsenbauer-Jambor C, Smythies LE (2005). Intestinal macrophages: unique effector cells of the innate immune system. *Immunol Rev* 206: 149-59.

Smythies LE, Sellers M, Clements RH, Mosteller-Barnum M, Meng G, Benjamin WH, Orenstein JM, Smith PD (2005). Human intestinal macrophages display profound inflammatory anergy despite avid phagocytic and bacteriocidal activity. *J Clin Invest* 115: 66-75.

Sutmuller RP, den Brok MH, Kramer M, Bennink EJ, Toonen LW, Kullberg BJ, Joosten LA, Akira S, Netea MG, Adema GJ (2006). Toll-like receptor 2 controls expansion and function of regulatory T cells. *J Clin Invest* 116: 485-94.

Szebeni B, Veres G, Dezsofi A, Rusai K, Vannay A, Mraz M, Majorova E, Arato A (2008). Increased expression of Toll-like receptor (TLR) 2 and TLR4 in the colonic mucosa of children with inflammatory bowel disease. *Clin Exp Immunol* 151: 34-41.

Toiyama Y, Araki T, Yoshiyama S, Hiro J, Miki C, Kusunoki M (2006). The expression patterns of Toll-like receptors in the ileal pouch mucosa of postoperative ulcerative colitis patients. *Surg Today* 36: 287-90.

Tomita T, Kanai T, Fujii T, Nemoto Y, Okamoto R, Tsuchiya K, Totsuka T, Sakamoto N, Akira S, Watanabe M (2008). MyD88-dependent pathway in T cells directly modulates the expansion of colitogenic CD4+ T cells in chronic colitis. *J Immunol* 180: 5291-9.

Torok HP, Glas J, Tonenchi L, Bruennler G, Folwaczny M, Folwaczny C (2004a). Crohn's disease is associated with a toll-like receptor-9 polymorphism. *Gastroenterology* 127: 365-6.

Torok HP, Glas J, Tonenchi L, Mussack T, Folwaczny C (2004b). Polymorphisms of the lipopolysaccharide-signaling complex in inflammatory bowel disease: association of a mutation in the Toll-like receptor 4 gene with ulcerative colitis. *Clin Immunol* 112: 85-91.

Ungaro R, Fukata M, Hsu D, Hernandez Y, Breglio K, Chen A, Xu R, Sotolongo J, Espana C, Zaias J, Elson G, Mayer L, Kosco-Vilbois M, Abreu MT (2009). A novel Toll-like receptor 4 antagonist antibody ameliorates inflammation but impairs mucosal healing in murine colitis. *Am J Physiol Gastrointest Liver Physiol* 296: G1167-79.

Vermeire S, Van Assche G, Rutgeerts P (2011). Inflammatory bowel disease and colitis: new concepts from the bench and the clinic. *Curr Opin Gastroenterol* 27: 32-7.

Vijay-Kumar M, Aitken JD, Sanders CJ, Frias A, Sloane VM, Xu J, Neish AS, Rojas M, Gewirtz AT (2008). Flagellin treatment protects against chemicals, bacteria, viruses, and radiation. *J Immunol* 180: 8280-5.

Vijay-Kumar M, Sanders CJ, Taylor RT, Kumar A, Aitken JD, Sitaraman SV, Neish AS, Uematsu S, Akira S, Williams IR, Gewirtz AT (2007a). Deletion of TLR5 results in spontaneous colitis in mice. *J Clin Invest* 117: 3909-21.

Vijay-Kumar M, Wu H, Aitken J, Kolachala VL, Neish AS, Sitaraman SV, Gewirtz AT (2007b). Activation of toll-like receptor 3 protects against DSS-induced acute colitis. *Inflamm Bowel Dis* 13: 856-64.

Waller S, Tremelling M, Bredin F, Godfrey L, Howson J, Parkes M (2006). Evidence for association of OCTN genes and IBD5 with ulcerative colitis. *Gut* 55: 809-14.

Watanabe T, Asano N, Murray PJ, Ozato K, Tailor P, Fuss IJ, Kitani A, Strober W (2008). Muramyl dipeptide activation of nucleotide-binding oligomerization domain 2 protects mice from experimental colitis. *J Clin Invest* 118: 545-59.

Wehkamp J, Salzman NH, Porter E, Nuding S, Weichenthal M, Petras RE, Shen B, Schaeffeler E, Schwab M, Linzmeier R, Feathers RW, Chu H, Lima H, Jr., Fellermann K, Ganz T, Stange EF, Bevins CL (2005). Reduced Paneth cell alpha-defensins in ileal Crohn's disease. *Proc Natl Acad Sci U S A* 102: 18129-34.

Yang Z, Fuss IJ, Watanabe T, Asano N, Davey MP, Rosenbaum JT, Strober W, Kitani A (2007). NOD2 transgenic mice exhibit enhanced MDP-mediated down-regulation of TLR2 responses and resistance to colitis induction. *Gastroenterology* 133: 1510-21.

Zhou R, Wei H, Sun R, Tian Z (2007a). Recognition of double-stranded RNA by TLR3 induces severe small intestinal injury in mice. *J Immunol* 178: 4548-56.

Zhou R, Wei H, Sun R, Zhang J, Tian Z (2007b). NKG2D recognition mediates Toll-like receptor 3 signaling-induced breakdown of epithelial homeostasis in the small intestines of mice. *Proc Natl Acad Sci U S A* 104: 7512-5.